MENTAL HEALTH
Psycho-Social Perspectives

VOLUME SIX: Women Mental Health

The Details of the Volumes: Mental Health

Volume 1: Issues and Interventions

Volume 2: Multigroup Analysis

Volume 3: Strength of Human Resources

Volume 4: Therapeutic Applications

Volume 5: Adolescents & Children Mental Health

Volume 6: Women Mental Health

About the Editors

Anubhuti Dubey is presently Professor and Head, Department of Psychology DDU Gorakhpur University, Gorakhpur and has been teaching here since 1998. Apart from publishing more than 60 research papers in journals, 40 chapters in edited volumes, she has written a book entitled 'Psychological Perspectives on Chronic Illness' (2012) and co-edited a series of mental health in 2015 (volume 1 & 2) and in 2017 (volume 3 & 4). Her research interests include Health Psychology, Positive Psychology, Gender issues, and Counselling. She is more interested in applying qualitative research methodology. She has carried out ICSSR research projects and 14 students have been awarded Ph.D. under her supervision and she has also guided 20 M.Phil. dissertation and more than 150 PG dissertations so for. She is also a Master Trainer and Supportive Supervisor for Training HIV/AIDS counsellors under GFATM-Round 7 Programme. E-mail: anubhutiddu@rediffmail.com

Aradhana Shukla (Ph.D.) is former Professor and Head, Department of Psychology and Dean (Arts) Kumaun University, Nainital. She is now Senior Fellow (ICSSR, New Delhi) at Department of Psychology, SSJ University, Almora. She has served here as a teacher for the last 35 years and before joining here she served as Research Associate (UGC,New Delhi), Gorakhpur University and Assistant Research Officer, at Department of Paediatrics, Banaras Hindu University. She guided 52 Ph.D. students and conducted five major research projects from NCERT, UGC, ICSSR and UNESCO. She served as a supportive supervisor in the GFATM Round 7 project. She has written 16 books and developed 15 psychological tests. She has published more than 200 research papers in national and international journals and edited volumes. Moreover, she has received 15 awards from the organisations of national and international repute. She has co-edited a series of mental health in 2015 (volume 1 & 2) and in 2017 (volume 3 & 4). She is an established motivational speaker and counselor. The major areas of her interest are Cross Cultural Psychology, Health Psychology, Positive Psychology and Mental Health Interventions. E-mail: aradhana.shukla5@gmail.com

MENTAL HEALTH
Psycho-Social Perspectives

Volume Six

Women Mental Health

Edited by

Anubhuti Dubey
Aradhana Shukla

CONCEPT PUBLISHING COMPANY PVT. LTD.
NEW DELHI-110059

ISBN: 978-93-5125-173-6 (Series)
ISBN: 978-93-5439-025-8 (Vol. VI)

First Published 2021

Published and Printed by

Concept Publishing Company Pvt. Ltd.
A/15-16, Commercial Block, Mohan Garden,
New Delhi-110059 (India)
T: 91 11 41101460, 91 11 25351460, 91 11 25351794
E: publishing@conceptpub.com, *W*: www.conceptpub.com

Cataloging in Publication Data--Courtesy: D.K. Agencies (P) Ltd. <docinfo@dkagencies.com>

Mental health : psycho-social perspectives / edited by Aradhana Shukla, Anubhuti Dubey.
volumes cm
Contributed articles.
Includes bibliographical references and index.
Contents: volume 5. Adolescents & childrens' mental health — volume 6. Women mental health
Volumes 5-6 received now.
ISBN 9789351251736 (series)
ISBN 9789354390173 (vol. V)
ISBN 9789354390258 (vol. VI)

1. Teenagers—Mental health—India. 2. Child mental health—India. 3. Women—Mental health—India. I. Shukla, Aradhana, editor. II. Dubey, Anubhuti, editor.

LCC RA790.7.I5M46 2021 | DDC 362.20954 23

Preface

We desire to live a healthy and happy life. It is a common and well accepted fact that everyone desires to live a healthy life. The mind and bodily functions are closely embedded hence, the relative significance of mental health along with physical wellness cannot be denied. As mind and bodily functions are closely embedded we cannot deny the relative significances of mental health long with physical wellness. Mental health is an integral part of health, mental health is more than the absence of mental illness, and mental health is intimately connected with physical health and behaviour. Mental health is the foundation for well-being and effective functioning for an individual and for a community. Good mental health is a sense of wellbeing, confidence and self-esteem. It enables us to fully enjoy and appreciate other people, day-to-day life and our environment.

Mental health is the sheer responsibility of a person himself. The mental health field aims to deal with: (1) mentally ill people, (2) people at risk, and (3) promoting mental health of normal people so that their normality can be sustained.

If we go back into the history of mental health we can see that it was treated either as "boon of God "(good or positive mental health) or "curse of God "(bad or negative mental health). Both the eastern and western evidences support the notion. Not only in abroad but our ancient evidences also support this notion. The western literatures on mental health were seen hallucinations as communication of humans with bad souls, ghosts and witches. Moreover, in the ancient Indian literature of Ayurveda, Mental disorders are represented as various forms. The aetio-genesis of these disorders was thought to be endogenous because of provoked humours like vat, Pitta & Kalph. Exogenously the causes were attributed to sudden fear or association with ill influence of certain mythological gods or demon. Charak Samhita listed Psychiatry as 'Bhuta Vidya'. Psychotherapy was known as Ilaj-I-Nafsani in Unani Medicine. But time never remains stable.

Years and years were passed and the outlook of people towards mentally ill people become more and more aversive and they were treated like an undesirable social being for whom only such behaviour was required that was only meant for animals or criminals. Even with the advent of modern scientific methods and practical thoughts, the stigma and discrimination against mentally illnesses prevails the society. However, the advocates of Psychology started to cola soft touch and healing approach for the mentally ill people. Again it took decades to develop behaviour and psycho therapies against tying mentally ill people with iron chain, and treat them like prisoners. A complete soft and medico-human environment under single roof was constructed for them and it was termed as asylum or mental hospital. Psychologists attempted such patients to get out from the boundaries and from the trap of ojhas, neem-haquims and other such traditional healers and placed them at asylum. The patients were properly medicated along with different psychotherapies and many of them got complete recovery. At first the asylums were established in abroad but in India the first asylum was established in 1787 by Surgeon Kenderline in Calcutta and thereafter many asylums were made. This period was relatively longer but it opened the doors of a new era for the support and care of mental ill-health. They not only paid attention to treat the mentally ill people but also concentrated on maintaining and nurturing public health, and trying to eradicate the stigma and discrimination faced by people with mental disorders. Psychologists and mental health care professionals are still trying to launch innovative programs for the same. The focal theme of these developmental programs is the utilization of community resources for mental health care. These programs have given new vision to the mental health care professionals to prevent mental disorders and promote mental health. This also needs a greater role for the non medical mental health care professionals and better utilization of cultural resources in terms of belief, practice and important social institutions like family and community groups. The contemporary world's realization about mental health and mental illness has come to a point where we find passionate discussions and caring mental health professionals to deal with mental disorder and promote well being.

Keeping these views into consideration the innovative thought of this series appeared in our mind and we decided to pool the thoughts of psychologists and health care professionals regarding various concerns of mental health. The basic aim of this series was: (i) to bring concepts, issues, strengths and treatment in a single jacket. (ii) bring a sense of mental health awareness in people so that they can make their health safe with additional attention on social health (iii) to carve the research competence in young researchers and (iv) to put forth the mental health policies before the readers, so that a better understanding of mental health can be developed.

About the Series Mental Health: Psycho Social Perspectives

It is a series on the psychology of mental health and we have tried to cover as many areas as possible and we could justify its name i.e. rethinking. Many traditional notions of mental health have been reconceptualised and many concepts in a new framework have been introduced. This series has six volumes:

1. **Mental Health: Psychological Issues and Interventions:** In this volume we have covered various issues that foster or hamper mental health. Also, strategies to minimize negative mental health and improve positive mental health are discussed.
2. **Mental Health: Multigroup Analysis:** This volume covers the conceptual background and psycho-social perspective of mental health in various social settings.
3. **Mental Health: Strength of Human Resources:** In this volume we have tried to throw light on the promotional strategies of mental health following which a person can be relieved from negative mental health.
4. **Mental Health: Therapeutic Applications:** This volume covers a range of behavioural therapies which were found effective to minimize or overcome mental ill health.
5. **Mental Health of Adolescents and Children:** This volume presents a wide spectrum of the mental health of children and adolescents which are seen in them.
6. **Women Mental Health:** This volume presents the mental health of women in different perspective

We have exercised our best attempt to seek out as many experiences as possible and we also anticipate that this will open new foresight for the researchers. However, we will be highly blessed to obtain the healthy and critical comments from our colleagues, seniors and friends and we will appreciate them from the bottom of our hearts.

Anubhuti Dubey
Aradhana Shukla

Acknowledgements

We, the editors, feel immense pleasure to present our series on mental health before the august readers. We hope that it will be admired by you all and the comments will be highly appreciated.

We fell our deep sense of gratitude and thankfulness to our respected contributors. If was their support that these volumes came in the shape. We are thankful to Mr. Abhishek and Mrs. Kavita Khawar for computer task.

Last but not least, we are thankful to Mr. Ashok Mittal, M/s. Concept Publishing Company Pvt. Ltd., New Delhi to shape our dreams in concrete form.

15 March, 2021

Anubhuti Dubey
Aradhana Shukla

Contents

Our Contributors

Aishwarya Jaiswal, Department of Psychology, Banaras Hindu University, Varanasi, U.P. India.

Akansha Pandey is ICSSR Fellow and Research Scholar of Psychology at Deen Dayal Upadhyay Gorakhpur University. She is a member of International Association of Premenstrual Disorders (IAMPD) and currently working in the area of women health as her part of research entitled as 'Relationship of Distress, Psychological Immunity and Coping with Premenstrual Syndrome and Polycystic Ovary Syndrome'. **E-mail:** akancha0994@gmail.com

Aparna Joshi is currently working as an Assistant Professor in Tata Institute of Social Sciences (TISS), Mumbai. She has been involved in designing and teaching courses for post graduate students of Applied Psychology at the School of Human Ecology and certificate courses in couple and family therapy for counselors and mental health professionals. Her areas of interest and expertise include counseling and psychotherapy, gender and mental health, violence against women, couple and family therapy and ethics in psychotherapy. She has been practicing as a psychotherapist for past 19 years. **E-mail:** aparna.joshi@tiss.edu

Amrita Joshi is presently Co-director, Project Sukoon and was previously an Assistant Professor at the School of Human Ecology, TISS, Mumbai. She has completed her Doctor of Psychology (Psy. D.) from University of Hartford, U.S.A. (Accredited by the American Psychological Association). She has received intensive practical experience dealing with issues such as stress, panic attacks, low self-esteem, grief, trauma and abuse, divorce, addiction, body image issues, and depression. She is a guest faculty in many universities in Mumbai and teaches various modules to undergraduate and post graduate students. She also has her own private practice and is actively involved in providing services such as individual psychotherapy, group therapy, couples counseling (pre- and post-marital and divorce) and family counseling. **E-mail**: dramritajoshi@gmail.com

Aneri Shah has completed her Masters degree from the Department of Psychology, The Maharaja Sayajirao University of Baroda and has also pursued Fellowship in Psycho-Oncology (PGDP) from the Center of Psycho-Oncology for Education & Research, Bangalore. She has been working as a Psycho-oncologist since October 2016 and has experience in the areas of Surgical, Oncological and Radiation Oncology in Clinical history taking, psychological screening and assessment and conducting interventions.

Ankita Ojha is pursuing her Ph.D. in Department of Psychology, DDU Gorakhpur University, Gorakhpur (U.P.). Her areas of interest are culture and identity.

Anubhuti Dubey is presently Professor of Psychology and has been teaching since 1998 at Department of Psychology, DDU Gorakhpur University, Gorakhpur (U.P.), India. Apart from publishing more than 45 research papers in journals, 33 chapters in edited volumes, she has written book entitled 'Psychological Perspectives on Chronic Illness' (2012) and also co-edited four volume series on Mental Health: Psycho-Social Perspective and also 'Psyche of Asian Society' (2018). Her research interest includes Health Psychology, Positive Psychology, Gender issues, and Psychological Counselling. She is more interested in applying qualitative research methodology. She has also carried out ICSSR research project and 11 students have been awarded Ph.D. under her supervision. She is a Master Trainer and Supportive Supervisor for Training HIV/AIDS counsellors under GFATM-Round 7 programme. **E-mail:** anubhutiddu@rediffmail.com

Anushree Puntambekar is working as Senior Research Assistant in Project Sukoon of TISS, Mumbai. She has completed her post-graduation in Social Work with a specialization in working with Children and Families from TISS, Mumbai. She has experience in working on issues of gender, youth and violence against women.

Aradhana Shukla (Ph.D.) is former Professor and Head Department of Psychology and Dean (Arts) Kumaun University, Nainital. She is now Senior Fellow (ICSSR) at Department of Psychology, SSJ campus, Almora. She is serving here since last 35 years and before joining here she served as Research Associate (UGC), Gorakhpur University and Assistant Research Officer, at Department of Paediatrics, Banaras Hindu University. She guided 52 Ph.D. students and conducted four major research projects from NCERT, UGC and ICSSR. She served as supportive supervisor in GFATM round-7 project. She has written 16 books and developed 15 psychological tests. She has been co-editor in 6-volume series of mental health. One edited volume on the Psyche of Asian Society is also co-edited by her. The major areas of her interest are cross-cultural psychology, health psychology and mental health interventions. **E-mail:** aradhana.shukla5@gmail.com

Chinmayee Kantak is a Senior Research Assistant at Project Sukoon of TISS, Mumbai. She has completed her Master's in Applied Psychology (Specialisation in Clinical Psychology) from TISS, Mumbai. She has been working with Sukoon, in the research division, for one and a half years and has over two years of research experience.
E-mail: chinmayee.kantak@tiss.edu

Dhananjay Kumar is presently Professor of Psychology and has been teaching since 1998 at Department of Psychology, DDU Gorakhpur University, Gorakhpur (U.P.), India. His areas of interest are culture and identity. **E-mail:** dk_ddugu@yahoo.co.in

Dhvani Patel is Assistant Professor in Maharaja Sayajirao University of Baroda. Her research interest lie in understanding the experiences of women. **E-mail:** patel.dhvani-psy@msubaroda.ac.in

Garima Singh is Assistant Professor of Psychology at St. Joseph's College for Women, Gorakhpur. She was awarded PhD from D.D.U. Gorakhpur University in the year 2019 on the topic 'Mental health and wellbeing of caregivers of chronically ill patients: Role of Psychological Resources'. She has published eight research papers in journals and also contributed five chapters in edited books. Her research interests include the areas of Health Psychology, Positive Psychology and Social Psychology.
E-mail: garima.keepintouch@gmail.com

Ipsita Chatterjee is the project co-ordinator of Project Sukoon, TISS, Mumbai. She has completed her post-graduation in Applied Psychology (Specialisation in Clinical Psychology) from TISS, Mumbai. She has a certificate in couple and family therapy from TISS, Mumbai. She has about three years experience in research pertaining to family courts, and an overall five years research experience and three years experience in the area of psychotherapy. She also has a small private practice and provides psychotherapeutic services to children, adolescents, adults, couples and families facing psychosocial distress.

Laxmi Vajpeyi is working as Associate Professor and Head of the Department of Humanities & Professional Communication at Babu Banarasi Das Educational Group, Lucknow. Her research interest includes counselling, health psychology, Indian Psychology. She is also Convener of Value education cell of the university and an active member of Value Education Cell, Dr. A.P.J. Abdul Kalam Technical University, Uttar Pradesh.
E-mail: headhumanities@bbdniit.ac.in

Manisha Gauniyal is working as Counseling Psychologist at Shanti Lal Natha Lal Kansagera School Rajkot. **E-mail**: manishagauniyal196@gmail.com

Monika Misra received her PhD from University of Lucknow. She is an Assistant Professor of Psychology at Indira Gandhi National Open University where she teaches Developmental Psychology, School Psychology, Environmental Psychology and Personality theories and assessment. She has been developing courses for undergraduate and post-graduate courses of psychology. **E-mail**: monikamisra@ignou.ac.in

Nandita Das is Associate Professor (Retired), Department of Psychology, Utkal University, Bhubaneswar, Odisha. **E-mail**: das.namita@gmail.com

Niharika Bisht is Senior Research Fellow, All India Coordinated Research Project, Child Development Unit, College of Home Science, G.B. Pant University of Agriculture and Technology, Pantnagar, Uttarakhand.

Parisha Jijina is a Clinical Psychologist trained at the Institute of Human Behaviour and Allied Sciences (IHBAS), New Delhi. She has been working as an Assistant Professor at the Department of Psychology, The Maharaja Sayajirao University of Baroda since 2013. She is a trained hypnotherapist and is currently the Assistant Director of the Post Graduate Diploma in Clinical and Applied Hypnosis being offered by the Dept. At present, she is pursuing her PhD on the topic 'Equanimity and its Psycho-social health concomitants'. **E-mail**: parisha.jijina@gmail.com

Pooja Suteri is working as Counselor in JNV, Bageshwar, Uttarakhand. **E-mail:** pooja251802@gmail.com

Priyanka Pathak is Assistant Professor, P.G. Department of Psychology, Veer Kunwar Singh University, Ara, Bihar. She was awarded Ph.D. in psychology from Banaras Hindu University, Varanasi. **E-mail**: priyankapathak456@gmail.com

Ram Kalap Tiwari is retired as Associate Professor from Department of Psychology, K.S. Saket P.G. College, Ayodhya, Uttar Pradesh, India. His research interest includes areas of social and cognitive psychology. **E-mail**: tiwarirk111@gmail.com

Ritu Singh is Associate Professor of Home Science and Principal Investigator, All India Coordinated Research Project, Child Development Unit, College of Home Science, G.B. Pant University of Agriculture and Technology, Pantnagar, Uttrakhand.

Rupali Joshi is serving as Assistant Professor at Indian Institute of Banking and Personnel Selection, Mumbai. Her major areas of interest is Counselling psychology. **E-mail:** kashi.bhu@gmail.com

Selene Khosla is a PhD Scholar, Discipline of Psychology at Indira Gandhi National Open University. She has been working in the area of Positive Psychology. She completed her Masters in Psycho-Social Clinical Studies from Ambedkar University, New Delhi and Graduation from Jesus and Mary College, University of Delhi.

Shikha Dixit is Professor of Psychology in Humanities and Social Sciences Department, Indian Institute of Technology Kanpur, Kanpur, Uttar Pradesh, India. Her research interest includes health psychology, social representation, illness narratives, social and organizational cognition, mental models. **E-mail:** shikha@iitk.ac.in

Shobhna Joshi is Professor, Department of Psychology, Faculty of Social Sciences, Banaras Hindu University, Varanasi, Uttar Pradesh. She did her M.Phil. and Ph.D. from Gurukul Kangri University, Haridwar, Uttarakhand. Her research interest includes developmental and sports psychology, personality, psychological wellbeing. She had published more than thirty research papers in journals of national and international repute.
E-mail: getshobhna@yahoo.com

Sucharita Maji is Research Scholar, Humanities and Social Sciences Department, Indian Institute of Technology Kanpur, Kanpur, Uttar Pradesh, India.

Suchismita Pramanik is Research Scholar, National Institute of Science Education and Research, Jatni, Bhubaneswar, Odisha.
E-mail: suchipramanik@gmail.com

Sukanya Chowdhury is Post Graduate in Psychology, University of Calcutta, Kolkata, West Bengal.

Tilottama Mukherjee is Associate Professor, Department of Psychology, University of Calcutta, Kolkata, West Bengal.
Email: tilottamamukherjee3@gmail.com

Turfa Ahmed is Post Graduate in Psychology, University of Calcutta, Kolkata, West Bengal.

Tushar Singh, Assistant Professor, Department of Psychology, Faculty of Social Sciences, Banaras Hindu University, Varanasi, U.P. India 221005.
E-mail: tusharsinghalld@gmail.com

Vibha Kriti is Research Scholar, Department of Psychology, Banaras Hindu University, Varanasi, Uttar Pradesh, India.

Yogesh Kumar Arya, Department of Psychology, Banaras Hindu University, Varanasi, U.P. India.

1
Introduction

Anubhuti Dubey and *Aradhana Shukla*

Mental health in broad sense, has been described either a level of cognitive and emotional well-being or the absence of mental disorders (Malhotra & Shah, 2015). On the basis of positive and holistic view mental health includes one's ability to relish the life, maintain the resilience and a balance between favourable and unfavourable events of life. On the other hand there is a grey shade of mental health where a person fights with mental disorders and develops a sense of depression, anxiety and many more negative features of the life. Moreover, prevalence of positive and negative mental health is directly visible in human behaviour on the basis of which he/she is regarded mentally healthy and/or ill.

A plethora of studies have shown that gender is a pivot and critical factor while assessing any process of humans. The pattern of psychological (mental) health in many women is highly different than men (Apte, 2005; Seligman & Csikzntmihalyi, 2000; Sovani, 2010). Gender differences occur particularly in the rates of common mental disorders wherein women predominate over men. Differences between gender have been reported in the age of onset of symptoms, clinical features, frequency of psychotic symptoms, course, social adjustment and long term outcome of several mental disorders. Girls from nuclear families and women married at a very young age are at a higher risk for suicide attempt and self-harm. Social and gender bias generates many mental health problems in them. In addition, not only in India but also in the world women are the victims of domestic violence. So many political policies and social reformulation attempts have been made but the magnitude of social change is remained more or less same.

Although gender does not play an important role while dealing with the prevalence of mental disorders or better mental health (Piccnelli & Homen, 1997; Freeman Arnold and McElroy, 2002) cross-cultural studies have shown that, "female gender" is associated with better course of schizophrenia in the developing countries.

However females are more associated with favourable outcomes, social consequences such as abandonment by marital families, homelessness, vulnerability to several abuses, exposure to the and other infections contribute to the difficulties of rehabilitation of women. In India, the absence of any clear policy regarding the welfare of severely ill women and the social stigma further add something more in the problem (Thara, 2001). This stigma has been reported to be more toward ill women as compared to men and many times female caregivers become a target of the schemes (Thara, Kamath and Kumar, 2003).

There are so many indicators of good mental health. Their presence/ absence up to the marked status decides the types of mental health that a person may have. It means whether the person is mentally healthy (having positive and desirable attributes) or mentally sick (having negative and undesirable attributes). Although a person cannot be always happy and cheerful and vice-versa. So, there is a need to be balanced in daily circumstances (as maximum as possible). But "all that glitters is not gold" Outer layer of a person may be healthy and elated but the inner one may be full of irritability, sleeplessness and emotional irregularities that is disguised by the person for impression formation and social adjustment, personal satisfaction and mobilization in the society. So there is a need to evaluate the person on the basis of his/her consistent behaviour and deep assessment is required.

Keeping these views in consideration it is surely fair to be claimed that women are not in such mental state as they should be still they are treated as second grade national. Therefore, there is a need to understand the psyche of women and place them respectfully in the mainstream of society. The present volume is the outcome of this thought.

There are twenty-two chapters in this volume the first one is "Introduction" of the volume and presented by Anubhuti Dubey and Aradhana Shukla. In this chapter the concept of mental health, current status of women's mental health and the contributions of the volume are discussed. The second chapter entitled as "Women and mental health" by Anubhuti Dubey and Aradhana Shukla have put light on the current status of women's mental health in Indo-Western perspective.

The third paper, written by Tilottama Mukherjee, Sukanya Chaudhary and Turfa Ahmed deal with the current scenario of COVID-19 with a gendered lens. In a review paper Sucharita Maji and Shikha Dixit have shed light on imposter phenomenon and women's mental health. Ramkalap Tiwari in his paper discussed health status and wellbeing of elderly Tharu women and Priyanka Pathak with Shobhna Joshi have discussed work-life balance difficulties among working women in India. Ritu Singh and Niharika Bisht studied reproductive health and psychological wellbeing of women from Agrarian families and Selena Khosla and Monika Mishra explored mental health and identity of the 21st century home makers.

Parisha Jeena and Aneri Shah have elaborated the concept of empty nest and explored it among employed and home-makers. Aradhana Shukla and Pooja Suteri studied learned helplessness in women of various age groups, marital status and having various cultural setup, Motherhood and mental health during Postpartum depression is described by Laxmi Vajpeyi and Polycystic Ovary Syndrome (PCOS) as determinant of women's mental health is described by Vibha Kirti and Shobhna Joshi. Ankita Ojha and Dhananjay Kumar have also studied Polycystic ovary syndrome (PCOS) and correlated it with psychological and life style behaviour. Akanksha Pandey and Anubhuti Dubey tried to understand mental health of women suffering from Post Menstrual Syndrome. Marital conflict, litigation and psychological distress in women is sketched by Aparna Joshi, Ipsita Chatterjee, Chinmayee Kantak and Anushree Puntambekar. Rupali Joshi and Aradhana Shukla have shed light on rape victims and psychological consequences of rape on them. Dhavni Patil and Manisha Gauniyal explored the notion of happiness in Indian women of middle adulthood and Garima Singh guided by Anubhuti Dubey described the mental health of women caregivers of chronically ill patients. Suchismita Pramanik and Nandita Das discussed ageism, psychological capital and life satisfaction in elderly women.

Similarly Anubhuti Dudey has shed light on the mental health risk factors in women. Aishwarya Jaiswal, Tushar Singh and Yogesh Kumar Arya have discussed the issue of menstrual menace in Indian context. In another paper the same trio has addressed notion of misogyny in comprehensive way.

In this way this volume has clustered twenty one papers in itself. All papers are thought-producing and they unravel the grassroots and future outcomes of women health studies. We are quite sure that these articles will facilitate the pertinent research and add some more in the vision, thought and practice of researchers, teaching and mental health professionals.

References

Apte, S. (2005). Stigma associated with schizophrenia coping in caregivers and efficacy of targeted intervention, *Unpublished Ph.D. thesis*, Department of Psychology, Mumbai University.

Freemans, M.P.; Arnold, L.M. and McElroy, S.L. (2002). Bipolar disorder. In: S.G. Korsteen and A.H. Crayfon (eds). *Women's Mental Health: A Comprehensive Text book,* N.Y. Guilford.

Malhotra, S. and Shah, R. (2015). Women and mental health in India: An overview. *Indian Journal of Psychiatry*, 57 (Supp 2).

Piccinelli, M. and Homen, F. (1997). Gender differences in the epidemiology of affective disorders and schizophrents. *Genera World Health Organization.* (Google Scholar)

Seligman, M. and Csikzntmihalyi, M. (2000). Positive psychology. *American Psychologist*, 55 (1), 5-14.

Sovani, A. (2010 b). *Naate Tujhe Maajhe* (Marathi). Pune Umesh.

Thara, R. Patel (2001). Women's mental health: A public health concern. In: Regional health forum-WHO South-East Asia (Google Scholar).

Thara, R., Kamath, S. and Kumar, S. (2003). Women with schizophrenia and broken marriages: doubly disadvantaged (Part I-Patients' perspective). *International Journal of Social Psychiatry*, 49, 225-232 (a).

2

Women: Psyche, Society and Mental Health

Anubhuti Dubey and *Aradhana Shukla*

Gender is always considered as an important factor to determine ones' behaviour. It is a significant variable in social science researches but in literature and other modes of knowledge have also narrated its relative significance in various perspective. In global scenario women is considered as the second grade national and discriminated and maltreatment has always come in her part. It is a common saying that, "ladies first or the better half" but all man proverbs reside only in words while the reality is very bitter. This second grade marginalinalized behaviour also, impacts the women. Bearing all cruelties, she keeps mum and does all household chores and so many times outer work also. This feelings of being neglected and rejected generates a kind of emotional insecurity, learned helplessness and depression and it detrimentally impacts her own mental health.

But this tendency turns into manifolds in thoughts, actions and behaviour of males and a considerable changes in the roles and status of women have taken place. Women are gaining the landmarks of education, security, financial status and many more walks of life from where they have achieved status and recognition. As a result the status of women health and wellbeing has slightly changed.

In present day situation gender equality and minimization of gender discrimination has become a foci of academic discourse. Not only in academics but also in daily life circumstances women hold similar and equivalent position to men. Also, in medical sciences special attention is focused on women. (Chaddha, 2010) Although, gender is described as critical determinant of mental health and illness (WHO, 1997).

Gender differences have been mentioned mainly in the prevalence of common mental disorders including depression, anxiety, somato form disorder, learned helplessness, emotional insecurity, lack of health awareness, stress and many more (Patel, Arya, Delima, Ludemir and Todd, 1999; WHO, 2000, Geeta, 2010; Joshi, 2018; Kharkwal, 2018; Shukla, 2020; Dubey & Tripathi, 2016; Dubey & Singh, 2014).

Gender role and women gender roles have been culturally prescribed through the prehistoric cultures to this date and highly technical societies. In hunter-gatherer societies, women were generally the gatherer of plant foods, small animal foods, fists and learned to use dairy products while men hunted big animals for meat. Due to the course of time and changed scenario of society gender roles of women have drastically changed. Traditionally, middle class women were found typically involved in domestic tasks emphasizing child care for rather poor women. Economic necessities and increasing daily requirements pushed them to go out from home and season employment out. In such conditions women had to stand on both platforms and serve sincerely. It was their sheer responsibility to take care the family members and deal successfully at office on the other side of the coin. Gradually there had been a change in the availability of employment to more respectable office jobs where more education was demanded. In this way, although a large section of women from all socio-economic strata are employed outside the home, this neither returned them from household chores or their social status is changed. For centuries the difference between gender and the roles (?) is socially defined and evaluated on the basis of sexism (gender bias) in which men use to assume superiority over women and maintain their dominance over women. In this way it is apparent that women and man differ in biological attributes, needs and vulnerabilities.

Although the status of women has slightly changed yet it is not so high. There has been an increasing recognition of the fact that women are at the receiving end due to the destructive effect of gender inequalities and the stress that differentially affects them. When we think about our own culture we find that our Indian culture is unique. Joint family system, patriarchy marriage, marriage imperative, marriage as sacrosanct union, subservient status of daughters-in-law at home, preference to the male child, practice of dowry, lower educational status of women, strict rigid and backward conduct code for women and considering women as a sole source of child bearing and child rearing, and the "Indian Paradox' (the married women with severe mental illness, subjected to domestic violence makes frantic efforts for restitution of conjugate rights rather than for separation or divorce, are the features of Indian culture (Sharma, Pandit, Pathak and Sharma, 2013; Sharma, 2015).

These factors significantly affect the occurrence, manifestations, treatment and outcome of mental disorders of women in India. In this way, women's mental health can be conceptualized as having a wide range of pertinent areas, including reproductive health, psychopharmacology, psychological determinants of mental health, legal and issues. However, traditionally, women mental health is considered in terms of reproductive health (Sharma & Pathak, 2015)

Malhotra and Shah (2015) have shed light on some psychological theories that shed light on a gender sensitive point called alpha bias and there are others that are gender neutral representing beta bias. Alpha bias proposes that men and women are different and opposite, as in beta bias differences between men and women are usually ignored. Alpha bias is clearly revealed in psychodynamic theories and therapies whereas in accordance with Freudian view point, male anatomy and masculinity in the most deserved and cherished goal. Certainly female anatomy and feminity are seen as a deviation. Moreover, cognitive theories, behavioural theories and existential theories have beta bias (Hare Mastin and Marecek, 1988).

Acquired Risk and Gender

It has been noted that males have more risk of negative mental health than females due to their jobs, financial burden, parental and parenting responsibilities, socialites etc. Women have more risks in two respects—from more contact with young children and emotional/physical pressure. Also, it has been noted that males have more risk in two respects-from more contact with children and from emotional distress. Women adopt more preventive health practices, vitamin supplements, drug prescriptions less alcohol consumption and frequent consultation form minor symptoms. Moreover, they feel more distress on day to day basis and over their life time rather than men do, and this, many time decreases their resistance in all perspectives. Also, women tend to be delighted less than men and more vulnerable towards stress with special reference to routine stress (Joshi, 2018; Shukla, 2020). But it is good than women feel and bear more responsibility of home and outer world than men. (Malik, 1993)

Concept of Health

In 1981 World Health Organization reported social dimensions of mental health and stated. "Mental health is the capacity of the individual, the group and the environment to interact with one another in ways that promote subjective wellbeing, the optimal development and use of mental abilities (cognitive, affective and relational) the achievement of individual and collective goals consistent with justice and the attainment of preservation of conditions of fundamental equality."

This definition has several advantages in relation to women's mental health because it:

— stress the complex web of interrelationships that determine mental health and that determine health operate on multiple level.
— goes beyond the biological and individual level
— acknowledges the critical role of the social context.
— highlights the importance of justice and equality while determining mental well-being.

It means to say that gender can lay its impact on the production of mental health of any and every level.

In general, health is the state of complete physical, mental and social well-being and not merely an absence of disease and infirmity" (WHO, 1978). It is the definition of good and positive health but goes beyond the mere absence of disease. Also, this definition is centred on the maintenance of good health rather then the treatment of different diseases. It covers four dimensions and components of health, physical, mental, social and spiritual (Dalal & Misra, 2012). Thus, it is surely fair to say that health refers to proper functioning of mind and body capacity to share the social activities role performing and abiding by the moral principles as well. Also, nutritional status, immunity from disease and better quality of socio-familial life are also a matter of consideration. In this way WHOs definition clearly emphasizes the positive side of mental health rather than negative but negative sides are also a matter to be studied and checked because they, surely affect mental health and may deteriorate. It is a commonly accepted view that the presence of mental illness is relatively less in India as compared to other nations. Perhaps it is caused by limited and rather low level of hi-tech culture and a feeling of affinity and belongingness. (Prabhu & Raghu Rama, 1987). The focus of mental health issue was based on direct treatment of illness rather than prevention or promotion. So far as the matter of role gender on mental health is concerned it can be said that throughout in the world women are supposed to be more mentally ill than men (Vindhya, Kiranmayi and Vijayalakshmi, 2012) but the psychological distress of women has not been articulated as a distinct agenda by the main stream psychological approaches. Almost approaches related to mental health model consider psychosomatic factors in their diagnosis and almost ignorance of socio-cultural impact is seen (Haslam, 2000). But the advocates of feminist psychological researcher have pointed out that consideration of women's mental health needs requires recognition of the impact of social context on mental health (Carmen, Russo and Miller, 1981). It has also noticed that most of the mental health problems is women are generated by their roles not by their biological complaints. It is mostly observed that the mental illness of a woman is always revealed in stress, social influences and sleetying, vulnerabilities and developmental pathways, rather than locating cause of any particular abnormality or illness (Nicolson & Ussher, 1992). Stroebe and Stroebe (1995) have stated that the feminist views on women's mental health and illness is in fact in line with the biopsychosocial perspective and social factors rather than focusing on aberrant somatic processes to identify the cause of an illness as revealed in the traditional biomedical model.

Women and Mental Health Problems

It is common fact that women have more frequent illness and disability but they are not taken seriously as compared to men. Certainly, men suffer from more life threatening experiences. It means that one sex is considered as sicker to other one, but only a smart part of "iceberg of morbidity" (White, 1961) is visible but bulk of "iceberg" comes in the part of women.

Obesity and risk: obesity in women is defined as the magnitude of more fat in any part of the body. It is emerged due to overeating, hypertension, atherosclerosis and sometimes diabetes. They are the major risk factors and they directly impact on coronary diseases.

Alcohol and drug Abuse: The magnitude of drug abuse is our country is less than western countries but it is prevailed in more or less magnitude. Prescription drug and over the counter drugs are consumed more by users (Malik, 1993). Two third of prescriptions for psychotropic drugs like Diazepam and Alprazolam are more used by women very frequently.

Illness behaviour: It most commonly perceived that women are more sensitive for body comfort than men. This may be able to socialization in early childhood. They are more apt to label their symptoms as physical illness and injuries more severe than men while men many times ignore their illness. Most of women show more sick behaviour and dependency towards men along with help seeking behaviour. Moreover, the concept of learned helplessness is more common in women (Suteri, 2016). So far as the matter of ability factor is concerned women are found comparatively more flexible with men. Also, more morbidity is shared by them. One most common thing that is almost visible in women is their tendency to share their pains to their friends' colleagues and neighbours. They, many times are based on the complaints of the family (Malik, 1993). They prefer to talk about very minor health problems and seek help and sympathy from others.

Violence against women: In accordance with National Statistics lot of women experiences any type of abuse by the partner (Yoshikawa, Agrawal, Poudel and Jimba, 2012; Abbot & Williamson, 1999; Coker, Hopenhayn, Desimone, Bush and Crofford, 2009). It has been noted that domestic violence can last the psychophysical capacity of women and cuts, bruises, bite marks, broken bones, miscarriages, joint damage, hypertension, heart disease and sexually transmitted infections are the main signs of a woman to be the victim of domestic violence. Although physical injury is harmful for a woman yet the imprints of psychological loss are comparatively more important and a reliable source of mental loss (Hill, Schroeder, Bradley, Kaplan and Angel, 2009). Psychological health is affected more by domestic violence and it has been noted by many psychologists that multiple health disorders like stress, anxiety, depression, alcohol and/or substance use, personality disorder, post-traumatic stress disorder, sleeping and eating disorders, social disfunction and even suicide (Abbot & Williamson, 2010; Gerlack, 1999; Howard, Trevillion & Agnew Davis, 2010). Preventing violence against women requires addressing causes and risk factors, which are complex and multiple, contextual and can stiff with broader social changes (Deshpandey & Chauthia Wale, 2017). Group or community based relationship level intervention appropriate policy, articles, 14, 15, 16 and 42, Protection of Women from Domestic Violence Act 2005 are the major sources following which domestic violence can be minimized.

Occupational Stress: With change in time women have established their roles and prestige in the outer world as they have crossed the boundaries of home and provide them as good worker at outer world. This life of women is just like oscillating between home and work place and it causes courses a sense of occupational stress. On the one side of a coin she performs the role of wife, mother, maintenance of extending family, caretaker of elderly relatives and the other side of the coin is related to work place. It has been noted that increase in the occupational stress generates multiple tension and heart disease in employed women. In the changing scenario of Indian society, although the women goes out from home and does the outer job along with the household chores the women face more difficulty and it impacts deleteriously their mental health. In a study Eaker (1989) reported that clerical workers who reported having as an unsupportive boss were at increased risk of developing heart disease also, meta-analytic, shades of job involvement and women have indicated that it is unrelated to a type—A personality—a constellation of personality traits that have been linked to heart disease in men (Booth & Friedman, 1987).

Women who smoke have two or four times more risk of heart attack (DHHS, 1981, 1988). Further, the risk factors for coronary outing disease (lipid disorders, hypertension, diabetes and smoking) tend to cluster in the same patients. In an country even though women take less alcohol, they tend to be more risk line for coronary heart disease than the women of western country (DHHS, 1988).

Schizophrenia: In early studies it has been noted that 50-60 % of men but only about one third of women have been admitted in regard to schizophrenia (Hafner et al., 1989; Goldstein, 1989, 1990, a, b; Lewine, 1988) with variation in cultural setting (Sartorius, 1986). Tekki (1992) has noted that schizophrenia females like male and female patients showed a significant seasonality of first admission with a peak of July. It was also noted that the outcome of schizophrenia tended to be better in females. Thara and Raj Kumar (1992) have reported that the gender differences in outcome were more pronounced in Schizophrenia than socio-affective and affective disorders.

Sucide in schizophrenia is more common in men (Brier & Astrachan, 1984). Part of better outcome in females in the short and mid-term may be explained by a better response to both drug treatment and family intervention (Seeman & Lang, 1990; Haas, 1990).

In Chestnut Lodge follow up study (MC. Glashan & Bardenstein, 1990) it was noted that Schizo- affective women were married more often than the men at index hospitalization. This study also found very less difference in global outcome, although the males achieved more education in comparison to females. Marital rates were not found to differ to an other study. Additional difference noted had a high prevalence, older age of onset and greater suicidal tendencies in women.

All findings cited above in general reveal that the status of the mental health of women is not found state at every time. As the advancements in life happened, the women decided her roles and responsibilities many time more and her status varied but many places the conditions of the understanding of women and their mental health is found in status quo, So, it is the duty of society to rethink over it and improve the status of women. Society can take some steps listed below:

- Society should understand that health policies are not only made for men. Women should also be privileged by them.
- Proper knowledge about health care system is also resumed.
- Provision of effective health services to women is also required.
- Preventive measure and reductions of risk factors should also be known by women.
- Establishment of women health equity act should also be take in comederale (Afroz & Tiwari, 2019)
- An interpretation between gender mainstreaming and women-focused holistic care, research and policy is also required.
- Evaluation and remaking of relevant health policies and research is also needed.
- Disaggregating all health data by sex, age and PSS is also a matter of attention.
- Exploring multisectoral response to women's health as more efficient, effective approach than relying solely or the health care system as the policy area responsible for general health and well-being are also a matter to think.
- Develop and increase the competence of primary health care provides to recognize and treat mental health consequence of disorganized home climate and cute work climate should also be taken to raise the mental health faculty of women.

References

Abbott, P. & Williamson, E. (1999). "Women, health and domestic violence", *Journal of Gender Studies*, 8,4, 83-102

Booth & Friedman (1987) Psychological predictors of heart disease: A quantitative review. *Psychological Bulletin*, 101, 343-362.

Breier, A. & Astrachan, B. (1984) Characteristics of schizophrenic patients who commit suicide. *American Journal of Psychiatry*, 141, 206-209.

Carmen, E.H., RUSSO, N.E and Miller, J.B. (1981). Inequality and women' mental health: An overview. *American Journal of Psychiatry*, 138,10, 1019-1030.

Chadda, R.K. & Sood, M. (2010) Indian research on women and psychiatry. *Indian Journal Psychiatry,* 52, Suppl, 53, 229-232

Coker, A.K., Hopenhayn, C., DeSione, C.P., Bush, H.M. and Crofford, L., (2009). "Violence against women raises risk of cervical cancer", *Journal of Women's Health,* 18, 8, 1179-1185.

D.H.H.S., U.S. Public Health Service (1981) *Women's Health* (Supplement). Public Health Reports.

D.H.H.S., U.S. Public Health Service (1988) *Women's Health* (Supplement). Public Health Reports.

Dalal, A.K. & Misra, G. (2012), *New Direction in Health Psychology,* New Delhi, Sage.

Deshpandey, V. & Chauthaiwale, J. (2017). Tackling Violence against Women: A study of state intervention measures, *(Unpublished Report)*. Bharatiya Stree Shakti, Government of India, New Delhi.

Dubey, A. & Tripathi, K.M. (2016). Health literacy and health practices in women of Sabia village of Kushinagar district: A qualitative analysis. *International Journal of Physical and Social Sciences*, 6, 2, 1-12.

Dubey, A. & Singh, S. (2014). Stress during infertility treatment process, *UJAS*, 8, 21, 1-12.

Eaker, K.I. (1969). Psychosocial factors in the epidemiology of coronary heart disease in women. *Psychiatric Clinics of North America*, 12, 167-173.

Garcia-Moreno, C., Jansen, H., Ellsberg, M., Heise, L. and Watts, C.H. (2006). "Prevalence of intimate partner violencea: Findings from the WHO Multi-country study on women's health and domestic violence", *The Lancet*, 368 (9543), 1260-1269.

Geeta (2010). Learned helplessness and depression in the student of different professional and nonprofessional courses. *Unpublished Ph.D Thesis*, Department of Psychology, Kumaun University, Nainital.

Gerlock, A.A. (1999). Health impact of domestic violence, *Issue in Mental Health Nursing,* 20, 373-385.

Goldstein, J.M. (1989). Gender and schizophrenia: Implications for understanding the heterogeneity of the illness. *Psychiatry Research*, 28, 243-253.

Goldstein, J.M. (1990a). Sex differences in the familial transmission of schizophrenia. *British Journal of Psychiatry*, 156, 819-826.

Goldstein, J.M. (1990b). The role of gender in identifying subtypes of schizophrenia: A latent class analytic approach. *Schizophrenia Bulletin*, 16, 263-275.

Haas, P.M. (1990). Gender and Schizophrenia outcome: A clinical trial of an inpatient family intervention. *Schizophrenia Bulletin*. 16, 277-292.

Hafner, H., Rossler, A.R. Muurer, K. and Loffer, W. (1989). How does gender influence age at first hospitalization for schizophrenia? A transnational case registers study. *Psychological Medicine*, 19, 903-918.

Haslam, N.(2002). Psychiatric categories as natural kinds: Essentialist thinking about mental disorder. *Social Research*, 67, 7, 1031-1058.

Howard, L.M., Trevillion, K. and Agnew Davis, R. (2000). Domestic violence and mental Health. *International Review of Psychiatry*, 22, 5, 526-534

Joshi, B. (2018), Effect of marital status, age and culture on life satisfaction, temperament and health related beliefs unpublished Ph.D. thesis, Department of Psychology, Kumaun University, Nainital.

Lewine, R J . (1988) Gender and schizophrenia. In H.A. Nasirullah (Ed.) *Handbook of Schizophrenia,* Vol 3. Amsterdam: Elsevier.

Malhotra, S & Shah, R. (2015), Women and mental health in India: An overview. *Indian Journal of Psychiatry* 57, 2, 205-211

Malik, S.C. (1993). Presidential address: Women and mental health. *Indian Journal of Psychiatry,* 47, 3-10.

McGlashan & Bardenstein (1990). Gender differences in affective, schizo-affective and schizophrenic disorders. *Schizophrenia Bulletin*, 16, 205-210.

Mustin, R.T. and Marecek, J. (1988) The meaning of difference. Gender theory, postmodernism and psychology. *Annual Review of Psychology.* 43,455-464.

Nicholson, P. & USSER, J.(1992). *The Psychology of Womens' Health and Healthcare*. Baringstoke, U.K. Macmillan.

Patel, V., Araya R, De Lima M.S., Ludermir A. and Todd, C.(1999). Women, poverty and common mental disorders in four restructuring societies. *Social Science Medicine*, 49,146-171.

Prabhu. G.C. & Raghuram (197). Mental health in India. In *Encyclopedia of Social Work in India,* 2, New Delhi, Ministry of Welfare.

P. Kharkwal, M. (2016). Developmental pattern of mental health among professional women: A comparative study. *Unpublished Ph.D Thesis*, Department of Psychology, Kumaun University Nainital.

Sartorius, N. (1986). Harly manifestations of first contact incidence of schizophrenia in different cultures. *Psychological Medicine*, 1 6, 609-628.

Seeman, M.V. & Lang, M. (1990). The role of oestrogen in schizophrenia: gender differences. *Schizophrenia Bulletin*, 16, 185-195.

Shukla, A. (2020). Mental health of Kumauni Women: An intervention based study in cultural perspective, *Senior Fellowship ICSSR No [2-33/19-20/Sf/ GEN] in Progress,* Department of Psychology, Kumaun University, Nainital.

Sharma, I., Pandit B, Pathak A, Sharma R. (2013). Hinduism, marriage and mental illness. *Indian Journal Psychiatry,* Suppl 2,5, 243-249.

Sharma, I. (2015). Presidential address: Violence against women: Where are the solutions? *Indian Journal Psychiatry,* 57, 17-25.

Sharma, I. & Pathak, A. (2015). Women mental health in India. *Indian Journal of Psychiatry*, 52,2, 201-204

Strobe, W. & Strobe, M.S.(1995). *Social Psychology and Health*, Milton Keynes, Buckingham: Open University, Press.

Takei, N. (1992) Seasonality of admission rates in psychosis: effects of diagnosis, sex and age at onset. *British Journal of Psychiatry*, 161, 506-511.

Thara, R. & Rajkumar, S. (1992) Gender differences in schizophrenia. Results of a followup study from India. *Schizophrenia Research*, 7, 1,65-170.

Vindhya, U., Kiranmayi, A. and Vijayalakshmi, V. (2012). Mental disorders in women, in A.K. Dalal & G. Misra (Eds.), *New Directions in Health Psychology*, New Delhi, Sage.

White (1961). 'The ecology of medical care. *New England Journal of Medicine*. 2,5, 885-892.

Suteri, P. (2016). *Unpublished Ph.D Thesis*, Department of Psychology, Kumaun University Nainital.

World Health Organization (1978). *Alma-Ata Declaration*, Geneva, World Health Organization.

World Health Organization (1997). *Nations for Mental Health: A Focus on Women*. Geneva: World Health Organization.

World Health Organization (2000). *Women's Mental Health: An Evidence Based Review*. Geneva.

Yoshikawa, K. Agarwal, N.R., Paudel, K.C. and Jimba, M.A. (2012). Life time experience of violence and adverse reproduction outcomes: Findings from population surveys in India. *Bio Science, Trends*, 6, 3, 115-121.

3

A Patriarchal Pandemic-Looking at COVID-19 through a Gendered Lens

Tilottama Mukherjee, Sukanya Chowdhury and *Turfa Ahmed*

The turn of this decade introduced the world to a new word COVID-19 or the Novel Corona Virus that very soon achieved a pandemic status worldwide. However, countries dealing with this crisis have not yet explored in detail its psychological implications. People are in a state of constant fear and deep anxiety as there is no final word on how long this pandemic will continue to haunt our lives. As per the World Health Organisation, people are now told to make up their minds to live with this virus for a long time without any clarity—the virus is reported to continuously change its design rendering it practically impossible to concur, there is no vaccine in sight or a definite cure that would help us breathe a sigh of relief. Protective guidelines have been dictated to help individuals keep the virus at bay and take care of their physical health in their limited capacity. However, little has been discussed about the more subtle and far-reaching impacts of this pandemic, especially the effect it has on girls and women all over the world. COVID-19 might be threatening to men and women in terms of physical health, but keeping the epidemiological effects aside, the outbreak of the disease impacts people and groups very differently. It wouldn't be unfair to say that the disease is a silent killer for women—increasing the rate of violence and abuse inflicted on them all over the world, exposing them to a far greater threat than just ailing physical health.

In 2000, the World Health Organisation (WHO) declared gender to be a critical determinant of mental health and mental illness, pointing out that gender dictates the differential power and control men and women possess over the socioeconomic factors that determine the state of their mental health and lives. Observing the grim nature of this pandemic, United Nations policy brief emphasized "Across every sphere, from health to the economy, security to social protection, the impacts of COVID-19 are exacerbated for women and girls". Inequalities related to the intersecting elements of our identities have always been present in the society, however, the arrival of this pandemic has made it extremely essential to understand and discuss the intersectional gendered implications—especially while talking about women empowerment, gender-based violence, the emotional and financial security of women. COVID-19 has given us an elaborate picture of the trauma that women across different race, nationalities, caste and socio-economic spectrum battle with daily to survive in a largely patriarchal world.

The present circumstances suggest that women are not only at risk of developing the disease by contracting the virus but are also at a greater risk of facing domestic abuse, experience an increased burden of care giving, housework and economic stress. In addition to this, the isolation measures imposed, resulting in reduced access to support services.

Unpaid Care Work and Domestic Responsibilities

Women are often the main caregivers in their homes, communities, and health facilities, which puts them at an increased risk of contracting COVID-19. In the UK, 77 per cent of the NHS workforce and the majority of informal carers are women. More broadly, an analysis of 104 countries revealed that women form 70 per cent of workers in the health and social sectors, and 50 per cent of unpaid carers. Lockdowns and self-quarantine measures across the world have led women to face increased responsibilities of workload in care giving due to various social, cultural and economic factors with even less physical and economic security. Data from the Organisation for Economic Cooperation and Development (OECD) shows that Indian women do nearly six hours of unpaid care work each day. Indian men, on the other hand, spend less than an hour on an average doing the same. Globally, women have been recorded to engage in 76.2 per cent of the total hours of unpaid care work. COVID-19 is shifting other household dynamics, too. Domestic responsibilities that women are expected to take up, like cooking and cleaning, looking after the kids have increased manifold. In addition to this due to schools and coaching centres shutting down because of the lockdown, in several families, women have also had to take up the additional responsibility of looking into the education of the kids. In an article published by *The Business Insider India*—a survey conducted by leading education resources and lesson plan experts Plan Bee revealed that mothers are picking up almost all the home teaching burden during the corona virus-induced lockdown with just 11.8 per cent fathers taking the lead on helping their children keep up to date with their school work. Many women working in the public sector have also been engaged in work from home during the lockdown phase. Having to work from home in addition to performing household chores has left women with little or no time to look after their selves.

There might be an argument in this context stating that women perform these activities under normal conditions as well, however, there are major differences between functioning in a pre- and post-COVID world, especially in developing countries. Even though a great number of women have spent considerable time engaging in these activities, but under normal conditions despite performing household work, women do manage to take some time out to tend to their own needs and care for themselves. But the constant presence of all family members due to the lockdown has led women to become neglectful of their needs and desires. This has had worse effects on women's mental and physical health in various ways. One instance is that women in several semi-urban and rural Indian families tend to eat only after the rest of the family has and consume the least amount of food; research has shown that financial strain and shortages in food tend to affect women's nutrition more than men's. The same pattern has been observed across the countries of the developing world, from Zimbabwe to Bangladesh. To make matters worse, the lockdown has cut off most formal and informal support systems for women. In developing countries, a lot of low-income families do not have access to television or cable connections and often share one smart phone, usually owned by a male member in the family. Hence, women's lack of digital access is making them more susceptible to misinformation and fake news. Women in the households are mostly conferred an inferior position where they do not get the financial opportunity of managing the family expenditure and as a result of their lack of decision-making capacity and autonomy, they have poor self-perception and thus more prone to experience abuse and exploitation.

To provide a solution to this, it might be helpful to turn to Jessica DeGroot (2008), quality of life theorist and founder of Third Path Institute, who introduced the concept of "shared care". It involves a radical unlearning of social conditioning and removing gender as a determinant of who does more work, honest sharing of domestic work and emotional labour between partners to chart out goals, equally share responsibility and increase gratitude so that both may thrive at home and work, and remain healthy and happy.

It is important to make inclusive and gender-sensitive social protection programmes for women to mitigate the effects of the overload of unpaid care work, for instance, providing paid sick or emergency care or lactation leaves, flexibility in work arrangements like tele-working at the time and place most convenient, flexi-time and reduced workload based on social dialogue and consultation with workers and their representatives. The aim should be on supporting workers to be as productive as possible in the context of additional care and family responsibilities.

Lack of Basic Health-Care Facilities for Women

The prevalent social norms in some contexts influence women's ability to receive timely care for COVID-19 because they are the last to receive medical attention when they become ill. This could have serious implications for those who are at greater risk of contracting COVID-19 such as older women or those with chronic conditions or weakened immune systems due to being infected with HIV, malaria, or tuberculosis (Sands, 2020) or for women and girls suffering from malnutrition. The gender inequality becomes stark when health resources that are crucial needs for women have been diverted away because of out-stretched health services such as lack of access to pre- and post-natal health care and contraceptives. Hurdles in accessing contraception, safe abortion and medication further perpetuate heighten the risks for women's well-being and health and lead to feelings of isolation, shame and lowered self-worth. These evident or veiled wounds of exploitation and abuse shall remain with women throughout their lives.

The Economic Hardships of Women During COVID-19

This pandemic has brought with it economic stress for women as well. The majority of women work in the informal sector, with low pay, limited protections against dismissal, unpaid sick leaves, non-existent or inadequate health insurance schemes, and inadequate or unpaid maternity leave. The lockdown has also led many women, from domestic helps to migrant labourers, to forego the public spaces and social interactions which were a source of their employment and hence lost their jobs. Hence, financial insecurity adds to a woman's burden of care. COVID-19 has amplified the pre-existing inequalities for women living in society and deepened the gaps for attaining economic independence. The pandemic has also exposed the gaps in pay that women have been experiencing for a long time. The pay gap between men and women has increased to 16 per cent and is as much as 35 per cent in a few countries. This inequality has left women to be underpaid and save less as a result and hence have become more vulnerable to being pushed into poverty, unable to fulfil their basic needs or sustain their families. For those working women working in the formal sector, the lockdown has disproportionately affected women because of layoffs and cuts in salaries.

Women at the Receiving End of Experiencing Gender-Based Violence

One of the most adverse effects of the lockdown period has been that many women are isolated at home with abusive spouses. The COVID-19 pandemic has been linked to spikes in domestic violence reports and crisis calls in China, France, U.K., Canada and India—to name a few countries. This reflects similar patterns that were observed in past disease outbreaks as well. In India, the National Commission for Women (NCW) has raised an alert about an increasing number of domestic and intimate partner violence cases since the national lockdown began. In Canada, women's shelters and organizations have also sounded alarms about the risk of increased violence. Rates of gender-based violence across the world have always been high, even before the pandemic. However, quarantines and social isolation mean that abusers and those they harm are in close proximity of each other around the clock and other people aren't around to see the signs of abuse and provide the necessary help. Women and girls all over the world are now exposed to an increased risk of facing emotional, physical or sexual abuse at home with COVID-19 isolation measures that have been implemented.

Restriction of movement and lockdown measures has confined victims of abuse at home. They may be punished by denying them their basic needs and items for engaging in health-protective behaviours such as soap or sanitizers, face coercion and manipulation or deliberately face harm to make ends meet. The abusers may frighten the women by sharing false information about the outbreak and withhold insurance plans to prevent them from seeking medical assistance if required. Even belittling and derogatory comments about their subordinate status are enough to make them feel inadequate, self-blaming and unable to protect herself. They even come to experience trauma bonding with the perpetrators where they associate affection with abuse. The stigma of seeking help and the lack of availability of social support during pandemic also make them internalize the abuse over time. They may eventually rationalize, defend or minimize the abuse and are less likely to report it.

These concerns can further exacerbate the mental health conditions of women. A range of symptoms may be experienced, that include negative self-perception, persistent low and anxious mood, erratic behaviour, inability to experience pleasure in usual activities, attention and memory difficulties, changes in bodily functions of appetite, sleep, fatigue or bodily pains and thoughts of inflicting self-harm and suicide.

There could be a host of reasons for this sudden increase in the rate of domestic violence. In a lot of homes history of emotional abuse already exists, that sometimes gets manifested in the form of a sense of control over the woman, possessiveness, doubtfulness, jealousy, and misogynistic attitudes. In addition to this various pandemic-related stressors can become triggers, including the loss of job and reduced income, fear of contracting the virus, food shortage and insecurity, ongoing physical and emotional stress, disrupted family routines. The lockdown has led to changes in relationship roles as well, for example, when one partner suddenly had to become the primary caregiver while the children are at home away from school and the other partner had to become the sole breadwinner when their partner lost their job. In most cases, it's the woman who takes up the role of the primary caregiver at home. Higher rates of conflicts may emerge or worsen when couples don't exercise the means of having better communication either because individual issues are going on or the couple is engaging in what is called situational couple violence, leading to an escalation in physical abuse. All of this points to male psychological distress resulting from the uncertainty of the present circumstances, and subsequent violent behaviour and/or confinement at home with abusive partners during the lockdown. As a result, in the long-run women's psychological well-being might be affected even more adversely than men's from financial and emotional stress, combined with physical violence.

Social isolation also makes it difficult for the victims of abuse to access support services that could take necessary interventions to rescue them from this plight. An initiative has been adopted in this particular regard, known as the "Signal for Help". This is a simple one-handed sign that someone can use on a video call, where the person faces their palm to the camera, tucks their thumb and then presses it with the other four fingers. It can help a person silently show they need help and want someone to check in with them in a safe way. The Signal for Help was launched by the Canadian Women's Foundation in response to COVID-19 and is now being shared by partner organizations around the world. Although a good initiative this has a very limited reach, as most women in developing countries do not have any access to technology or awareness of how to use it.

COVID-19 and a Threat to Education

COVID-19 has also disrupted the lives of thousands of young adolescent girls all over the world, snatching away from them their chance of a bright future. According to the UN education agency—United Nations Educational, Scientific and Cultural Organization (UNESCO), the pandemic has disrupted the education of some 154 crore students worldwide, as schools have been shut down. UNESCO reports stated that girls will be the worst affected as it will lead to increased drop-out rates and further entrench gender gaps in education. Stefania Giannini, UNESCO's Assistant Director-General for Education, in an interview to the Press Trust of India said that shutting down of schools due to the COVID-19 pandemic comes with a warning of "potential for increased drop-out rates which will disproportionately affect adolescent girls, further entrench gender gaps in education and lead to increased risk of sexual exploitation, early pregnancy and early and forced marriage". In the third world developing countries, families in rural areas are reluctant to send their daughters to school. In most cases, the girls drop out of school at a very young age and are forced into marriage or take up jobs to support their families. Nevertheless, developments made in the last few decades had brought with them a series of positive changes. Many governmental and non-governmental organisations now work actively for the education of the girl child. Families are now compelled to send their daughters to school and allow them to complete their education. But the arrival of the pandemic has brought with it another new fear, with jobs being lost and financial conditions worsening many families with fragile socio-economic conditions may force their daughters to drop out of school. Particularly for women and girls in countries where limited social protection measures are in place, economic crisis often leads families to consider the financial and opportunity costs of educating their daughters as opposed to their sons. Hence it is not unfair to assume that a similar picture will be observed in a post-COVID world.

This crisis is bringing to light a lot of existing societal divides in the way it is disproportionately impacting lower-income communities. While many girls, especially from the upper socio-economic strata will continue with their education once the school gates reopen, others will never return to school. According to Giannini, the situation is even more critical for girls living in various refugee camps across the world, or who are internally displaced. Suspension of schools for an indefinite period will hinder any progress made to uplift their condition as they are already at a disadvantage and education responses must prioritise the needs of adolescent girls' at the risk of reversing 20 years of gains made for girls' education. Refugee girls at the secondary level have a lower probability to enrol as their male peers. The UNESCO has called for policy-makers and practitioners to look into lessons from the crises that the world has faced in the past to tackle the challenges faced by these young girls, as the governments of various countries prepare for indefinite school closures.

What can be done to Mitigate the Gaps in Services for Women?

Amid the global crisis, a diverse approach has to be considered when dealing with the situation and acknowledge the gender-differential impact of the pandemic. The United Nations has supported gender analysis and sex-disaggregated data collection, so that women's needs and realities during a pandemic, such as heightened susceptibility to infection, increased burden of care giving, economic hardships and lack of access to basic health facilities, do not fall through the cracks. Equal pay and equal opportunities need to be ensured for enabling the full participation of women in the workforce. Hence, the programmes have aimed at building women's economic resilience and preparedness for such crises by providing them with the resources they need for themselves and their families. Efforts have been taken to leverage existing networks of women-led organizations so that women are included and represented in economic and emergency response planning and policy decision-making. For instance, in China, UN Women has focussed on economic recovery solutions to mitigate the negative economic impact of the pandemic by supporting small and medium businesses owned by women. When aids such as loans, credit or grants are in place, an industry can stabilize the economic shocks of a crisis. It has also supported outreach programmes and campaigns to promote women's participation in leadership and planning during the COVID-19 response.

Moreover, a gender-focused response has been implemented by UN Women also expected for women's health and appropriate steps have been taken by collaborating with local governing bodies and mental health organizations to ensure women's safety and prevent the harm that has already been done. Also, help-lines are insufficient and unequipped to handle the rise in the number of cases and for providing the right kind of counselling support for women and children. These help-lines are also not widely known to all and are not advertised by police and government at regular intervals. Raising awareness, community outreach and training programmes can ensure that women, especially from marginalized sections, can receive public health messages to access basic reproductive and menstrual health services. With limited access to education and therefore having low levels of literacy in some settings, messaging must be accessible, culturally appropriate and understandable by all.

Moving services online and creating social networks for survivors where local women speaking to other women via different media, including radio and text messaging can ensure the flow of vital information from the concerned authority through a trusted source. Increasing awareness and advocacy campaigns can prioritize and prevent adversities against women such as the Shadow Pandemic campaign focusing on the global increase of domestic violence during the COVID-19 health crisis. Initiatives need to be undertaken to establish shelters for victims of domestic violence by converting existing public buildings such as hotels or schools and colleges into new shelters that can be accessed easily. Designating safe spaces to anonymously report abuse, such as grocery stores or pharmacies can alert the authorities and protect victims such as using code words for seeking help. Initiatives taken by other nations can serve as models for implementation such as establishing hotlines and making denunciation through WhatsApp and e-mails possible 24/7 and allowing for easy localization of the victim, circulating pamphlets, or social media campaigns to call out the abusers.

Psychological first aid can be a useful tool to assess the pressing concerns of the women and offer them practical or informational assistance where required. Community, as well as frontline health care workers, can be trained for providing psychological first aid for dealing with women's issues, especially those who have faced gender-based violence by regularly following up with them. Moreover, psychological first aiders can also provide them with an empathic understanding of their distress by offering to just listen to them reflectively and maintaining confidentiality. They can also help in stabilizing the myriad of emotions that the uncertainty of the lockdown has invited.

Even with the presence of a host of modern technology services and disaster management schemes, it'll be fair to say that the COVID-19 pandemic has halted the progress that the human race has made over the last few decades, especially in areas concerning the development and safety of women. The factors discussed above have already had a disproportionate impact, causing an overnight upheaval in the lives of many young girls and women all over the world. If we are to make any recovery in our efforts to achieve gender equality and make the world a safe place for women, social and economic reforms must take a feminist approach-ensuring their safety and empowerment with an inclusive leadership of, for and by the women of the world.

References

1.54 bn students out of school over Covid-19; girls to be worst hit: UNESCO. Available at: https://www.business-standard.com/article/current-affairs/1-54-bn-students-out-of-school-over-covid-19-girls-to-be-worst-hit-unesco-120042200741_1.html. COVID-19 and the impact on women. Available at: https://www.theigc.org/blog/covid-19-and the-impact-on-women/

De Groot, J. (2008). Personal correspondence with Gerson, K. *The Unfinished Revolution How a New Generation Is Reshaping Family, Work and Gender in America*. New York: Oxford University Press.

How COVID-19 is amplifying gender inequality in India. Available at: https://indianexpress.com/article/opinion/coronavirus-gender-inequality-india-6414659/

Love under Lockdown-How couples can cope during Covid-19. Available at: https://www.unlv.edu/news/release/love-under-lockdown-how-couples-can-cope-during-covid-19.

Mothers pick up almost all home teaching burden during lockdown in UK. Available at: https://www.businessinsider.in/international/news/mothers-pick-up-almost-all-home-teaching-burden-during-lockdown-in-uk/articleshow/75576044.cms.

Sands, P. (2020). COVID-19 Threatens The Poor And Marginalized More Than Anyone. The Global Fund to Fight AIDS, Tuberculosis and Malaria. Available at: https://www.linkedin.com/pulse/covid-19-threatens-poor-marginalized-morethan-anyone-peter-sands-1f/.

Scarred Minds: There is More to the Psychological Impact of Covid-19 Crisis Than Meets The Eye. Available at: https://www.news18.com/news/opinion/scarred-minds-there-is-more-to-the-psychological-impact-of-covid-19-crisis-than-meets-the-eye-2630607.html.

Signal For Help. Available at: https://canadianwomen.org/signal-for-help/

The Facts: Women and Pandemics. Available at: https://canadianwomen.org/the-facts/women-and-pandemics/

United Nations (UN). (2020). Policy Brief: The Impact of COVID-19 on Women. Available at: https://www.un.org/sexualviolenceinconflict/wp-ontent/uploads/2020/06/report/policy-brief-the-impact-of-covid-19-on-women/policy-brief-the-impact-of-covid-19-on-women-en-1.pdf

United Nations Women (UN Women). (2020). Family-Friendly Policies and other

Good Workplace Practices in the Context of COVID-19. Available at: https://www.unwomen.org/-/media/headquarters/attachments/sections/library/publications/2020/family-friendly-policies-and-other-good-workplace-practices-in-the-context-of-covid-19-en.pdf?la=en&vs=4828

What Covid-19 teaches us about women's mental health. Available at: https://timesofindia.indiatimes.com/blogs/uterus-diaries/what-covid-19-teaches-us-about-womens-mental-health/

4

Imposter Phenomenon and Women's Mental Health

A Review

Sucharita Maji and *Shikha Dixit*

Introduction

> '*People occasionally fall ill precisely because a deeply-rooted and long-cherished wish has come to fulfilment.*'
>
> (Freud, 1915; p. 324)

Greek myths of Oedipus, Phaeton, and Icarus remind us that the legends of triumph and victory often end up in the tragedy of guilt, annihilation, and retribution. Success, even being the most desired life outcome, often leads to undesired psychological consequences. This conundrum of success has, therefore, been a matter of inquest for the psychologists from a considerable length of time. Psychoanalytic theorists, beginning from Freud (1915) to Fenichel (1945), Lorand (1950), and Schuster (1955) have thoroughly explored and analysed the negative emotions associated with success; which they referred as success neurosis or success phobia. Consistently, psychoanalytic theorists have attributed this success neurosis to the guilt stemming from the unresolved oedipal dilemma. Achievement-motivation theorist Atkinson (1964) advocated that individuals often avoid success since it might lead to the anxiety associated with failure; i.e., individuals avoid failure rather than success. The fear of defeating others and losing the affection from others might also be at the base of fear of success, as Bierce (1911) mentions success to be "the one unpardonable sin against one's fellows" (p. 333).

Finally, Matina Horner, in 1972, popularised the concept of fear of success. In her study, fear of success was more prominently observed among women than among men, which was in contradiction with the existing psychoanalytical theories. Horner's (1972) work also suggests that the scope of fear of success is not limited to expectancy-value theory and neither it is devoid of the dominating social stereotypical representation of success. Horner's work, undoubtedly, initiated a research tradition to investigate the link between gender and achievement. Deaux (1976) for instance, came up with the notion that women attribute temporary success to external factors rather than something internal. Clance and Imes' (1978) concept of imposter phenomenon (IP) is one such construct that links the notion of gender hierarchy and success.

Imposter Phenomenon (IP)

Based on their research with a large sample of high-achieving women, Clance and Imes (1978) observed that most of these successful women, despite being objectively successful in their lives, frequently experience a perception of intellectual phoniness. They believe that all their achievements are the outcomes of some discounts or luck or anything but their own potentials or intelligence. Harvey and Katz (1985) summarised IP as "a psychological syndrome or pattern based on intense, secret feelings of fraudulence in the face of achievement tasks and situations" (p. 2).

Broadly, IP has the following characteristics—

1. The main feature of IP is the feeling of intellectual fraudulence. No matter how many objective achievements one has in his\her life to prove his\her capability, the person would continue believing that all the achievements are outcomes of some factors other than their talents. They often develop different theories to explain their success. Some people might believe that their success has come out of their hard work, some people might believe in some magical thinking and reason that their repeated imagination of failure helps them avoid failures. Therefore, they develop worrying rituals. Some people with IP might accredit their achievements to their charm, impression management, or their conduct (Clance, 1985).

2. Individuals with IP measure their success or failure in the context of others rather than having an objective assessment of it. Clance's Imposter Phenomenon Scale also has few items which measure the extent to which the individuals with IP compare their success with others. This is also associated with the factor that IP sufferers tend to have an external locus of control (Sightler & Wilson, 2001). Also, to evaluate and validate one's performance in terms of others, IP sufferers also have a very high level of achievement orientation. Clance (1985) refers to this need as 'the need to be special, to be the very best' (p. 24). Such individuals have a high striving

for perfectionism (Sakulku & Alexander, 2011; Cowman & Ferrari, 2002; Henning, Ey, & Shaw, 1998).

3. IP has been found to originate from a sense of low self-esteem (Dahlvig, 2013; Cusack *et al.*, 2013).

4. The perception of intelligence is also different among individuals with IP. They have a notion that intelligence is a fixed entity. Dweck's (1988) model suggests that there are two types of perceptions about intelligence. Some people believe that intelligence is malleable, and they tend to engage in learning-oriented behaviours, whereas individuals who thought that intelligence is a fixed entity engage in performance-oriented actions. Midgley and colleagues (1998) referred to these behaviours as ability-approach goals. Individuals with IP focus more on performance rather than on learning. Langford and Clance (1993) found that individuals with IP often feel helpless at the end of an achievement task since they focus on performance rather than learning. IP is predicted by fear of failure concerns (Fried-Buchalter, 1997).

5. Some researchers found a personality pattern among people with IP. Most consistently associated personality traits are introversion (Holmes, Kertay, Adamson, Holland, & Clance, 1993), narcissism (Gibson Beverly & Schwartz, 2008), and neuroticism (Chae *et al.*, 1995).

6. IP has a developmental origin. Two common upbringing patterns are observed among individuals with IP, either they are brought up in a family with a lack of cohesiveness among the family members or they have an over-protective environment (Li, Hughes, & Thu, 2014; Want & Kleitman, 2006).

7. IP is also characterised by the intense feeling of anxiety and worry. Some studies report a significant positive correlation between trait anxiety and IP (Langford *et al.*, 1993). The concern of being discovered as an imposter also bothers them.

8. One important characteristic feature of IP is imposter cycle. When a task is assigned to a person with IP, there might be two forms of responses. First, the person will procrastinate in the beginning and then work even harder to reach the goals; second, the person works hard from the start. Imposter cycle is a critical source of anxiety.

IP is not free from the societal structure and the gender-based hierarchy, where women are placed at a lower position in society than men. The perception of femininity generally does not go in coherence with the traits associated with success and ambition, such as competitiveness, independence, and power. Since the social definition of success and femininity contradict each other and therefore, most of the women choose to keep success away from their awareness (Clance, Dingman, Reviere, & Stober, 2008) by discounting their achievements. J.B. Miller (1991), in her book, for example, remarked that success, for women is "psychic equivalent of being a destructively aggressive person. This is a self-image that few women can bear. In other words, for many women, it is more comfortable to feel inadequate" (p. 202). Judith Jordan's (1997) self-in-relation theory states that women's self is relational in nature where they define their self-concept in terms of the relationships they have. This relational/feminine trait is also in counter-statement with ambitiousness, which requires one to defeat others. The fear of being too different from others develops some conflicts, and IP is a strategy to distort that ambition to avoid the resultant conflicts.

In terms of the social location of a person, the social status of a group one belongs to also determines one's vulnerability to IP. McIntosh (1985), for instance, reports "people feel fraudulent especially when ascending in hierarchies in which by social definition they do not belong at the top of the pyramid" (p. 3). IP has been consistently found to be higher among members of lower status groups (Bernard, Hoggard, & Neblett, 2017; Ewing, Richardson, James-Myers, & Russell, 1996). In consonance, Harvey (1981) found that IP is determined by the perception that a person is out of place. Therefore, it is related to the discrepancy that one experience between the ideal and the real self (Hirschfield, 1982). This also explains why women are more likely to have IP in comparison to men (Cusack, Hughes, & Nuhu, 2013; Prata & Gietzen, 2007; Oriel, Plane, & Mundt, 2004). Clance and O'Toole (1988) suggest that "we believe that women are more likely to be limited, and, limited more powerfully by imposter phenomenon" (p. 53).

Imposter Phenomenon and Mental Health

Since IP involves negative cognitive and affective states, it is very obvious that IP would have some hazardous effects on the mental health status of a person. The present chapter included the following inclusion criteria to locate the studies which address the mental health consequences of IP. Articles that were only published in English, were published online, involved qualitative or quantitative or mixed methodology to understand the link between mental health and IP were reviewed for the present work. To identify the primary studies, three databases PubMed, PsychNet, and EBSCO Host were searched using the combination of 'Imposter phenomenon', 'impostor phenomenon' (since both spellings are used in literature) and mental health. The search was done on 15th May, 2019.

Search Word	*PubMed*	*EbscoHost*	*Scopus*
Imposter Phenomenon	30	26	74
Impostor Phenomenon	82	26	121
Mental health	312191	88136	297337
Combining 1 & 2	0	1	1
Combining 1 & 3	3	3	6

After comparing these three databases, a total of twelve unique articles were found which connected IP with mental health. Also, there were articles which studied IP in the context of specific mental disorders like depression, anxiety etc. Therefore, it was necessary to combine 'Imposter phenomenon', 'Impostor Phenomenon', 'imposterism', 'Imposter Syndrome' with 'depression', 'depressive disorder', 'mood disorder', 'anxiety', 'anxiety disorder', 'personality disorder' in all these three databases. This search, further adds 10 articles in the list. The connection of IP with these disorders is discussed in detail in the following section.

IP and Anxiety

> "*The girl who maintains qualities of independence and active striving (achievement-orientation) necessary for intellectual mastery defies the convention of sex-appropriate behaviour and must pay a price, a price in anxiety*".
>
> (Maccoby, 1963; Quoted in Clance & Imes, 1978; p. 5)

Psychoanalytic theorists have considered anxiety as the core of neurosis (Endler & Kocovski, 2001); Freud (1936), for instance, mentioned anxiety as the "fundamental phenomenon and the central problem of neurosis" (Freud, 1936, p. 85). Besides being placed as a different category of a bunch of diagnosable and clinically significant disorders in the Diagnostic and Statistical Manual of Mental Disorders (DSM-I), anxiety is a symptom of a number of mental disorders. These are the reasons why anxiety is often referred to as the 'most pervasive psychological phenomenon' (Hoch & Zubin, 1950).

Anxiety has consistently been studied in the context of IP. Looking at the core theoretical underpinning of IP, it becomes evident that the fear of getting discovered by others as incompetent, the pressure to maintain an impression, and the excessive efforts made to win the competition, make one vulnerable to anxiety. In fact, the imposter cycle, which is a defining characteristic of IP revolves around anxiety, hard work, and procrastination. Imposter cycle begins with a feeling of anxiety or fear of getting discovered at the beginning of any achievement-related task. Then the person might choose either to work hard till the deadline or to procrastinate in the beginning and work frenziedly right before the deadline. If, at the end of the task the person succeeds, in the first situation, the person attributes his/her success to the relentless hard work. In the second situation, the person attributes it to luck, charm, or discount. Therefore, the person cannot internalise the achievement. The anxiety perpetually emerges every time there is a project. Therefore, anxiety is an undercurrent of IP.

Now, one might be puzzled by the direction of cause and effect between anxiety and IP. Topping and Kimmel (1985) found that trait anxiety has a significant positive correlation with IP. Trait anxiety locates anxiety at an individual-difference level; Spielberger and colleagues (1971) defined trait anxiety as "the general tendency to worry, especially in social situations that pose some threat to self-esteem" (p. 147). Moreover, individuals with IP tend to have high scores in the anxiety facet of neuroticism (Ross, Stewart, Mugge, & Fultz, 2001; Chae, Piedmont, Estadt, & Wicks, 1995). This might suggest that it is the neurotic personality disposition which makes individuals more vulnerable to IP. Oriel and colleagues (2004) found that IP was significantly correlated to both the state and trait anxiety among a sample of family medicine residents; this might suggest that IP is determined by the disposition of trait anxiety and also lead to elevated state anxiety in an evaluative situation. In a different setting, among the patients of Bulimia Nervosa, social anxiety was positively related to the perception of fraudulence (Striegel-Moore, Silberstein, & Rodin, 1993). This study is in consonance with the finding of Kolligian and Sternberg (1991), who also found perceived fraudulence to be a significant determinant of social anxiety. However, IP cannot be simplified as only perception fraudulence, it is the perception of intellectual fraudulence, however, it is difficult to generalise that IP would always be associated with social anxiety. Chrisman and colleagues (1995), studied the correlation between IP and fear of negative evaluation and social recognition. They found a significant correlation between social anxiety and IP. Harvey and Katz (1985) suggested IP be a significant cause behind the panic disorder and obsessive-compulsive disorder (Winson, 1992). Harvey and Katz (1985) suggested that there are one type of IP where individuals rely on some form of magical thinking where they believe that they would not experience failure at a task if they ritualistically worry about the failure or develop some anxious preoccupation with the failure. However, due to defensive pessimism (Norem & Cantor, 1986), the performance does not get affected as a consequence of IP.

Following Dweck's (1988) model, also, one can assume that since individuals with IP have performance goals rather than learning goals, they are more likely to experience anxiety and shame and helplessness when they experience failure (Langford & Clance, 1993). There is also one study which found no association between anxiety and IP (Mattie, 2007).

Therefore, based on all these works, it is difficult to come to a conclusion regarding the dynamics between IP and anxiety. Future work should attempt to understand the link between anxiety and IP at the clinically significant anxiety disorder level.

Depression and IP

Depression is often considered as the 'common cold of psychiatry' (H. Miller, 1969) since the epidemiological studies reveal a huge prevalence rate of depression across the world. There has been a huge account of debate regarding the gender gap in depression, i.e., women are approximately twice more likely to have depression than men (Alexandrino-Silva *et al.,* 2013). The biological differences could not satisfactorily resolve this puzzle. There are a number of social and psychological factors which might increase women's vulnerability towards depression. The connection between IP and depression among women has also been explored considerably well.

Imposter phenomenon has low self-esteem issues and perceived inadequacy (Clark, Vardeman, & Barba, 2014) at its core. Low self-esteem issue is so ineludibly for IP that some theorists question the independent existence of the IP construct and suggest it to be understood as an extension of self-esteem (Sonnak & Towell, 2001; Cozzarelli & Major, 1990). On the other hand, Beck's theory (2002) emphasises three basic tenets at the foundation of depression. Notably, a negative view of the self (low self-esteem), along with the negative perception of the experience and negative view of the future build the 'cognitive triad' for the development of depression. Among a sample of doctoral students, IP was found to be a predictor of self-efficacy (Jostl *et al.,* 2012). This might provide an explanation of why IP significantly predicts depression (Spinath, 2011; Clance & Imes, 1978).

However, it must be noted that most of the studies have conceptualised depression as a level of the individual emotional state rather than a clinically significant diagnosable disorder. In terms of depression, as a facet of NEO PI-R neuroticism scale (Costa, & McCrae, 2008), depression was found to be significantly correlated to IP (Ross *et al.,* 2001). Sakulku and Alexander (2011) also observed IP sufferers have the personality traits of neuroticism and depressiveness.

Brauer and Wolf (2016) tested the attribution style of individuals with IP and its association with depression. Abramson and colleagues (1978) theorised depression as a cognitive disorder where one attributes the bad events of life to internal, stable, and global factors. It was found that there was a significant negative correlation between positive performance and internal and stable attribution style (Brauer & Wolf, 2016). The connection of IP with helplessness also explains the connection between IP and depression (Cromwell, Brown, Sanchez-Huceles, & Adair, 1990).

McGregor and colleagues (2008), in consonance with these findings, found a positive correlation between Beck Depression Inventory scores and IP. However, this study suggests that there is no impact of gender in the relationship between IP and Depression, i.e. both the genders have similar connection between IP and depression. Also, IP sufferers might experience symptoms of mild depressive disorders; however, one must be cautious since depression does "not always accompany the IP experience" (Terry, 1991; p. 43).

Mental Health Status

Some studies have aimed to discover how IP determines the overall mental health status of a person. Cusack and colleagues (2013), for instance, found a negative correlation between IP beliefs and overall mental health status among the participants of their study. It is also found that IP is a predictor of the status of mental health and wellbeing of a person compared to the distress generated from minority status among racial minor college students (McClain *et al.,* 2016; Coklay, McClain, Enciso, & Martinez, 2013). Similarly, it has been found that the racial identity and gender work as moderators in the relationship between mental health and IP (Bernard *et al.,* 2017). In a recent study, Hu and colleagues (2019) found that people with a high level of IP scores have negative feelings like shame, embarrassment, and inadequacy which deteriorate mental health. The anxiety and pressure caused by the demand for high performance lead to psychological maladjustment and distress (Henning *et al.,* 1998). Peteet and colleagues (2015) found that environmental mastery, which is a component of psychological wellbeing, is negatively related to IP.

Therapeutic Intervention

Since the mental health struggles associated with IP are real, clinical psychologists must work towards developing suitable therapeutic interventions. The first caution one needs to consider while developing a therapeutic intervention is the distinction one needs to make between the neurotic imposter and the genuine fakes (De Vries, 2005). Since there might be some people around us who genuinely masquerade and exploit their charm or passive compliance to gain success, but they are not neurotic imposters. The entire discussion in this chapter is based on the neurotic imposters who genuinely perceive intellectual fraudulence and therefore, suffer from the bunch of mental ailments and struggles mentioned in the previous section.

The second issue in developing therapeutic interventions for neurotic imposters is to differentiate IP from other clinical disorders. Individuals with IP might come for psychotherapeutic help with the symptoms similar to anxiety disorders, depressive disorders, or an overall deteriorated mental health. Therefore, the psychotherapist needs to reach the underlying cause of these psychological symptoms and identify the source, which might not be a simple task due to the defensive mechanisms used by them (Wilson, 1992). Clance and Imes (1978) suggested that there are two common themes of complaints that the women with IP come up with, the first theme is the anxiety and pain associated with achievements and second theme is lack of ambition even when one is performing reasonably well in professional front. Women with IP, also, often fail to bring achievement-related or career-related aspects in their counselling sessions. Moreover, women with IP often seems to go through isolation since most of the people discount their struggles and fears by providing examples of their real, objective achievements. Therefore, the first attempt made by the counsellor should be to believe their emotional journey without providing proof against it.

Since the notion of IP is based on a clear distinction between the real self and false self, Langford and Clance (1993) prescribed that both Rogers' (1995) and Kohut's (1984) strategy of strengthening the real-self will be beneficial therapeutic strategies. Rogers (1995) emphasises on three basic factors in his client-centred therapy might be used as a foundation while working with IP.

First, Unconditional positive regard, which Rogers (1995) defined as '*an acceptance of and regard for his attitudes of the moment, no matter how negative or positive, no matter how much they may contradict other attitudes he has held in the past*' (p. 34).

Second, empathic understanding, which '*enables me* (the therapist) *to see his private world through his eyes'* (p. 34).

Third, Congruence or genuineness of the therapist, which is the 'feelings the therapist is experiencing are available to him, available to his awareness, and he is able to live these feelings, be them, and able to communicate them if appropriate' (p. 61).

Langford and Clance (1993) also considered the mirroring strategy by Kohut (1984) to be effective for individuals with IP. Mirroring is defined as "acceptance and confirmation of the self in its grandness, goodness, and wholeness" (Wolf, 1988, p. 184). Mirroring is very similar to Rogerian unconditional positive regard however is not unconditional in nature (Kahn & Rachman, 2000).

Moreover, Clance and Imes (1978) also emphasised on the developmental origin and family-related variables since there are two distinct patterns found; i.e., either they have been told throughout their lives that they are the brightest one and therefore they felt the compulsion to develop a false self or they have been provided with the information that they are the weak ones.

Clance and Imes (1978) have relied on empathetic relating along with the cognitive restructuring process as a therapy for individuals with IP. Cognitive behavioural therapy has been proven to be beneficial for treating maladaptive perfectionism (Chand, Chibnall, & Slavin, 2017). Langford (1990) and Imes and Clance (1984) also recommended cognitive therapies to be effective for treating IP since it is a result of the maladaptive notion that intelligence is a fixed and inherent quality which cannot be developed over time and practice.

Clance and colleagues (2008) prescribed group therapy to be effectual for women. As it has been mentioned earlier, women with IP tend to suffer from loneliness and isolation. Therefore, group therapy will provide them with the opportunity to be aware of the similar struggles and eventually satisfy their relational self. There are three steps through which theme-centred imposter phenomenon groups' function,

First, individuals with IP are introduced to and made aware of the IP and how different family and social factors might function as an origin of IP. At the beginning of group therapy, women become very supportive of each other however, they become defensive when it comes to sharing their journey with IP with others. However, eventually, they come out of these self-protective mechanisms in a group setting since they fear that other group members might feel rejected as a result of their lack of disclosure.

Second, individuals of this group develop an identity and solidarity, when they listen to the stories of each other, they realise how these individuals with IP have successfully discounted their success and achievements and that also make them aware of their own biases in the attribution of success.

At the third phase, IP sufferers take risks and become aware of their goals and also learn to celebrate their success. Clance *et al.* (2008) recommend feminist therapy as an appropriate therapeutic strategy for women IP sufferers. Feminist therapy is defined as "the complex unfolding of a woman's story woven back and forth through past and present experiences, set in the context of patriarchal culture-provides us with a richness and depth of female life" (Rosewater & Walker, 1985; p. 22). Feminist therapy follows a three-step approach. In the beginning, women are made aware of the social aetiology of the mental health issue of women. This stage is followed by working on the three key aspects of feminist therapy, i.e., power, dependency, and responsibility. In the final stage, the person exercises more autonomy, power, and responsibility while letting go of the dependency. Similar to client-centred therapy, in feminist therapy, clients take the sole responsibility of deciding what is good for her.

Conclusion

It becomes evident from the present chapter that imposter phenomenon is one of the un-identified threats to women's mental health and wellbeing. Apart from having anxiety issues and low mood issues, IP sufferers, in general, experience deteriorated mental health. The chapter discusses a number of therapeutic interventions which might be used to deal with IP among women. Rogerian psychotherapy, feminist therapy, as well as cognitive behavioural therapy might be of help. However, the most crucial issue with IP is that often the sufferers are not aware of their attribution fallacy and they end up struggling with IP throughout their life. A huge impact of IP can be visible among the organisational settings, especially in the sectors that involve high-achieving careers. Mental health professionals, therefore, must consider working exhaustively in IP.

References

Alexandrino-Silva, C., Wang, Y.P., Viana, M.C., Bulhões, R.S., Martins, S.S., and Andrade, L.H. (2013). Gender differences in symptomatic profiles of depression: results from the Sao Paulo Megacity Mental Health Survey. *Journal of Affective Disorders*, *147*(1-3), 355-364.

Atkinson, J.W. (1964). *An Introduction to Motivation*. New York: American Book.

Beck, C.T. (2002). Postpartum depression: A metasynthesis. *Qualitative Health Research*, *12*(4), 453-472.

Bernard, D.L., Hoggard, L.S., and Neblett Jr, E.W. (2018). Racial discrimination, racial identity, and impostor phenomenon: A profile approach. *Cultural Diversity and Ethnic Minority Psychology*, *24*(1), 51.

Bierce, A. (2003). The Devil's Dictionary. 1911. *Unabridged republication*. Ed. Philip Smith.

Brauer, K., and Wolf, A. (2016). Validation of the German-language Clance impostor phenomenon scale (GCIPS). *Personality and Individual Differences*, *102*, 153-158.

Chae, J.H., Piedmont, R.L., Estadt, B.K., and Wicks, R.J. (1995). Personological evaluation of Clance's Imposter Phenomenon Scale in a Korean sample. *Journal of Personality Assessment*, *65*(3), 468-485.

Chand, S.P., Chibnall, J.T., and Slavin, S.J. (2018). Cognitive behavioural therapy for maladaptive perfectionism in medical students: A preliminary investigation. *Academic Psychiatry*, *42*(1), 58-61.

Chrisman, S.M., Pieper, W.A., Clance, P.R., Holland, C.L., and Glickauf-Hughes, C. (1995). Validation of the Clance imposter phenomenon scale. *Journal of Personality Assessment*, *65*(3), 456-467.

Clance, P.R., and Imes, S.A. (1978). The imposter phenomenon in high achieving women: Dynamics and therapeutic intervention. *Psychotherapy: Theory, Research and Practice*, *15*(3), 241.

Clance, P.R., and OToole, M.A. (1987). The imposter phenomenon: An internal barrier to empowerment and achievement. *Women and Therapy*, *6*(3), 51-64.

Clance, P.R., Dingman, D., Reviere, S.L., and Stober, D.R. (1995). Impostor Phenomenon in an interpersonal/social context: Origins and treatment. *Women and Therapy*, *16*(4), 79-96.

Clark, M., Vardeman, K., and Barba, S. (2014). Perceived inadequacy: A study of the imposter phenomenon among college and research librarians.

Cole, E., and Rothblum, E.D. (2014). *Treating Women's Fear of Failure: From Worry to Enlightenment*. Routledge.

Cozzarelli, C., and Major, B. (1990). Exploring the validity of the impostor phenomenon. *Journal of Social and Clinical Psychology*, *9*(4), 401-417.

Cromwell, B., Brown, N., and Adair, F.L. (1990). The impostor phenomenon and personality characteristics of high school honour students. *Journal of Social Behaviour and Personality*, *5*(6), 563.

Cusack, C.E., Hughes, J.L., and Nuhu, N. (2013). Connecting Gender and Mental Health to Imposter Phenomenon Feelings. *Psi Chi Journal of Psychological Research*, *18*(2).

Dahlvig, J.E. (2013). A narrative study of women leading within the Council for Christian Colleges and Universities, Christian Higher Education, *12*(1/2), 93-109.

Deaux, K. (1976). *The Behaviour of Women and Men*. Wadsworth Pub Co.

Dweck, C.S., and Leggett, E.L. (1988). A social-cognitive approach to motivation and personality. *Psychological Review*, *95*(2), 256.

Endler, N.S., and Kocovski, N.L. (2001). State and trait anxiety revisited. *Journal of Anxiety Disorders*, *15*(3), 231-245.

Ewing, K.M., Richardson, T.Q., James-Myers, L., and Russell, R.K. (1996). The relationship between racial identity attitudes, worldview, and African American graduate students' experience of the imposter phenomenon. *Journal of Black Psychology*, *22*(1), 53-66.

Fenichel, O. (1945). *The Psychoanalytic Theory of Neurosis*. New York (Norton) 1945.

Freud, S. (1915). Some character-types met with in psychoanalytic work. *Collected Papers* (Vol. 4). London: Hogarth, 1949, 318-344.

Freud, S. (1936). Inhibitions, symptoms and anxiety. *The Psychoanalytic Quarterly*, *5*(1), 1-28.

Gibson Beverly, G., and Schwartz, J.P. (2008). Attachment, entitlement, and the impostor phenomenon in female graduate students. *Journal of College Counseling*, *11*(2), 119-132.

Harvey, J.C., and Katz, C. (1985). *If I'm so successful, why do I feel like a fake?: The impostor phenomenon*. St. Martin's Press.

Henning, K., Ey, S., and Shaw, D. (1998). Perfectionism, the impostor phenomenon and psychological adjustment in medical, dental, nursing and pharmacy students. *Medical Education*, *32*(5), 456-464.

Hirschfield, M.M. (1982). The impostor phenomenon in high achieving women. *Dissertation Abstracts International*, *48*, 1772A.

Hoch, P.H., and Zubin, J. (1950). *Anxiety*, New York, Grune & Stratton.

Holmes, S.W., Kertay, L., Adamson, L.B., Holland, C.L., and Clance, P.R. (1993). Measuring the impostor phenomenon: A comparison of Clance's IP Scale and Harvey's IP Scale. *Journal of Personality Assessment*, *60*(1), 48-59.

Horner, M.S. (1972). Toward an understanding of achievement-related conflicts in women. *Journal of Social Issues*, *28*(2), 157-175.

Jordan, J.V. (Ed). (1997). Women's growth in diversity: More writings from the Stone Centre. New York: Guilford. Jordan, J.V., Kaplan, A.G., Miller, J.B., Stiver, I.P., and Surrey, J.L. (Eds.). (1991). *Women's Growth in Connection: Writings from the Stone Centre.* New York: Guilford.

Jostl, G., Bergsmann, E., Luftenegger, M., Schober, B., and Spiel, C. (2012). When will they blow my cover? The impostor phenomenon among Austrian doctoral students. *Journal of Psychology*, *220*(2), 109.

Kohut, H. (2009). *How does Analysis Cure?*. University of Chicago Press.

Langford, J., and Clance, P.R. (1993). The imposter phenomenon: Recent research findings regarding dynamics, personality and family patterns and their implications for treatment. *Psychotherapy: Theory, Research, Practice, Training*, *30*(3), 495.

Li, S., Hughes, J.L., and Thu, S.M. (2014). The Links between Parenting Styles and Imposter Phenomenon. *Psi chi Journal of Psychological Research*, *19*(2).

Lorand, S. (1950). *Clinical Studies in Psychoanalysis*. New York: International Universities Press.

Rosewater, L.B. and Walker, L.E. (1985). *Handbook of Feminist Therapy: Women's Issues in Psychotherapy*. Springer Publishing Company.

Mattie, C.N. (2007). *The Imposter Phenomenon: A Study of Self Assessment and Competency to Perform as a Physician Assistant in the Continental United States*. Pacific University, Oregon, Research Repository.

McGregor, L.N., Gee, D.E., and Posey, K.E. (2008). I feel like a fraud and it depresses me: The relation between the imposter phenomenon and depression. *Social Behaviour and Personality: an International Journal, 36*(1), 43-48.

McClain, S., Beasley, S.T., Jones, B., Awosogba, O., Jackson, S., and Cokley, K. (2016). An examination of the impact of racial and ethnic identity, impostor feelings, and minority status stress on the mental health of Black college students. *Journal of Multicultural Counselling and Development, 44*(2), 101-117.

McClelland, D.C., Atkinson, J.W., Clark, R.A., and Lowell, E.L. (1953). *The Achievement Motive.* New York: Appleton. Century, Crofts.

McIntosh, P. (1985). (1985). *Feeling like a fraud*. Stone Centre for Developmental Services and Studies. Wellesley College.

Midgley, C., Kaplan, A., Middleton, M., Maehr, M.L., Urdan, T., Anderman, L.H., and Roeser, R. (1998). The development and validation of scales assessing students' achievement goal orientations. *Contemporary Educational Psychology, 23*(2), 113-131.

Miller, J.B. (1991). *The Development of Women's Sense of Self.* Guilford, New York.

Norem, J.K., and Cantor, N. (1986). Defensive pessimism: Harnessing anxiety as motivation. *Journal of Personality and Social Psychology, 51*(6), 1208.

Prata, J., and Gietzen, J.W. (2007). The imposter phenomenon in physician assistant graduates. *The Journal of Physician Assistant Education, 18*(4), 33-36.

Rogers, C.R. (1995). *On Becoming a Person: A Therapist's View of Psychotherapy*. Houghton Mifflin Harcourt.

Ross, S.R., Stewart, J., Mugge, M., and Fultz, B. (2001). The imposter phenomenon, achievement dispositions, and the five factor model. *Personality and Individual Differences, 31*(8), 1347-1355.

Sakulku, J. and Alexander, J. (2011). The imposter phenomenon. *International Journal of Behavioural Science*, 6 (1), 73-92.

Schuster, D.B. (1955). On the fear of success. *Psychiatric Quarterly*, 29, 412-420.

Oriel, K., Plane, M.B., and Mundt, M. (2004). Family medicine residents and the impostor phenomenon. *Family Medicine-Kansas City, 36*(4), 248-252.

Sonnak, C., and Towell, T. (2001). The impostor phenomenon in British university students: Relationships between self-esteem, mental health, parental rearing style and socioeconomic status. *Personality and Individual Differences, 31*(6), 863-874.

Striegel-Moore, R.H., Silberstein, L.R., and Rodin, J. (1993). The social self in bulimia nervosa: Public self-consciousness, social anxiety, and perceived fraudulence. *Journal of Abnormal Psychology*, *102*(2), 297.

Terry, R.M. (1991). *The Imposter Phenomenon as related to Depression and Causal Attributes for Success.* Unpublished master's thesis. Georgia State University, Atlanta, GA.

Thompson, T., Foreman, P., and Martin, F. (2000). Impostor fears and perfectionistic concern over mistakes. *Personality and Individual Differences*, *29*(4), 629-647.

Topping, M.E., and Kimmel, E.B. (1985). The imposter phenomenon: Feeling phony. *Academic Psychology Bulletin*, *7*(2), 213–226.

Want, J., and Kleitman, S. (2006). Imposter phenomenon and self-handicapping: Links with parenting styles and self-confidence. *Personality and Individual Differences*, *40*(5), 961-971.

Wilson, G.S. (1999). Personality variables in levels of predicted and actual test anxiety among college students. *Educational Research Quarterly*, *22*(3), 3.

Wolf, E.S. (1988). *Treating the Self: Elements of Clinical Self Psychology*. New York: The Guilford Press.

5

Health Status and Wellbeing of Elderly Women of Tharu Tribe

An Investigation

Ram Kalap Tiwari

Introduction

As per the census of 2011 the tribal population consists of 8.6 per cent while it was 8.2 per cent according to the census of 2001 in India. The tribes are known for the simplicity, truthfulness, honesty, love of freedom, uprightness, hospitality and love of nature. They live in forest, hills and naturally isolated regions. They are different in physical appearance as compared to the other common people.

The Tharu is well known scheduled tribe of Uttar Pradesh declared in 1967 along with four other tribes: Raji, Bhotia, Jaunsari and Buxa. They live in terai belt of Uttar Pradesh. The region covers five districts of Uttar Pradesh namely, Lakhimpur Kheri, Balrampur, Baharaich, Shravasti and Maharajganj. The Terai or Tarai (Hindi: तराई; Nepali: तराइ) is a lowland region in southern Nepal and northern India that lies south of the outer foothills of the mighty Himalayas, the Shiwalik Hills, and north of the Indo-Gangetic Plain. This lowland flat belt is distinguished by tall and large grasslands, scrub savannah, sal jungles and clay rich swamps. In northern India, the Terai stretches from the river Yamuna eastward across states of Himachal Pradesh, Haryana, Uttarakhand, Uttar Pradesh and Bihar. The 2001 census showed the data that 77.4 per cent of the total tribal population of Uttar Pradesh with a population of 83,544 belongs to Tharu tribe. Mainly, the Tharu people are engaged in agriculture, hunting and fishing, forestry-related works which forms their economy. Tharu tribe have a deep affiliation to forest and rivers. An interesting thing about this tribe is that historically it was found that only this tribe survived from mosquito-borne *malaria* in the jungles and tarai regions.

Later, only when mosquito control measures became successful only then many other communities have migrated into these tribal areas. Hence, due to the affiliation with nature and hard working life style in jungles and living at riverside overall the health status of Tharu people are good but certain hygiene related, reproductive health, alcoholism issues emerges. Although, in Tharu community women are main work force and centre to economy but they are generally less aware about their health and hygiene.

The phenomenon of population aging is becoming a major concern for policy-makers all over the world, for both developed and developing countries, during last two decades. But the problems arising out of it will have varied implications for underdeveloped, developing and developed countries. Aging of population is affected due to downward trends infertility and mortality i.e. due to low birth rates coupled with long life expectancies.

Elderly or old age consists of ages nearing or surpassing the average life-span of human being. The boundary of old age cannot be defined exactly because it does not have the same meaning in all societies. Government of India adopted 'National Policy on Older Persons' in January 1999. The policy defines 'senior citizen' or 'elderly' as a person who is of age 60 years or above. People can be considered old because of certain changes in their activities or social roles.

In India the size of the elderly population i.e. persons above the age of 60 years is fast growing although it constituted only 7.4 per cent of total population at turn of the new millennium. Entailing almost a tripling of the population over the ages of 60 years (i.e. the elderly) (Government of India, 2011). This pattern is poised to continue. It is projected that the proportion of Indians aged 60 and older will rise from 7.5 per cent in 2010 to 11.1 per cent in 2025 (UNDESA, 2008). For a developing country like India, this may be pose mounting pressures on various fronts like health and wellbeing. Aging this segment of population faces multiple medical/ health and psychological problems. There is an emerging need to pay greater attention to aging-related issues and to promote holistic policies and programmes for dealing with aging society (Srivastava, 1994).

Aging is considered as natural and universal process. It is regarded as an biological phenomenon. Elderly people are suffering from various physical, mental, social and economical problems (Chaudhary, 2001; Dandekar, 2004).

Large-scale studies of the health behaviour of this growing elderly Indian population are scarce. Aging mainly associated with social isolation, poverty, apparent reduction in family support, inadequate housing, impairment of cognitive functioning, mental illness, loss and dependency towards end of life (Gore, 2004). Generally, at household level, cultural norms and practices and socioeconomic factors determine the extent of health problems among women. Change in socio-economic status and various health problems adversely affect an individual's way of life during old age.

According to the World Health Organization (WHO), the definition of health is a state of complete physical, mental and social wellbeing and not merely the absence of disease or infirmity. The health status of any community is influenced by the interplay of health consciousness of the people, socio-cultural, demographic, economic, educational and political factors. The common beliefs, traditional customs, myths, practices related to health and disease in turn influence the health seeking behaviour of people (Balgir, 2004). Health is an essential component of the well-being of the mankind and is a prerequisite for human development. In general heath of an average non-tribal Indian is inferior to western counterparts, the health of an average Indian tribal is found to be much poorer compared to the non-tribal counterparts (Barry, 2002). The health status of tribal population is very poor and worst of primitive tribal because of the isolation, remoteness and being largely unaffected by the developmental process going on in India (Soudarssanne *et al.*, 2009).

There were about 635 tribal groups and subgroups including 75 primitive communities who have been designated as 'primitive' based on pre-agricultural level of technology, low level of literacy, stagnant or diminishing population size, relative isolation from the main stream of the population, economical and educational backwardness, extreme poverty-dwelling in remote areas, constant touch with natural environment and unaffected by the developmental processes undergoing in India (Chakravarti, 2007). India is home to almost half the tribal population of the world. Tribals are characterized by a distinctive cultural, primitive traits, and socio-economic background (Panda, 2005).

Although tribals are accorded special status, their status on the whole, especially their health still remains unsatisfactory. They are highly disease-prone. Also they do not have required access to basic health facilities. They are more exploited, neglected and highly vulnerable to diseases with high degree of malnutrition, morbidity and mortality (Balgir, 2004). Their misery is compounded by poverty, illiteracy, ignorance of causes of disease, hostile environment, poor sanitation, lack of safe drinking water and blind belief etc.

Some of the preventable disease such as tuberculosis, malaria, gastro, measles, whooping cough, skin disease etc. is also high among tribes. Some of the genetic origin diseases are also prevented in tribes. Night blindness, sexually transmitted diseases are well-known public health problems of tribes in India.

Wellbeing is a way of life, especially in terms of life ideally inclined to health and wellness; unifying body, mind, and soul; individually full of purposeful attitude and aim to live life more fully; and a functional life in all social, personal, and environmental aspects (Myer, 2003). Health and wellbeing, and life style of an individual are closely related. Wellbeing aims to determine factors strengthening health and change individual's lifestyle in that direction.

Psychological health of individual depends on his positive functioning in certain aspects of his life. Individual should have a positive relationship with others, should be dominant over the environment, should accept himself and his past; should have a goal and meaning in life. But in tribes these characteristics are not properly developed and cultivated since long time.

The present investigation examines the health problems and well-being of the elderly in Tharu tribal woman. It also explores the accessibility and availability of public health services to these disadvantaged women in the tribal population at Bahraich district of Uttar Pradesh.

Objectives

- To study the health status and wellbeing of tribal elderly women of Bahraich district of Uttar Pradesh.
- To examine and understand the major health problems faced by the elderly tribal women.
- To study the status of the support receiving by the tribal elderly women from their family.
- To study the sociodemographic characteristics of the elderly Tharu women.
- To highlight the role of social worker in creating awareness of various health services available from the government for these women.

Research Design

Descriptive research design has been adopted for this study. The purpose of this investigation was to examine the health status and wellbeing of the respondents and elicit new information about elderly tribal women in the study area through the above objectives.

Area of the study: Based on the data available with the government regarding the numerical concentration of the tribals in Uttar Pradesh, Bahraich district was selected for the present study.

Sample: The sample consisted of 60 females belonging to age group between 60-70 years. All the elderly in the study area were taken as the sample and hence no sampling method was used.

Tools and Techniques of the data collection: Based on the objectives of the study an interview schedule was prepared to elicit the fact and details from the respondents selected for the purpose of the study. For the collection of primary data from the selected elderly tribal women in Bahraich district, semi-structured interview schedule was used. It was constructed after reviewing the past researches on elderly conducted in India with the tribal's covering the various health aspects.

Results and Discussion

Socio-demographic characteristics of the elderly tribal women: The sample consisted of elderly tribal women (N = 60), out of this total number 60 per cent were between the age group of 60-64 years, 20 per cent between 65-67 years and remaining 20 per cent between 68-70 years. This was purposefully done to examine the change in the nature of health problems with increase in age. These figures are presented in Table 5.1.

Table 5.1: Socio-demographic characteristics of the elderly tribal women

Socio-demographic Variables		*Percentage*	*N*
Age	60-64 years	60	36
	65-67 years	20	12
	68-70 years	20	12
Literacy	Literate	05	03
	Illiterate	95	57
Martial Status	Married	90	54
	Widow	10	06
Living Conditions	Hut Houses	95	57
	Pucca Houses	05	03

The total number of respondents were Tharu. 90 per cent of respondents were married and remaining 10 per cent women were widows. 95 per cent respondents were illiterate and rest 05 per cent were literate and had signature capability. Majority of these women living in joint families and 95 per cent living in hut houses with their children. The remaining 05 per cent lives in pucca or Khaparail houses with children.

Economic status: In the present investigation income of the elderly women was taken as a parameter to determine the health status and wellbeing of the respondents. The elderly women all of them were housewives and had very small income. They fetch wood from the forest and sell them in the market. They depended on their family members for food and shelter. They work hard in forest and agricultural areas. Majority of the elderly women reported that they are getting financial assistance from their sons.

The forest based, tribal economy in most parts of the study area is women-centred. Women make provision for the basic necessities like food, fuel, medicine, housing material etc. from the forest produce. Food was obtained from sifting cultivation and from minor forest produce like flowers and fruits collected from forest. Extraction from herbs, roots and animals were used for medicine. All these efforts incurred an excessive workload on women (Salil, 2000).

Health Aspects: All the respondents had some health problems, the most common being hypertension (40%), arthritis (20%), diabetes (5%), constipation (80%), and other included skin problems (63%), and vision problems (42%). Vitamins deficiency was common in all respondents. It was observed that all respondents had more than one health problem.

With increasing age, the health problems increase but the financial resources of the elderly women usually show a decline. 60 per cent of the tribal elderly reported that the doctors were not present in the PHC most of time because of remote area.

Previous studies show that almost 20 per cent of the PHCs (Public Health Centres) in tribal areas are not staffed with doctors and 15 per cent of the post of paramedical workers are vacant (Sondarssanane *et al.* 2012). Most of the tribal use Desi (local and native) medicine for their ailments as the first choice. They feel that medical services are expensive. They have developed a habit of getting health services free because of the poverty and family was not willing to pay for their health purposes. Elderly tribal women could not gain access to medical care services due to lack of communication and unavailability of transportation. Analysis of perception of their own health is presented in Table 5.2.

Table 5.2 clearly shows that most of the respondents from three age categories have minor as well as major health problems. When comparison was made it was found that 68-70 aged categories have more serious health problems followed by 60-64 age categories and 65-67 age categories respectively. The highest proportion (45%) of total respondents states that they were suffering from minor illness.

Table 5.2: Perceived health status of the elderly women

Age	Perception of health			
	On the whole good	Have minor illness	Have major illness	Total
60-64	10 (27.77%)	18 (50.00%)	8 (22.22%)	36 (100%)
65-67	3 (25.00%)	7 (58.33%)	2 (16.66%)	12 (100%)
68-70	1 (8.33%)	2 (16.66%)	9 (75.00%)	12 (100%)

The health status of the poverty stricken tribal aged is unquestionably the worst. The health care facilities to the aged are hardly availed due to utter ignorance, poverty and belief system that the failing of health is normal occurrence of life.

Apart from all the difficulties and problems respondents were asked to report on their specific health problems. The respondents overlooked some minor illness and reports only the main serious problems. Some of respondents had multiple illnesses. Distribution of the tribal elderly by the nature of ailments is presented in Table 5.3.

Table 5.3: Nature of illness in elderly women of Tharu tribes

Nature of illness	Age Groups		
	60-64 years	65-67 years	68-70 years
Back Pain	10%	50%	00%
Blood pressure	20%	30%	10%
Asthma	20%	30%	10%
Digestion	05%	30%	25%
Skin disease	15%	30%	15%
Body pain	10%	40%	10%
Headache	15%	40%	05%
Wellbeing	Unsatisfactory 85%		Satisfactory 15%

It was observed in the analysis that with increasing age, the percentage of respondent's ailments had increased. With increasing age, older tribal women usually showed serious and multiple illness and health problems. Expensive medical treatments in private clinics discouraged elderly women from paying attention to their health needs, inadequate facilities of mobilization and illiteracy in many instances, they neglect health. Wellbeing of 85 per cent elderly women was found unsatisfactory. Only 15 per cent respondents represented satisfactory conditions of wellbeing.

Occupational status: Nearly 30 per cent of the elderly women were housewives. They work in other houses for earning some money.

60 per cent of elderly women do not have any occupation because of their old age. They take care of their grandchildren. Some elderly women were engaged in agricultural areas and construction work on daily wages.

Role of social workers: In India, due to the elite structure of health care facilities, the poor and elderly women are often neglected. In the present investigation it was observed that once the elderly fall sick, they don't visit the PHC or private clinic.

Social work is mainly believed to be problem-oriented but while working with elderly it may be process-oriented. Social work can be conducted in hospital or through NGO or community-based rehabilitation centres. The useful intervention strategies for social worker may be:

1. Creating awareness for regular check-up, nutrition, and health related problems.
2. Counselling and training of local women in disease prevention, tribal women should be trained in healthy food habits through educational programmes.
3. Participation of local community and NGO worker to work in thc health area for elderly.
4. Health care units should be established for the elderly in their nearest approaches.

Suggestions

A mobile van to cater to the needs of the community every month on the fixed date and time should be available for tribes. Social and economic incentives should be provided to tribes for their health and wellbeing. Using these and more strategies the quality of life of tribes can be improved. The results of the study showed that there is a need for counselling centres that can take care of their physical and psychological needs.

References

Bala, S.M. and Thiruselvakumar, D. (2009). Overcoming the problems in practice of public health among tribal in India. *Indian Journal of Community Medicine*, 34 (4), 283-287.

Balgir, R.S. (2004). Dimension of rural tribal health, nutritional states of Kondha tribe and tribal welfare in Orissa: A biotechnological approach. Proceeding of the UGC sponsored national seminar on human health and nutrition: A biotechnological approach, Lead lecture, Thane, pp. 47-57.

Barry, A.M. (2002). *Understanding health*. New Delhi: Sage Publications.

Chakravarti, S. (2007). *Tribal welfare and development in India. Past present and strategies with special reference to agriculture and forestry*. New Delhi.

Chaudhary, A. (2001). *Active Aging in New Millennium*. New Delhi: Anugraha.

Dandekar (2004). *Aged in India*. New Delhi: Anmol Publications.

Gore (2004). *Aged in India*. New Delhi: Anmol Publications.

Panda, A.K. (2005). *Elderly Women in Megapolis: Status and Adjustment*. New Delhi: Concept Publishing Company.

Salil, B. (2000). Dimensions of tribal health in India. *Health and Population-Perspectives and Issues, 23*(2), 61-70.

Srivastava, R.C. (1994). *The Problem of the Old Age*. New Delhi: Classical Publication Company.

6

Work-Life Balance Difficulties among Working Women in India

Priyanka Pathak and *Shobhna Joshi*

Introduction

Work and life were integrated from ancient times. 'Work-Life Balance' is not a new concept it has developed over a long period. Day to day life activities like family members cares, personal involvement in different household tasks, social responsibilities, and public involvement combine along with work. Anne-Marie Slaughter said that why women still can't have it all and forced a discussion that involves educational, corporate, and political circles and quantity and time when women can balance their personal lives with their work.

Before 1950, only a few women participated in professional work outside the home. Education was limited to only some areas, and most of the male was authorized for education but not female. The main priority for women was to care about their husbands, children, and elderly persons and to fulfil social responsibilities. Most of the women were uneducated, and those who educated, many of them did not involve in paid work and those who engaged in work, most of them focused on primary teaching, nursing and other traditional female occupations. Very few women in the profession held authority, power and status in the work setting. The scenario of India has changed radically since twenty-first century (Claramma, 2007). Women's participation in different areas had been increased and they are making substantial progress towards their work and established an identity of their own and created a space for them in different sectors. Educational institutions started different types of plans for empowered women and trained them to enter new arenas and to enable them to move away from traditional roles. Families started to expect women not only to involve in household tasks with higher education but also to use their knowledge and talent in any profession they were interested. It is very common, after spending so many years in education and obtaining professional degrees, they became interested in using their efficiency and knowledge acquired productively and wealth. So in the age of globalization, Indian women made their presence in different sectors, which were unthinkable for women in the past. The number of working women is increasing and they are making substantial progress in their workplace. In the modern era, Indian women are well-educated with high proficiency, efficiency and skills. So the government of centre and state tried to change the socio-cultural setup.

The Indian scenario has been changed unpredictable ways due to globalization, urbanization, industrialization and high degree of competition. The structure of Indian families is also changed in this modern era. Nuclear families are increasingly in high rate, and joint families are broken rapidly. Indian women from all classes have entered into different occupations. Exposure of educational opportunities is substantially higher among women of urban areas as compared to women of rural areas. This is due to increased awareness and raised aspirations of personal growth, economic pressure, etc.

Today, working women in India keeping up two types of responsibilities in which they are continually challenged by the demands of full-time work and responsibilities and commitment of home. These dual responsibilities increasing anxiety, stress, conflict, guilt, and frustration among working women where they have to manage the duties of their family and work and need to make a balance between their work life and the personal life.

History of Work-life Balance

Work-Life Balance involves practices in maintaining a balance between the demands of work at the workplace and demands of family. The demands and pressures of work make difficult to extend time for balancing work-life activities. Organizations also have workplace culture and climates that affect employees' lives outside of workplace. Employees' physical health and psychological health is also very important for any organization's output, so the organization must concern about the time to time review of current work processes and practices to determine which factors play an important role in employees' stress and efficiencies. The purpose of the present study is to determine the work-life balance issues and problems faced by working women in India.

The main origination of the work-life balance word is in the Western world during World War-II. During World War-II, government encourages women to join the paid workforce in U.S. and U.K. But after World War-II women were asked to return home and resume their family roles. A work-life balance metaphor is a social construct located within a particular period and place. Research in work-life balance started at a time when many women entering the labour market. At that tlme, researches mainly focus on working mothers and dual-earner families. It is also known as work-life balance and work-family integration. Researchers began to show interest in the interaction between work and family because of the changing nature in gender roles resulting from these social dynamics (Mac Dermid, 2004). The period after World War-II was known as an idealization of the American family in which husband as the main breadwinner and the wife as housewife and mother. In this period, a movement was started with purpose of securing the rights of working women. On the other hand, during the 1960s and 1970s, a strong feminist movement started, which exert force on critical evaluation of the traditional gender roles. It became clear that women were taking on the burden of dual roles. Instead of being liberated from traditional gender roles in 1980, during the 1990s, the focus was on the expansion of work-family research to previously less studied populations in the U.S. such as ethnic groups, single-parent families, and poor working families, as well as on the organization's role to reduce the pressures of work and family faced by the employees (Rapoport *et al.*, 2002).

During the mid of 1970, research on work and family issues started in India. It was the time when research on working women was also increased, in which different issues include the socio-economic impact of women's work on the family, power relationships within the family, quality of marital relationship and impact on children. However, In India, work and family research has undertaken two separate tracks. One is the track in which the main focus of researches on the main role of patriarchy society of country in subordination of women at work and at home. On the other hand researchers of psychosocial areas examined the work and family relations within urban settings from a role theory perspective. There has been little difference between these two streams, which is lack of cross-preferences in published studies. Most studies conducted on Indian women were obsessed with the concerns of status, societal recognition and perceptions towards working women, inoluding working women's views about non-working women and non-working women's views about working women. Research also focuses on stresses and strains of balancing work and home roles and their impact on the psychological and physical health and well-being of women. Other studies examined the changing roles of women, values, demands and expectations of urban middle-class families. During recent times, research on work and family indicated that working status was not a guarantee to equitable relationships within the family, especially in Indian society where it is expected from working women to fulfill all the responsibilities related to home at any cost.

Definition of Work-Life Balance

Historical pieces of evidence show that work-life balance is not a new phenomenon. The main theory behind the work-life balance is that every individual is unique and varying, but sometimes they need to fulfil mutually exclusive demands due to the roles that they play in the different aspects of their lives, for example, mother versus worker (Ford *et al.* 2007). According to McCartney (2002), work-life balance can be described as the fit between multiple roles in a person's life. It is essential for all individuals to achieve and maintain the balance between their work and their personal life (Lockett, 2008). Work-Life Balance involved not one single ultimate experience, but it is a series of individual experiences unfolding over time (www.essay.uk.com).

Greenhaus and colleagues (2003) defined work-family balance as the extent to which an individual is equally engaged in and equally satisfied with his or her work role and family role. It means work-life balance involves satisfaction and good functionality at work and home with a minimum of role conflicts (Clark, 2001). They also suggested that work-life balance includes three interconnected, components such as time balance, involvement balance, and satisfaction balance. When imbalance or interference occurs between work and family roles for an individual who creates conflict, these three components should be considered as important factors to achieve work-life balance.

The most popular definition of work-family conflict states that it is a type of integral conflict in which the role pressures from the work and family facets are mutually incompatible in some respect (Greenhaus & Beutell, 1985). According to this definition, work-family conflict can occur in two directions: the first one is family can interfere with work (family-work conflict), or work can interfere with family (work-family conflict).

According to Guest (2001) work-family balance implies that there is a balance between the demands of work and family. Clark (2001) defined work-family balance as an absence of work-family conflict or increasing levels of work-family enrichment. Work-Life balance involves compatibility of roles and their promotion of growth, satisfaction between multiple roles, perceived control between multiple roles and relationship between conflict and facilitation (Kalliath & Brough, 2008; Clark, 2001). It is an art of managing both the work and family domains effectively.

A number of women working, particularly working in banks, factories and hospitals, complaining that they do not have enough time to look after and give care to their babies and family members. The efficiency of a working woman is always suspected by most of the people, especially their male colleagues. It is generally seen that after all qualifications remaining similar, men are usually preferred. Authorities are doubtful whether women would be able to handle male subordinates, make independent decisions, cope with crisis and manage their duties properly (Andal, 2002). Even though women prove they are efficient, authorities think twice before promoting them and even if women are given a chance, there is always a remark that they were given the position because they were women. Apart from this, working women suffer from sexual harassment. It is another serious problem faced by working women (illiterate, low paid workers or highly educated, highly paid executives) in different areas (organized or unorganized sector) at one time or the other by their male colleagues or their superiors. Although women have sufficient skills to perform higher-level jobs despite this, they tend to hold lower-level positions than men.

Issues Related to Working Women

It is very important to find out where a woman exists in this Indian society in current scenario. There is no single theory, model and approach that are right for everyone for their whole life (businessballs.com). In India women have struggled to establish their existence, identity, and place and trying to create a space for themselves in their workplace. Although in the age of globalization, women have more time-saving devices and facilities, the biggest problem is that they have less time to utilize this device. They continuously work longer hours and take fewer holidays. They are more contactable than ever before, often interrupted during dinner with family or other important events fulfil by a mobile phone ring (Chakravarty, 2000).

Work-life balance is more likely to create negative influences in the family-related domains, which increases anxiety, stress, frustration, internal conflict and lower life satisfaction. Studies have identified several variables that influence the level of work-life balance, which includes types of family, size of family, the age of children, support of spouse and family members, social support, work hours, and the level of organizational support, work environment, etc. These variables play important role in the development of the physical and psychological well-being of working women.

Super (1980) identified six common life roles for every individual in their whole life. He indicated that it is reality that every individual needs to balance these different roles simultaneously at various stages throughout their lives rather than transitional sequence from one role to another. It is required for women to perform an accretion of disparate roles simultaneously in which each role with its unique pressures (Kopp & Ruzicka, 1993). Every role has both positive and negative effects on the physical health, mental health, and well-being of working women. Studies also reported that in certain instances, women with multiple roles have better physical and psychological health than women with less role involvement (Doress-Wortes, 1994). However, multiple roles have also been found to cause a variety of adverse effects on women's mental and physical health (Hughes & Glinsky, 1994).

In the current scenario, women work as administrator, scientists, bankers, teachers, doctors, managers, lawyers and politicians also, etc. There are many professions today where women are employed or involved. They rise successfully in different fields like technology, politics, and business, etc. Society has started seeing women from a different perspective especially in India. But it is also true that majority of the women still face gender bias and discrimination also. Society has started seeing women from a different perspective. From the ancient time women have been subjected to physical, sexual and mental exploitation and torture. They faced uncounted challenges and problems at home and workplace both. It is reported that generally women face sexual harassment, mental stress, discriminatory practices, safety and security issues, etc. in the workplace (Martin, 1989). The traditional thoughts of India's patriarchal society are that women are only homemakers and sexual objects and generally are subjected to exploitation and torture (Dube, 2001).

Historically, in India, patriarchal society is dominating and women have suffered oppression and faced many problems and challenges by the patriarchal society. Since childhood, through socialization process, women were taught to accept their position and all rules and regulation which made only for women. They are also taught that they should be made obedient, daughter, wives, and sisters and also to respect and care their elders. They are neither considered as human being nor do they have any personal life. Their identity depends upon their father's identity before marriage, and after marriage husband identity is based on their identity. In traditional Indian society, the position of women is due to many reasons like early marriage and illiteracy etc. In many cultures, women have no right to make any decision because men think that they have not enough capacity to make a good decision. Not only in India, but women of all over the world face challenges, and sometimes these challenges are place and context-specific. Studies on the challenges and problems show that women face challenges not only in unorganized sectors but organized sectors also. Not only in India, women of various countries, trying to contribute to their best performance in the development of quality of life of their families and thereby to the economies of their country through hard work. Generally women are involved in temporary work as compared to men. In many organizations women employees do not have any social security or health care benefits. As a result, work-related illnesses such as mental pressure and other health problems, remain hidden. As per available literature, different type of problems and challenges faced by working women in the workplace such as balancing between work and family care, work-related stress, physical harassment, unfair treatment in the workplace, tolerance of abuse, violence, mental pressure and safety problems, prejudiced and stereotyped thinking, etc. This creates or increases fatigue, headaches, back pain, circulatory disorders, frustration, stress, and mental and emotional problems among women employees at workplace.

In the history of women's studies, which is not very long, various approaches have been adopted in order to understand women's problems, challenges and find solutions to them (Somjee & Somjee, 1989). Fiksenbaum *et al.* (2010) examined the relationship of the perceived presence of organizational practices, work attitudes, work satisfaction and psychological well-being among 286 women in managerial and professional jobs working in a big Turkish bank. The finding shows that women reporting more supportive organizational experiences and practices were more engaged in their work, more job satisfaction and greater levels of psychological wellbeing.

Wentling (2003) conducted a study on working women in Delhi. The study indicated that due to social structure, which is still more male-dominant creates tension and conflict among working women. It also indicated that the traditional authoritarian setup of Hindu social structure never changed and continues to be the same and women still face the problem of role conflict change in attitudes of men.

In a study, Ali (2011) investigated the challenges faced by women in their respective career development. He found that most of the women employees were dissatisfied with their career development programmes and they also experienced discrimination in career development opportunities. Ali's study recommended that organizations should strive to ensure that career development programmers were set to enhance career development amongst women employees. The management should ensure that career development of women employees is taken care of with utmost priority and introduce affirmative action to urgently address the career development of women.

In another study, Skinner and Pocock (2008) examined the relationship between work overload, work schedule control, work hours and work-life conflict among full-time employees. In their study, they observed that the strongest relationship among work-life conflict and work overload, followed by work schedule control, work hours and work hours fit. They found that to address work-life conflict effectively, time-based work-life policies, procedures and interventions were very necessary, but only this was not sufficient. They prescribed for managing work overload effectively to have a healthy and balanced work-life relationship.

Lilly *et al.* (2006) focus on work-family conflict occurs for both (men and women) which means that anyone with job demands and family demands needs to cope simultaneously. Delgado and Canabal (2006) also blamed work role for impacting family as well as work, which in turn ultimately causes Job spill over. It has been observed that working for late hours in many organizations affect severely appropriate parenting (Wood & Newton, 2006). Particularly in case of the banking sector of almost every economy, long work hours hampers good parenting as parents are away from their children for longer hours for six days a week and even on Sundays also.

To cope with never-ending demands of family and workplace, women need to become superpower or at least act like one, or they should find other ways of handling the workload at work and home simultaneously (Gordon & Whelan-Berry, 2005). Macdonald *et al.* (2005) conducted studies on adult Canadian women and men and found that women's greater hours of unpaid work contributed to more stress among women as compared to men and success in the workplace as superwomen in balancing work and family may come at a high cost in the form of stress. If this stress not handled carefully, then it may have adverse effects on women's health as well as their roles and responsibilities towards their families and work.

According to Elvin-Nowak and Thomsson, (2001) a working woman always exposed to the constant risk of her position. Especially, when she chooses employment for her well-being rather than being forced by external circumstances (Hakim cited in Easton, 2007) focuses on 'preference theory,' a new theory which indicates 'explaining and predicting women's choices between market-work and family work.' According to Hakim, women with adaptive tendencies always prefer on combination of employment and family work and these women are prepared to prioritize their work as men.

Work-life Balance Difficulties among Working Women

Most researches of married working women show that financial need as being the primary reason given for working women in India (Srivastava, 1978, Ramanna & Bombawale, 1984). Campbell *et al.* (1994) studied the effects of family life on women's job performance and work attitudes. Results revealed that women with children were significantly lower performance in workplace than women with no children. It was also found that women with younger children outperformed than women with older children. Makowska (1995) examine psychosocial determinants of stress and well-being among working women, and results revealed that work-related stressors were evidently significantly greater effect than the stressors associated with the family function and relationship between family functioning, stress and well-being were also significant.

India women are supposed to take care of kids and performing household chores as still thought by many. According to Delgado and Canabal (2006) gender is considered as most significant reason affecting jobs negatively because women in most cases are expected to excel at home as well as workplace. Moreover, sense of feeling guilty about responsibility towards their children, women are demotivated and fail to cope up with the demands made on them from all spheres of life. Most studies focus on married working women than on unmarried working women (Karl, 2009). Shalz (2011) focuses on organized sector rather than unorganized sector of working women. Eggins (1997) gave suggestions for more facilities to women in the workplace and suggests that it is an important part of developmental strategy as well as an act of social justice. It is estimated that Indian women make up one-third of the labour force (World Bank, 1991). According to Singhal (1995) for development of economy and population planning of any country, the participation of women is essential in workforce.

Samuel and Vivienne's (1996) studies show that men can identify their roles in work and family simultaneously but for women balancing their work and family identity by trading-off one role for the other.

Hyman and Summers (2004) studies on Work-Life Balance among employees at UK and classified seven major problems in which first is unevenness of adoption across different sectors and organizations, second is lack of formalization of policies at organizational level, third, restricted employee voice over the introduction and implementation of policies, fourth, policies are primarily to meet business needs, fifth, there is no evidence of reduction in working hours. Sixth, tangible and intangible work intrusions into domestic life and finally, domestic responsibilities are still conducted primarily by women irrespective of their employment status. It is concluded that many employees continue face difficulty in making up their work and domestic responsibilities.

In relation to this, Doherty (2004) also researched the UK hospitality industry to discover the effectiveness of Work-Life Balance helping women progress to senior management. Based on findings, it is concluded that the principal deterrents to these women from exploring career advancement opportunities are the lack of flexibility and very long hours.

Elizabeth *et al.* (2005) examine the role of gender and tenure status in balancing parenthood and job. The results revealed that women reported greater family stress and career stress as compared to men. It was also reported that women perceive less organizational support for balance of work and family as compared to men. In applied way it involves adjusting work patterns so everyone, regardless of gender, age, or race or can find a rhythm that enables them more easily to combine work and their other responsibilities and aspirations (Pillinger, 2001).

Ahmad and Aminah (2007) conducted a study on 239 married female production operators in dual-career families and examined the work-family conflict experienced by them, the social support they received, and the coping strategies they used to manage the conflict. The results revealed that women experienced more work interference with family than family interference with work. It was also found that intensity of work interference with family was significantly higher in the earlier life stage than in the later life stage. About two-thirds of the women reported that they intended to leave their job upon having another child due to the rising cost of child-care services. They received the least social and moral support from their supervisors as compared to other sources and tended to cope with conflict by using reactive role behaviour and personal role redefinition strategies.

Gunavathy and Suganya (2007) identify the causes, consequences of work-life imbalance and interventions for work-life balance among married women employees of BPO companies. More than two-thirds of the women employees stated that the primary reason for work-life imbalance is work interference with personal life. The causes for work-life imbalance were classified as organizational factors (including work-related, time-related and relationship-related factors) and personal factors (including marital conflict, lack of family support, and frequent change in sleeping patterns). According to this study, there are three main consequences of work-life imbalance were stress or burnout, ill-health, and poor work performance. The employees also experienced guilt of not being able to spend time with children and family, anxiety about poor performance, displacement of negative emotions on family members and co-workers.

Ming (2007) conducted a study among 109 married women in middle management at eight private manufacturing companies located in Bangi and Nilai and examined the relationship between self-efficacy, work-family conflict, social support, gender role attitude, role model and career aspiration. The main purpose of the study is to determine the contribution of each factor to career aspiration. The results revealed that self-efficacy; social support, gender role attitude and role model were significantly related to career aspiration. Specifically, self-efficacy and gender role attitude was the most significant antecedents of career aspiration among married working women in this field.

Doble and Supriya (2010) have highlighted Work-Life Balance across gender and found that not only women but men also experience work-life imbalance. Though after Liberalization, many organizations in India have been introducing various work-life balance practices like part-time work, flexi times and provision for childcare facilities, which are facilitated in various developed countries. It is also found that imbalance still exists among men and women both in every organization.

Rincy and Panchanatham (2011) revealed the main factors related to family which causes imbalance in work and personal life of women entrepreneurs. These factors including role overload, dependent care issues, quality of health, problems in time management and lack of proper support from the family. Santhi and Sunder (2012) also focus on different factors which play primary and secondary role in balancing work and personal life. Supporting environment in the organization, provision of welfare measures play a primary role and childcare and recreation and alternative working time play a secondary role in balancing work and personal life.

Kadam (2012) defines work-life balance is a broad concept including proper prioritizing between Work (such as career and ambition) and Life (such as health, pleasure, leisure, family and spiritual development). It is a subject, in which increased interest in academic literature, legislation and public discloser. It means meaningful daily achievement and enjoyment in each of four life quadrants work, family, friend and self.

According to Pandey (1996), work-life balance is a state of equilibrium in which the demands of a person's job and personal life are both equal. An employee with better work-life balance will contribute more meaningfully towards organizational growth and success. Effective work-life balance policies are valuable to organizations for many reasons, including reduced staff turnover rates, becoming a good employer or an employee, increased return on investment in training as employees stay longer, reduced absenteeism, improved morale or satisfaction, greater staff loyalty and commitment and improved productivity.

Padma *et al.* (2013) define the term Work-Life Balance (WLB) as a satisfactory level of involvement between the multiple roles of a person's life. This term attracted by all including individuals and organizations all over the world. It involves person's control over the responsibilities between their family and workplace as well as self-control. It is also a comfortable state of equilibrium, which is achieved by individuals between their primary priorities at their family as well as private life and their work life. In every person's life, there are so many people are involved like family members, friends, supervisors and peer groups, etc. The support gained from such people in any one's life plays a vital role in leading life comfortably.

Fu and Shaffer (2001) investigated the influence of multiple forms of family and worked specific determinants, which create conflicts between work and family. The results show that parental demands and hours spent on household work were important determinants of family-work conflict and role overload, role conflict and hours spent on work influenced work-family conflicts. It was also seen that spouse support, domestic support, and superior support at workplace were played moderate role in the work-life conflict. Supporting this, Greenhaus *et al.* (2003) suggested three aspects of work-family balance, which are time balance, involvement balance, and satisfaction balance. In turn, according to Frone (2003), work-family balance consists of work-family conflict and work-family facilitation.

Based on the literature review, it is found that work-life balance is not a new concept; it came into picture since 1986. It is not only balance between work and life, but it is an appropriate mixture of all the roles (like, daughter, homemakers, mother, daughter-in-law, manager, supervisor, worker, etc.), which played by working women from typical homemakers to successful business leaders. But it is also true that working women especially married working women are continuously trying to do their best to manage both work and life till today from past. They perform many responsibilities of family and work which is more stressful for any women, so due to this they face a work-life imbalance in their day to day life.

Discussion

With the advent of 21st Century and in this new era of globalization, scenario at the workplace is changing on daily basis due to neck to neck competition. New generation is focused on their career than probably never before. Women are no less than men in any field we name it, rather they are ahead, and their dominance can be easily observed. With increasing focus on work, interest in studying conceptual relationships between work and family domains is also increasing strongly with a research history that dates back to the early 1930s. Due to remarkable changes in the world of work over preceding years, the ability to take care of oneself and one's family and meet other obligations towards friends and society has been affected. Changing work has made life of women tougher in particular due to limitations or absence from home. Work-family issues primarily evolve from increased qualitative and quantitative job requirements, due to globalization, mobilization and new technologies, growing service sector or increased employment rate of women. The aim of this article is to define work-life balance, issues related to working women and consequences of poor work-life balance, etc. For working women balancing a challenging career with life outside work is a complex task and they have to maintain a balance between family, career, health, and society.

Researches on Work-life balance suggests that work should not hinder other important aspects in people's lives, such as spending quality time with family, personal development and involvement in creative activities etc. The ideal work-life balance may vary across the different phases of one's life, like before marriage, after marriage, with children, when starting a career or after retirement. It seems appropriate today may seem inappropriate tomorrow so, there is no one-size-fits-all or picture-perfect work-family balance. Many factors related to work increases excessive stress and strain among workers. As a result, due to work demands, work domination is seen in family life which creates work-family imbalance. To achieve success in both aspects, with the help of adjustment and accommodation, women can organize and balance their work and family life.

During earlier days, women were subjected to face fences, created by their relatives, they could barely cross but now women are breaking all fences around them and are playing vital roles in different sectors. Women today are breaking all the boundaries to get recognized not only for their work at home only but also at workplace. They are playing the dual role of balancing domestic life as well as professional life, giving a boost to their societal status in the process. However, with this advancement in their life women are facing challenges in making balance between dual responsibilities of domestic work as well as office work. Though more and more women are coming out of home for work and their families are also being benefitted from their income, the attitude towards women and their role in the family has not undergone much change. Women continue to be perceived to be primarily responsible for looking after the family and children. Schwarts (1992) said that most of those who entered in work force have no solid family support at home. During the past 30 years, women have increased their participation in paid employment, but men have not increased their participation from house to work (Evertsson & Nermo, 2004).

Women perform the same work as men at workplace and are equally paid, yet women are challenged by inequality in the workforce (Andal, 2002). Social, economic and political empowerment of women is necessary for the development of any society. The biggest challenge faced by women comes at home when they bear the responsibility of household work without any help and support of men. This creates extra workload on women and needs to be understood and addressed by their male counterparts.

Workplace characteristics play important role in higher levels of Work-Family conflict. Researchers have found that number of workplace characteristics such as the number of hours worked per week, the amount and frequency of overtime, an inflexible work schedule, unsupportive supervisor and colleagues and an intolerable organizational culture increase the conflict between family roles and work role among women (Greenhaus & Beutell, 1985, Galinsky *et al.*, 1996, Frone, *et al.*, 1996). Baruch and Barnett (1987) found in their study that married women who play different roles were less depressed and had higher self-esteem and more satisfied compared to women who were not married, unemployed or childless.

It is also reality that every woman has different perception of their needs, different levels of fears, anxiety, stress, and frustrations, etc. Some are happy with their job; some are frustrated because of mental stress and physical stress both. Some women have a good job environment; on the other hand, some women are highly depressed because of issues with their colleagues, stressed work environment, less job satisfaction, etc.

In India, there are some stereotyped thinking that persists is whether women, who are crossing the four walls of their homes for work or jobs, are capable enough to compete with others, and at the same time, they are also capable of making appropriate balance between family life and professional life. They fulfil their all responsibility of family and work at the cost of their physical and mental health deterioration. But the serious issue arises as to why only women have to balance both lives and why they have all these burdens thrust on them. Is it only women's responsibility to take all the burdens? These are serious questions that need to be addressed.

Conclusion

Women have been playing vital roles in household works since ancient times. In this new era of technology or development, women have created their niche in every field apart from work at home. Every country should make a society where every woman can breathe freely without any fear, oppression, gender bias, discrimination, and exploitation. It is very important to ensure a better future for the next generation. It is presumed that as compared to uneducated women, educated women especially urban women to be more aware of the opportunities and challenges of the workplace. They have better understanding of their roles and limitations in the workplace. They are also perceived to be bold enough to develop their personalities, with or without support from their families. It is a fact that women have to face problems just by their being women. Although women make their place in this traditional society where males always dominated by their hard work and proficiency but It is also a fact that women have to face problems just by virtue of their being women and social attitude to the role of women hidden in the frame of laws and governance, but this attitude can be seen at the time of recruitment of female employees.

Future Directions

It is very critical and difficult for research related to work, family, and life to fully understand the conditions under which the married working women experience conflict, stress, and frustration between their roles in family and work settings. There is a need to consider spouse support; family members' support, good working environment, job satisfaction, number of working hours in future research. To attain in-depth knowledge and understanding of any women's work and family life, researchers in work—family-related fields should include various perspectives such as physical health, mental health, quality of life, job stress, family-related demands, and work demands. It is also important to explore multiple waves of data collection over a longer period to better understanding the changing nature of family and work roles over time. There is needed to be conducted longitudinal studies to examine how the different stages of life affect family and work domains. It is clear from a review of literature that married working women indeed experience work-life imbalance while attempting to balance their work and family lives.

References

Ahmad, A. (2007). Work-family conflict, life cycle stage, social support and coping strategies among women employees. *The Journal of human Resource and adult learning, 3*(1), 70-79.

Ali, S.J. (2011). Challenges facing women employees in career development: A focus on Kapsabet municipality, Kenya. *International Journal of Current Research, 3*, 196-203.

Andal, N. (2002). *Women and Indian Society: Option and Constraints.* New Delhi: Rawat Publications.

Baruch, G.K., and Barnett., R.C. (1987). Role quality, multiple role involvement and psychological well-being in midlife women. *Journal of Personality and Social Psychology. 51*, 578–585.

Campbell, D.J., Campbell, K.M., and Kennard, D. (1994). The effects of family responsibilities on the work commitment and job performance of non-professional women. *Journal of Occupational and Organizational Psychology, 67*, 283–296.

Chakraborty, S. (2013). Empowering the Tribal Women through Education: Issue of Social Justice with Reference of West Bengal. *Afro-Asian Journal of Anthropology and Social Policy, 4*(1), 24-28.

Claramma, T.K. (2007). *Work-life Balance: A Sociological Study of Women Professional in Kerala.* Ernakulum: Department of Sociology, St. Teresa's College.

Clark, S.C. (2000). Work/Family Border Theory: A New Theory of Work/Life Balance. *Human Relations, 53*(6), 747-770.

Clark, A.E. (2001). What really matters in a job? Hedonic measurement using quit data, *Labour Economics 8*, 223-242.

Delgado, E.A., and Canabal, M.E. (2006). Factors associated with negative spillover from job to home among Latinos in the United States. *Journal of Family and Economic Issues, 27*(1), 92-112.

Doble, N., and Supriya, M.V. (2010). Gender differences in the perception of Work-Life Balance. *Management, 5* (4), 331-342.

Doherty, L. (2004). Work-Life Balance Initiatives: Implications for Women. *Emerald, 26*(4), 433-452.

Doress-Wortes, P.B. (1994). Adding elder care to women's multiples roles: A critical review of the caregiver stress and multiple roles literature. *Sex Roles, 3,* 597–613.

Dube, L. (2001). *Anthropological Explorations in Gender: Intersecting Fields.* New Delhi: Sage Publications Pvt. Limited.

Easton, C. (2007). *Coping Mechanisms of South African Women Balancing managerial and motherhood roles.* Unpublished master's dissertation, University of Pretoria, South Africa.

Eggins, S., and Slade, D. (1997). *Analysing Casual Conversation.* London: Continuum.

Elizabeth, M., and O'Laughlin, L.G. (2005). Balancing Parenthood and Academia Work/Family Stress as Influenced by Gender and Tenure Status. *Journal of Family Issues, 26* (1), 79-106.

Elvin-Nowak, Y., and Thomsson, H. (2001). Motherhood as idea and practice: A discursive understanding of employed mothers in Sweden. *Gender and Society, 15,* 407-428.

Evertsson, M., and Nermo, M. (2004). Dependence within families and division of labour: Comparing Sweden and United States. *Journal of Marriage and Family, 66,* 1272-1286.

Fiksenbaum, L., Koyuncu, M., and Burke, R. (2010). Virtues, work-experiences and psychological well-being among managerial women in a Turkish bank. *Equality, Diversity and Inclusion, 29* (2), 199-212.

Ford, M.T., H.B. (2007). Work and Family Satisfaction and Conflict: A Meta-Analysis of Cross Domain Relations. *Journal of Applied Psychology, 92*(1), 57-80.

Frone, M.R., Russell, M., and Barnes, G.M. (1996). Work-family conflict, gender and health-related outcomes: A study of employed parents in two community samples. *Journal of Occupational Health Psychology, 1,* 57-69.

Frone, M.R. (2003). *Work-Family Balance. Handbook of Occupational Health Psychology*. Washington, DC: American Psychological Association.

Frone, M.R., Yardley, J.K., and Markel, K.S. (1997). Developing and testing an integrative model of the work—family interface. *Journal of Vocational Behaviour, 50,* 145–167.

Frone, M.R., Russell, M., and Cooper, M.L. (1992). Antecedents and outcomes of work—family conflict: Testing a model of the work-family interface. *Journal of Applied Psychology. 77,* 65–78.

Frone, R.M., Russell, M., and Cooper, M.L. (1992). 'Prevalence of work-family conflict: Are work and family boundaries asymmetrically permeable?'. *Journal of Organizational Behaviour, 13,* 723-729.

Fu, C.K., and Shaffer, M.A. (2001). The tug of work and family: direct and indirect domain-specific determinants of work-family conflict. *Personnel Review, 30*(5), 502-522.

Galinsky, E., Bond, J.T., and Friedman, D.E. (1996). The role of employers in addressing the needs of employed parents. *Journal of Social Issues,* 52, 111–136.

Gordon, J.R., and Whelan-Berry, K. (2005). Contributions to family and household activities by the husband of midlife professional women. *Journal of Family Issues, 26*(7), 899-923.

Greenhaus, J.H., and Beutell, N.J. (1985). Sources conflict between work and family roles. *Academic Manage Review. 10,* 76–88.

Guest, D. (2001). *Perspectives on study of work-life balance.* Discussion paper presented in 2001 ENOP Symposium, Paris, 29-31 March, http://www.ucm,es/info/Psyap/enop/guest.htm

Gunavathy, J.S., and Suganya, N.P. (2007). Work-life imbalance among married women employees of BPO's. *Indian Journal of Training and Development, 37* (1), 157-168.

Hyman, J., and Summers, J. (2004). Lacking Balance. *Personnel Review, 33* (4), 418-429.

Hughes, D.L., and Glinsky, E. (1994). Gender, job and family conditions and psychological symptoms. *Psychological Women Quart, 18,* 251–270.

Kadam, B.S. (2012). Work-Life Balance: Dilemma of Modern Society, A Special Reference to Women Bus Conductor in Maharashtra State Road Transport. *ZENITH International Journal of Business Economics and Management Research, 2.*

Kalliath, T., and Brough, P. (2008). Work-Life Balance: A review of the meaning of the balance construct. *Journal of Management and Organization, 14*(3), 323-327.

Karl, M. (2009). Inseparable: The Crucial Role of Women in Food Security Revisited. *Women in Action. 1,* 8-19.

Kopp, R.G., and Ruzicka, F.M. (1993). Women's multiple roles and psychological well-being. *Psychological Report, 72,* 1351–4.

Lilly, J.D., Duffy, J.A., and Virick, M. (2006). A gender-sensitive study of McClelland's need, stress, and Turnover intent with work-family conflict. *Women in Management Review, 21*(8), 662.

Lockett, K. (2008). *Work-Life Balance for Dummies.* Milton, AU: Wiley Publishing.

MacDermid, S.M. (2004). (Re)considering Conflict between Work and Family. In: Kossek, E.E. and Lambert, S. (eds.), *Work and Life Integration in Organizations: New Directions for Theory and Practice.* Elbraum, Mahwah, NI.

Maskowska, Z. (1995). Psychosocial characteristics of work and family as a determinant of stress and wellbeing of women: A preliminary study. *International Journal of Occupational Medicine and Environment Health, 8,* 215–222.

Padma, S., and Reddy, M.S. (2013). Role of Family Support in Balancing Personal and Work-Life of Women Employees. *International Journal of Computational Engineering and Management. 16*(3), 93-97.

Pandey, M. (1996). Professionalism versus socialism: A study of women employment. *Indian Journal of Psychometry and Education, 27*(2), 77-80.

Pillinger, J. (2001). *Work-Life Balance: Towards a New Politics of Work and Time.* The Industrial Law Society Annual Conference, Conference Proceedings.

Ramanna, A., and Bombawale, U. (1984). Transitory status images of working women in modern India. *Indian Journal of Social Work, 45,* 189–202.

Rapoport, R., Bailyn, L., Fletcher, J.K., and Pruitt, B.H. (2002). *Beyond Work-family balance: Advancing Gender Equality and Workplace Performance.* San Francisco, CA: Jossey-Bass.

Rincy, V.M., and Panchanatham, N. (2011). An exploratory study on work-life balance of women entrepreneurs in south India. *Asian Academy of Management Journal, 16* (2).

Samuel, A., and Vivienne, L. (1996). Balancing Two Major Parts of Adult Life Experience: Work and Family Identity among Dual-Earner Couples. *Human Relations, 49*(4), 465-487.

Santhi, T., and Sundar, K. (2012). A Study on the Work-Life Balance of Women Employees in Information Technology Industry. *ZENITH International Journal of Business Economics and Management Research,* 82-96.

Schwatrz, S.H. (1992). Universals in the content and structure of values: Theoretical advances and empirical tests in 20 countries. *Advances in Experimental Social Psychology, 25,* 1-65.

Skinner, N., and Pocock, B. (2011). Flexibility and Work-life Interference. *Journal of Industrial Relations, 53*(1), 65-82.

Somjee, G., and Somjee, A.H. (1989). *Reaching Out to the Poor: The unfinished rural revolution.* Revolution. Macmillan. London.

Srivastava, V. (1978). *Employment of educated women in India: Its causes and consequences.* New Delhi: National Publishing House; [Google Scholar]

Super, D.E. (1980). A life-span, life-space approach to career development. *Journal of Vocational Behaviour, 16*, 282–290.

Wentling, R.M. (2003). The career development and aspirations of women in middle management-revisited. *Women in Management Review, 18*(6), 311-324.

Wood, G.J., and Newton, J. (2006). Childless and women managers: 'Choice', context and discourses. *Gender, Work and Organization, 13*, 338-358.

Work-Life Balance from http://www.essay.uk.com.

7

Reproductive Health and Psychological Well-being of Females from Agrarian Families of Districts Udham Singh Nagar and Nainital

Assessment and Intervention

Ritu Singh and *Niharika Bisht*

Introduction

Reproductive health has been a great concern for every woman. It is a pivotal part of general health and a primary feature of human development. Reproductive health is defined as: "A state of physical, mental, and social well-being in all matters relating to the reproductive system. It addresses the reproductive processes, functions and system at all stages of life. Reproductive health, therefore, implies that people are able to have a responsible, satisfying and safe sex life and that they have the capability to reproduce and the freedom to decide if, when and how often to do so (Reproductive Health in the Western Pacific).

Reproductive health is critical to an individual's growth and development. It is a paragliding notion composed of several separate yet linked issues such as conception, contraception, abortion, child birth, sexuality, conception, contraception and maternal mortality, menstruation, menopause, infertility etc.

Reproductive health is often considered a private issue, so individuals sometimes feel reluctant to ask for precise information about it. This may be a valid reason why these problems are still not publicly discussed and services are scarce and fragmented in relation to them.

Nearly 75 per cent of the population in India lives in rural regions. These rural females, who belong to farm families in particular, are mostly involved in farming operations and also as workers. The nature of the women's job generally involves drudgery and they are expected to do all domestic chores. Not only do they deal with child-bearing and child-rearing responsibilities but also struggle with managing the family's daily demands through cooking, cleaning, poultry and livestock care. They also provide the sick, elderly and disabled in the family with nursing care. All of these variables lead to health issues in women. Women in rural areas often carry triple job loads, in their homes, in agricultural activity and in their reproductive role (Pujar *et al.,* 2017).

According to studies, it is estimated that 47 per cent of girls in India are married before their 18th birthday (Nambiath, n.d). A common result of early marriage is that girls enter marriage and become mothers without sufficient information on issues of reproductive and sexual health, including sexual intercourse, conception, contraception, sexually transmitted diseases (STIs), pregnancy and childbirth, infertility issues.

Girls who are even quipped with information are probably denied access to secure motherhood, contraceptive and illness prevention facilities because of cultural norms and limitations that restrict their mobility and access to data and resources (Mathur *et al.,* 2003, Jejeebhoy, 1998). For unmarried women, social obstacles are even bigger. In some areas of India, many women experience "eve teasing," and sexual assault in extreme instances. Girls are denied access to reproductive and sexual health information, and it is anticipated that they would not ask questions about such problems because they are unmarried and female.

While reproductive health impacts both males and females, females bear the brunt of reproductive ill health, not only because of their biological status, but also because of a broader social, financial and political disadvantage. In determining reproductive health biological, social, cultural, economical and behavioural factors also play an important role.

Women's role in reproductive health is influenced and could have an impact on their personal status and empowerment. Women's choice of livelihood, where to reside, who to marry, number of kids, liberty of motion, and selection of friends are critical choices that can empower them to become family matriarchs.

Gynaecological circumstances influence the health and wellbeing of women in physical and mental health. Stress owing to white vaginal discharge, unintended pregnancies and unsafe abortion causes severe mental illness (Patel & Oomman, 1999). Perinatal depression is one of the most prevalent and severe complications of pregnancy and childbirth (WHO, 2009). Miscarriage is strongly linked with depression (Beaurepaire, 1994). These mental health problems that arise during pregnancy or after childbirth not only hamper mother's mental, physical and social well-being, but also child care and general child development (Rintoul *et al.,* 1998). Because of the thinner vaginal wall, young females are susceptible to sexually transmitted infections than older females. Women's subordination, poverty, lack of education, substance abuse and economic dependence on males make it hard for women to insist on safer sex, leaving females more susceptible to STIs, including HIV (WHO, 2009). Early marriage, and desire for a male child results in frequent child bearing during the reproductive years.

Most females of reproductive age have little or incorrect reproductive health information. Learning about the course of reproductive life, how to stay healthy and how to access care when required offers a strong foundation for future health choices, although many studies report large gaps in this aspect.

Reproductive health is often linked to psychological well-being. Psychological well-being is a wide ranging, multifarious concept. It includes different aspects of everyday experience. According to many researchers (Andrew & Withey, 1976; Najman & Levine, 1981; Campbell & Converse, 1971) psychological well-being is considered to be the composite measure of physical, mental and social well-being as perceived by each individual. Psychological well-being has been and still is usually inconspicuous, peripheral and marginal as an element of reproductive health. Due to the immense contributions of mental and reproductive health to the worldwide burden of disease and disability, the absence of attention it has received is unfortunate. Reproductive health and psychological well-being are two constructs that form an integral part of overall health and are interconnected throughout the course of life. As they form a fundamental part of overall health, therefore the present study was conducted to study these two important aspects of health.

Knowledge Gap

Numerous studies have been conducted to assess the reproductive health awareness among women; however, intervention studies on this pertinent area are relatively few. The impact evaluation of such interventions has also been so far underrated, inadequate and has scant database. Not many researches in India and in particular in Uttarakhand have worked on women's own perceptions of their well-being and their knowledge, attitude and practices regarding reproductive health. The present study is in the direction to fill this gap.

The objectives of the study were:

1. To assess the knowledge, attitude and practices of females from agrarian families on reproductive health.
2. To assess the psychological well-being of females from agrarian families.
3. To implement an intervention to enhance the reproductive health knowledge and psychological well-being of females from agrarian families.
4. To conduct the impact evaluation of the intervention on reproductive health and psychological well-being.

Methodology

Locale: The present study was part of the All India Coordinated Research Project on 'Parenting and Reproductive Health Care in Agrarian Families' of G.B. Pant University of Agriculture & Technology, Pantnagar, India. As per the mandate of the university, different departments of the University adopt some nearby villages for carrying out developmental and welfare activities through research. The sample for the present study were selected from the seven adopted villages of the department viz. Buksora, Durgapur I, Durgapur II, Anjaniya, Pateri village of District Udham Singh Nagar and Dogra, Suryajala village of District Nainital, Uttarakhand.

Sample: The sample for the present study comprised of a total of 300 respondents from two groups of population, viz. adolescent girls and married women.

Tools

1. Structured socio-demographic and socio-economic questionnaire: A questionnaire was developed to assess the socio-demographic and socio-economic profile of participants.

2. Self-structured Questionnaire was developed to assess the knowledge, attitude and practices about reproductive health. The questionnaire was divided in to three parts i.e. knowledge, attitude, practice each comprising of 20 items. The knowledge part was answered on a two point rating scale i.e. Yes, No. The attitude part was answered on a three point Likert scale i.e. Agree, Doubtful, Disagree. The questions pertaining to practice part were answered on two point rating scale i.e. Yes and No.

3. Well-being Assessment Tool: This tool was an adapted version of the well-being tool of McKinley Health Centre at the University of Illinois. The test was translated into Hindi language. This test measures well-being across 5 components viz., Physical, Social, Emotional, Spiritual and Intellectual. Each subscale encompasses of 10 items. The responses are rated on a four point Likert scale i.e. rarely ever, sometimes. Most of the time, always (Wellbeing Assessment Tool adapted from McKinley Health Centre at the University of Illinois, 2005).

4. Intervention Module: The various issues are dealt with, in detail, intermingled with games, along with appropriate visuals to make the learning enjoyable. Issues like menstruation; adolescent pregnancy, abortion, contraception, conception, reproductive tract infections; sexually transmitted diseases/HIV/AIDS, infertility related issue has been discussed and dealt within these modules.

This module has sessions on purpose of training, anatomy and physiology of male and female reproductive system, physical changes during and after puberty, menstrual cycle, pregnancy, antenatal care, safe motherhood and delivery, early pregnancy, contraceptive methods, repeated pregnancy, safe abortion, supportive supervision, gender-based sensitization, infertility issues, various government schemes related to sexual and reproductive health, individual and group counseling, relaxation techniques, effective coping techniques, games etc. Programme included lectures, presentations, group discussions, brainstorming sessions. Audio-visual aids such as power point presentation using LCD projector, video films, charts, posters were also used. The lectures were followed by interactive session with the participants.

The intervention was delivered by research team along with experts from concerned field, community/frontline workers, volunteers, health workers and social workers.

(a) Direct interventions with adolescent girls and women: The direct intervention with adolescent girls and married women focused on individual counseling and group counseling through personal visits and group discussions, lectures on health and economic benefits of delaying pregnancy, safe-motherhood and delivery, early pregnancy, contraceptive methods, repeated pregnancy, safe abortion, infertility issues prevention of RTI/STI and improving reproductive healthcare by involving husbands.

(b) Interaction with the expert: This exercise was used to organize open sessions on stress, factors affecting it, its implication, strategies for coping with the help of experts in the concerned field through use of drama, video clips and discussion etc.

(c) Discussions with family members and community: The interventions with family and community attempted to influence the decision-makers and gatekeepers of the primary target group of women and adolescent girls. These strategies ranged from consultations with key community members, parents, other decision-makers and youth before the intervention started; the creation of community-based groups.

(d) Life Style Skills: Lifestyle skills help to enhance our knowledge of the world around us and prepare us with the abilities required to achieve a more productive and satisfying life. A number of sessions were taken by the team to foster positive life-style skills like.

(i) *Relaxation techniques*: It includes exercising regularly, practicing relaxation techniques. For example, in tense situations, slowly breathe in and out for several minutes.

(ii) *Positive self-talk*: Using positive and encouraging statements for self. These are sometimes referred to as positive assurance that is helpful in establishing self-confidence and challenging adverse ideas. For instance, "Yes I can do this, I can do it" or "I'm going to try my best.

(iii) *Time management*: Pre-planning and avoiding delay is useful in decreasing stress.

(iv) *System of support*: It basically means having one or more friends with whom you can share personal matter.

Pilot Testing

The tools were translated into local language and a pilot study of questionnaires was carried out with 30 women (not part of the study) to test the clarity of questions. Necessary modifications were done.

Intervention Module: After constructing the intervention module, it was mailed to the experts of Psychology, Human Development, Extension Education, and Social Work of different Universities and modified in the light of suggestions given by them.

Procedure for Data Collection

The investigators were familiar with the objectives of the study, tools for data collection and ethical protocols. A standardized protocol was followed to build rapport with the women and to conduct the interviews and discussions. Respondents who met the inclusion criteria were selected and briefed about the purpose of the study. The investigators then took a written consent. The study was conducted in five phases. In the first phase, the pilot testing of the research tools was done to test the clarity of the questionnaires. In the second phase, the pre-test data was collected. In the third phase, the intervention module was implemented. In the fourth phase, which apparently took place after a gap of 6 months from the third phase, a repeat assessment, i.e. post-test data collection was carried out. Throughout the data collection confidentiality was maintained. The responses of the personal interviews were tape recorded and later transcribed.

Data Analysis Plan

Results were reported in terms of frequencies and percentages to find out the distribution of respondents over knowledge, attitude and practices towards reproductive health and psychological well-being before and after intervention.

Results

Table 7.1 depicts the socio-demographic and economic profile of the respondents which elaborates on age, family type, caste, marital status, education, occupation and income. Around 35 per cent of the respondents were in the age group of 20-25 years followed by 29 per cent in the age group of 15-20 years and 24 per cent were between of 25-30 years of age. The table further elucidates the family type of respondents and it was reported that around 54 per cent hailed from joint families followed by 46 per cent of who were nuclear family setup.

On throwing light on the data relating to caste, it is evident that around 40 per cent belonged to upper caste followed by 36 per cent who were from other backward classes (OBC). Data on marital status revealed that majority (74%) of the respondents were married. On analyzing the trend of educational level, it was observed that nearly half (49%) of the respondents were graduates followed by 30 per cent who were educated up to senior secondary level. Around 10 per cent and 11 per cent of respondents had studied till matriculation and post graduation respectively. Data on occupation reveals that nearly half (44%) of respondents were housewives and 21 per cent, 20 per cent were reported to be in service and self-employed, respectively. Since the sample for the study consisted of women and adolescent girls, therefore there were around 14 per cent respondents who reported to be students and were pursuing education.

Table 7.1: Socio-personal profile of respondents (N = 300)

Variables	*Frequency*	*Percentage*
Age		
15-20 years	88	29
20-25 years	106	35
25-30 years	72	24
30-35 years	34	11
Family type		
Joint	163	54
Nuclear	137	46
Caste		
Upper caste	119	40
OBC	107	36
Dalits	42	14
Tribal	32	11
Marital Status		
Married	221	74
Unmarried	79	26
Educational Qualification		
Matriculation	29	10
Senior Secondary	91	30
Graduation	146	49
Post Graduation	34	11
Occupation		
Housewife	132	44
Self-employed	61	20
Service	65	21
Student (Pursuing education)	42	14
Monthly Income (Rs.)		
>50000	1	0
20000–49999	16	5
10000-19999	100	33
5000–9999	125	42
2500–4999	47	16
1000–2499	9	3
<1000	2	1

The data on monthly income revealed that around 42 per cent of respondents family income was between Rs. 5000-9999 followed by 33 per cent who had monthly family income ranging from Rs. 10000-19999. Around 16 per cent and 5 per cent of the respondents reported having family income of Rs. 2500-4999 and Rs. 20,000-49999 respectively.

Reproductive Health Knowledge

Fig. 7.1 elucidates reproductive health knowledge of the respondents. The data reveals that during pre-test, majority (64%) of the respondents had moderate level of knowledge followed by 36 per cent who reported having good knowledge.

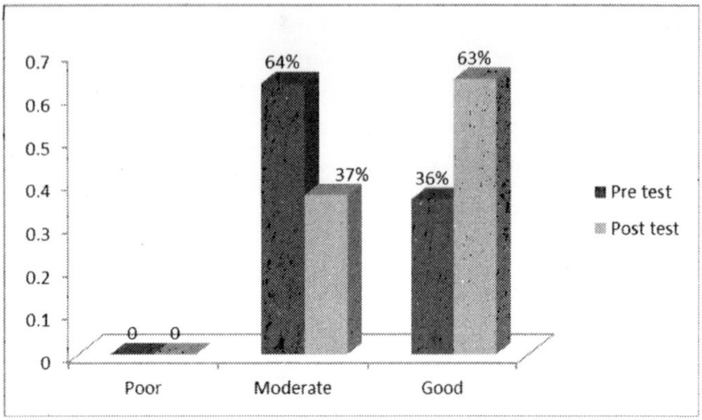

Fig. 7.1: Per cent distribution of respondents on reproductive health knowledge

Post-intervention, a shift was witnessed as majority (63%) of the respondents came under the good level of knowledge followed by 37 per cent who had moderate knowledge of reproductive health. A comforting sign of relief is the fact that not even a single respondent had poor knowledge of reproductive health.

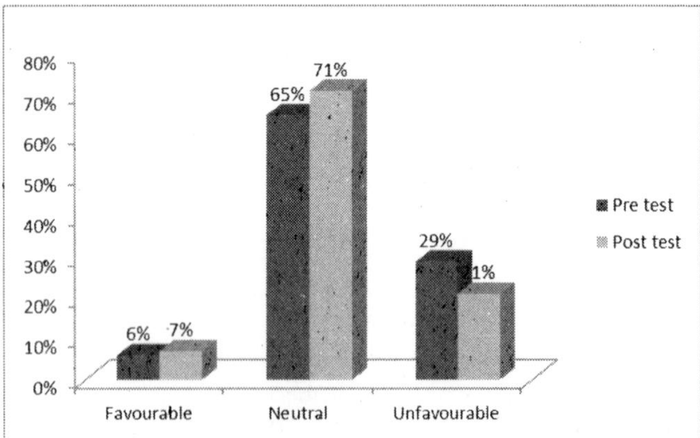

Fig. 7.2: Per cent distribution of respondents on attitude regarding reproductive health

Figure 7.2 depicts the attitude of respondents towards reproductive health. As can be seen from the graph, the percentages in pre- and post-tests are quite similar in the category of favourable attitude. In the pre-test phase, around 29 per cent of respondents had unfavourable attitude towards reproductive health which reduced to 21 per cent post intervention and 65 per cent respondents who had neutral attitude in pre-test phase rose to 71 per cent post-intervention.

From the percentages in Figure 7.3, it appears that during the pretest nearly half (46%) of the respondents reported to follow unhealthy practices followed by 54 per cent who followed healthy practices relating to reproductive health. The scenario changed after the intervention as majority (73%) of the respondents started to follow healthy practices followed by 27 per cent who still followed unhealthy practices relating to reproductive health.

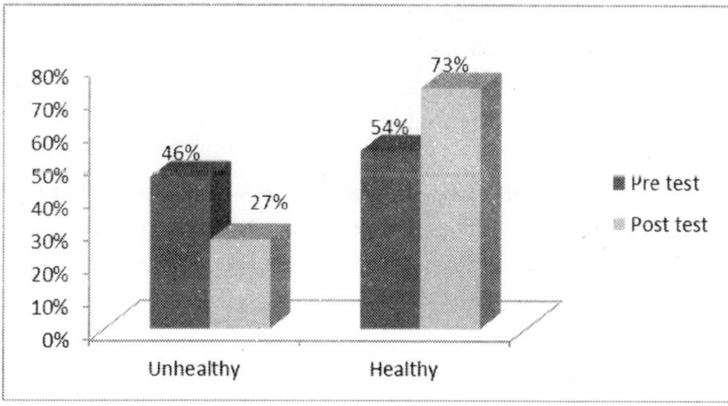

Fig. 7.3: Per cent distribution of respondents on practices followed relating to reproductive health

Psychological Well-being

Figure 7.4 depicts data on psychological well-being of respondents on different components viz. physical, social, emotional, spiritual and intellectual. It is apparent by looking at the data of pre-test that majority of the respondents scored average across all the components of wellbeing.

The results of the post-test indicate that although majority of respondents still had average scores across all the components, however the number of respondents falling in category good of well-being improved slightly as compared to the pre-test phase.

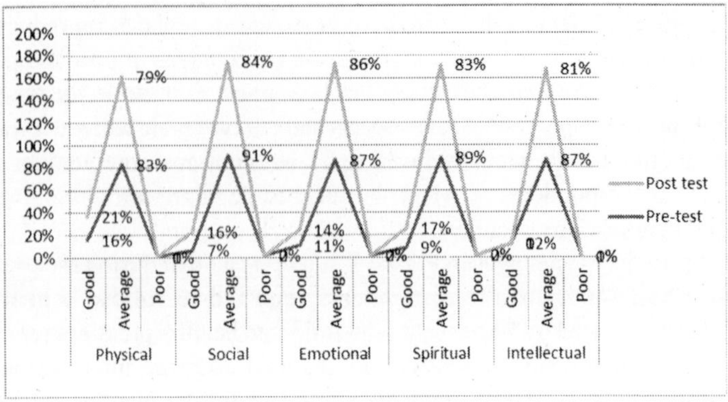

Fig. 7.4: Per cent distribution of respondents on different components of psychological well-being

Figure 7.5 highlights the per cent distribution of respondents as per levels of their psychological well-being. In the pre- test phase, it was found that majority (96%) of respondents had average level of psychological well-being. It was rather sad to witness just a meagre (4%) proportion of sample was on the good level of psychological well-being. The data of post-test revealed that although the majority (88%) still falls in the average level of psychological well-being but around 12 per cent reported having good psychological well-being as opposed to just 4 per cent during the pre-test stage.

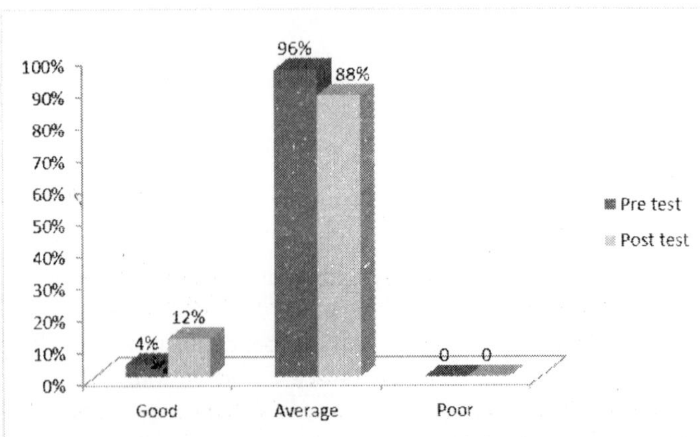

Fig. 7.5: Per cent distribution of respondents on overall psychological wellbeing (N = 300)

Discussion

This study evaluated the knowledge, attitude and practices of adolescent girls and women towards reproductive health. Striking enhancement was observed in the knowledge of respondents regarding reproductive health. Prior to intervention, the major proportion of population had moderate knowledge regarding puberty, menstrual cycle, physiological anatomy of reproductive organs, conception and pregnancy related complications, modern methods of contraception, transmission and prevention of STDs. The intervention tried to discuss all these topics through varied means. The impact of the intervention was clearly evident which elucidate in the post-test as majority of the respondents reported having good level of knowledge. The results are concurrent with an intervention study on adolescent girls which reported that a significant increase in overall knowledge regarding menstrual cycle, ovulation, fertilization and pregnancy, knowledge about transmission and prevention of STDs was observed. It concluded that a comprehensive reproductive health education intervention programme improves the knowledge and attitude among rural adolescent girls regarding reproductive health (Malleshappa *et al.,* 2011). Various studies have also shown the effectiveness of intervention in increasing the knowledge of reproductive health (Shetty & Kowli, 2001; Mandal, 1998).

The remarkable shift in the level of knowledge was also apparent in the focus group discussions, observations of the sessions that took place during and after the intervention. One of the participants during one such FGD said that "*Earlier I just knew that menstrual cycle is about the removal of impure blood as told by elders and it is essential for women to have menses in order to get pregnant. But, now I understand the process of menstrual cycle. That pictorial presentation of anatomy has helped me understand it clearly.* Another participant said "*My husband and I never stayed together after marriage for a long period as he was working in other city and used to visit home once in a month. One year after marriage everyone started suggesting me to conceive and we succumb to that pressure and started trying with no results. Now when I look back and think if I knew how much unnecessary stress I took thinking what is wrong in my body, will I be able to conceive? Now I get to understand that we may never have cohabited during the ovulation phase which is necessary to conceive. I wish I knew it earlier.*

Some adolescent girls also expressed their concern about finding it difficult to discuss the topics related to reproduction in schools and colleges. They said that the chapters of reproduction were completely skipped because teachers were hesitant in discussing them. They felt it is the biggest barrier on the way to gain knowledge. A research study highlighted the need for schools to introduce sex education. Adolescents lack correct and scientific knowledge on sexuality and their fears and concerns related to their sexuality are not being addressed. There are no forums where they can discuss sexuality issue without fear and guilt. They concluded that lack of knowledge particularly about sexually transmitted infections pose a serious health problem which the policy-makers of the nation need to take up seriously on an urgent basis (Sathe & Sathe, 2005).

Further the results relating to attitude regarding reproductive health revealed that post-intervention, the change in attitude was not remarkable and it can be justified because attitude is a construct that cannot be changed overnight. More so, it cannot be directly observed, it is often inferred from what people say and do. However, knowledge does play an important role.

During one subsequent session after the intervention one of the participant said "*I still don't touch container having pickles during menses, although I know it's just a myth, I even tried to convince my grandmother after learning about it from that programme but she was firm that I must follow it. It's very hard to convince her*".

There were some other respondents who too shared that it's difficult to break the age-old practices in such a short span. This is in agreement with a study which revealed that women are often aware of benefits of family planning but the decision related to it family planning methods are affected by their perceptions of contraceptive risks and benefits, and assessment of how particular methods may affect relationships with partners or other family members (Marchant *et al.,* 2004; Finger & Ndong, 1998). So, it can be inferred that significant changes in attitude can take place overtime and more of such interventions and exposures could help in this process.

The practices relating to reproductive health like consulting a gynaecologist when dealing with complications associated with menses, pregnancy, menopause etc., use of sanitary pad over cloth, consumption of adequate fluid and enriched diet improved significantly after the intervention.

One of the respondents shared *"I used to avoid going to doctor thinking that everyone faces some problems like abdominal cramping, burning sensations, itching in genitals. But when we were explained about the symptoms of infection in the programme, I could relate to them. So then I decided to go to the public health centre of our area to consult doctor. She diagnosed me with a urinary tract infection and gave me medicines and suggested to complete the course which I did. Now things are fine."*

This paradigm shift in the outlook of the respondents towards reproductive health practices can be attributed to the intervention which enhanced their level of awareness on different aspects, lack of which generally leads to uncertainty and feelings of helplessness.

The results pertaining to psychological well-being depict an enhancement in the level of well-being of the respondents post-intervention. This improvement suggested the importance of a structured psychosocial intervention programme involving counselling in enhancing the quality of life. The pedagogy used for intervention programme included informative presentations and group exercises such as role plays, games, relaxation exercises were practiced at the end of each morning and afternoon session. The counselling sessions were focused on making them identify the stressor and teaching them positive coping strategies for dealing with it. The reading material was also provided which helped participants to understand repercussions of taking unnecessary stress in day to day life. It seemed that some participants were able to transfer the knowledge acquired during the sessions to their daily lives. Group sessions which included listening and sharing stories, problems helped them realize that their issues are not unique. The results are supported by a study that reported that interventions which focus on "group interactions" act as a preventive strategy that seek to reduce future mental health problems and to promote well-being (McWhirter & McWhirter, 2010). Another study reported that the psychological and social benefits of intervention are based on open and anticipatory dialogues with adults and adolescents, community along with the professionals. It reported that rather than focusing on just an individual, facilitating supportive interactions among peers, professionals and family members might be an asset underpinning mental health interventions with children and adolescents (Seikkula & Arnkil, 2006).

Some respondents shared their before and after experience of intervention. Some stated that the relaxation exercises helped to improve their general health. One participant said "*I always had a problem while sleeping at night, the quality of sleep was very poor and felt lethargic for the entire day but after I started doing some of these exercises, the quality of my sleep has improved.*"

Conclusion

The findings from study on reproductive health and psychological well-being indicated that interventions proved to be beneficial for the respondents. Such interventions can contribute in screening and intervening in mental health and reproductive health conditions which can improve quality of life. The study also pointed out greater provision for the professionals to educate the rural women on the issues of reproductive health. Interventions should aim to involve the parents, teachers and community into discussing reproductive health issues to eliminate stereotypes at all levels, in particular acknowledging and challenging stigmas that start early in life and which are reinforced throughout the life-course. Adequate information can help to address the gaps in knowledge, eliminate misconceptions and foster skills for healthy behaviour. This would in turn help to bridge the gap between knowledge acquisition and behaviour modification. Embracing a rational outlook can help to change conventional attitude and practices attached with reproductive and mental health.

[**Acknowledgement:** The authors express their sincere thanks to all the participants of this study. There is no conflict of interest in this study. Financial funding by Indian Council of Agricultural Research and data collection by Dr. Neera Agarwal and Ms. Huma Parveen is duly acknowledged.]

References

Andrew, F.M. and Withey, S.B. (1976). *Social Indicators of Well-being. American's Perception of Life Quality*. Plenum Press, New York.

Beaurepaire, J. (1994). Psychosocial adjustment to infertility and its treatment: male and female responses at different stages of IVF/ET treatment. *Journal of Psychosomatic Research, 38*(3), 229-240.

Campbell, A., and Converse, P. (1971). Monitoring the Quality of American Life. A Proposal to the Russell Sage Foundation. Survey Research Centre, University of Michigan.

Finger, W.R. and Ndong, I. (1998). Male responsibility for reproductive health. *Network, 18*(3), 4–6.

Jejeebhoy, S.J. (1998). Adolescent Sexual and Reproductive Behaviour: A Review of the Evidence from India. *Social Science and Medicine, 46*(10), 1275-90.

Malleshappa, K., Krishna, S. and Nandini, C. (2011). Knowledge and attitude about reproductive health among rural adolescent girls in Kuppam mandal: An intervention study. *Biomedical Research*, 22 (3), 305-310.

Mandal, K. (1998). Teaching adolescent school girls about menstrual hygiene. *Indian Journal of Nursing Midwifery*, 1, 19-26.

Marchant, T., Mushi, A.K., Nathan, R., Mukasa, O., Abdulla, S. and Lengeler, C. (2004). Planning a family: Priorities and concerns in rural Tanzania. *African Journal of Reproductive Health*, 8, 111-23.

Mathur, S., Greene, M. and Malhotra, A. (2003). Too Young To Wed: The Lives,

Rights, and Health of Young Married Girls. International Centre for Research on Women, Washington, D.C.

McWhirter, P.T., and McWhirter, J.J. (2010). Community and school violence and risk reduction: empirically supported prevention. *Group Dynamics*, 14, 242–256.

Nambiath, S. (n.d). Retrieved from http://younglives-India.org/node/797.

Najman, J.M. and Levine, S. (1981). Evaluating the Impact of Medical Care and Technologies on the Quality of life. *Social Science Medicine*, 15F (2-3), 107-115.

Patel, V. and Oomman, N. (1999). Mental health matters too: Gynaecological symptoms and depression in South Asia, *Reproductive Health Matters*, *7*(14), 30-38.

Pujar, L., Chanda, K. and Morab A. (2017). Knowledge on reproductive health of rural farm women. *International Journal of Home Science*, *3*(1), 229-233.

Reproductive Health in the Western Pacific (n.d.). Retreived from https://www.who.int/westernpacific/health-topics/reproductive-health.

Rintoul, B., Thorne, J., Wallace, I., Mobley, M., Goldman-Fraser, J. and Luckey, H. (1998). *Factors in Child Development*. Part 1: Personal characteristics and parental behaviour. Retrieved from http://www.rti.org/pubs/child-development.pdf

Sathe, A.G. and Sathe, S. (2005). Knowledge, Behaviour and Attitudes about Sexuality amongst Adolescents in Pune: A Situational Analysis. *Indian Journal of Family Welfare*, 51, 49-60.

Seikkula, J., and Arnkil, T.E. (2006). *Dialogical Meetings in Social Networks*. Karnac Publishing, London.

Shetty, P., and Kowli, S. (2001). Family life education for non-school going adolescents: An experiment in an urban slum. *Journal of Family Welfare*, 47, 51-58.

Wellbeing Assessment Tool adapted from McKinley Health Centre at the University of Illinois (2005). Retrieved from http://www.mckinley.uiuc.edu/units/health_ed/he alth_education.ht

WHO (2009). *Mental Health Aspect of Women's Reproductive Health: A Global Review of Literature*. WHO Press, Geneva.

8

Exploring Mental Health and Identity of the 21st Century Home-makers

Selene Khosla and *Monika Misra*

Introduction

Advancing population health and enhancing economic prosperity are quintessential to developing nations, but come with the pre-requisite goal of dismantling gender inequality and empowering women. Among 17 Sustainable Development Goals (SDG) set by United Nations (UN), it may said that all the SDGs can be achieved and are in a way dependent on the SDG 5. UN SDG 5 aims to *achieve gender equality and empower all women and girls.* There are nine targets that are subsumed under SDG 5, each pertaining to eliminate inequality, discrimination and violence against female gender. One of the specific targets that are related to the theme of the present paper is *recognizing and value unpaid care and domestic work through the provision of public services, infrastructure and social protection policies and the promotion of shared responsibility within the household and the family as nationally appropriate.* In the wake of the 21st century where such issues are much talked of, the work being done to improve well-being of women still remains scanty and in adept. It is not only about changing the structures on which organizations operate, but also by understanding the position of women in the society and bringing about change at the grassroot level, i.e. at the individual level *per se.*

The identity of the woman being confined to the domestic front emerged as the "norm" in cultures throughout the world. Be it as a house wife, or as an aristocrat, this confinement has very subliminally and sometimes out rightly denied the entry of women into the work domain. Employment is a term which is often weighed in terms of the monetary advantages it brings to an individual, but has deeper connotations when looked into. It denotes freedom, strength, ability, value, and self-dependence. By virtue of the development of masculinity fostered by the society, these terms are associated with men, which make the entry of a woman into this arena even tougher. The deterministic life course for women set forth by first the father and then the husband or brother, is challenged when a woman tries to enter the space where free-will is fostered, i.e. employment. The ability to choose where to work, what to do, how to do it, and thereby being appreciated for it in itself is a great threat to the boundaries between man and woman. Masculinity has grounded itself on the foundation of superiority, not by virtue, but through dominance of the "weaker" sex which stands threatened with the influx of women in the labour force.

From the rise of aristocracy in the West, emerging importance of household helpers, to the idea of palace maids and "Dasis", a certain sub-section of "excluded" or "underprivileged" women did enter the arena of work and wages which came at the cost often borne by the loss of self-respect. Economic demands forced a certain stratum of women to cross the boundary and venture into the workplace, whereas the elite were pushed back harder into the domestic front. Corsets and well-groomed women were not only a symbol of aristocracy, but also the defining features that distinguished a "proper" woman, who stayed at home and raised the children from the working-class women. It is imperative to understand the discourse of women in the workplace to understand the inequality that existed in the societal norms, its manifestations in the current scenario and impact on mental health.

Gendering

The household is an important component when one talks of gendering because much of the practices that shape gender normative behaviours stem very early in developmental years. The cornerstone of research on well-being has centred itself on the experiences of men and women in the society along with the child-rearing practices that exist. Demarcation of attributes, values, and appropriate behaviours and inculcated in the forms of colours, toys, dressing styles and so on from a very early age. This in turn affects the traits one uses to identify as a male or female. Slowly, such values become a part of one's identity and is also used to label others based on these markers of identity which we often term as gender norms. Ram *et al.* (2014) shed light on the gendered nature of the socialization experience with respect to the representation of the social world for them. They showed how female youth expressed greater gender-egalitarian attitudes and were more likely to be impacted by gender discrimination in the family. Digressing from gender-specific norms further, leads to increase in mental health issues for both men and women, who are why more often than not, one tends to stick to them.

Masculinity is associated with *power* and *authority*, whereas femininity is synonymous to *submission*. Needless to say, men deem fit to exert undue authority by virtue of their gender, and often by being the sole bread-earners for the family. But when this notion is challenged by women entering the work arena, either such women are considered 'misfit' with respect to their role of a woman, as neglectful mothers, rebellious daughters, or ungovernable wives who bring shame to the family. This reflects a radical shift in the position. The *psychoanalytic theory* suggests that gender roles are acquired by identification with the same-sex parent. Bandura's (1956) social learning theory comes into play at the most rudimentary level by instructing the 'appropriateness' of behaviour and code of conduct that must be followed. Both reinforcement and modelling help in the acquisition of gender role appropriate behaviour. The modern versions of this school of thought emphasize on the significance of all relationships in early formative years. The *gender-role socialization theory* states that people and objects in the child's environment shape behaviour to fit gender-role norms while as, *social role theory*, a variant of the former suggests that the differences in women's and men's behaviour are a function of the different roles that women and men hold in our society. Often, the kind of role models present in the family dictates the course of development for both men and women, by virtue of observation. Social-role theory also examines those forces at a higher level, for instance that the division of labour between men and women, that is primarily, men working outside the house (Agentic role) and women caring for children (communal role). On the contrary, cognitive development theory emphasizes that the child as an active processor of the environment rather than a passive recipient of modelling and reinforcement. *Gender schema theory* contends that children acquire gender roles due to their propensity to process information into sex-linked categories. Gender schema theory combines the principles of social learning theory and gender-role socialization with cognitive development. A paradigm shift has been proposed by Deaux and Major (1987) that emphasize the characteristics of the perceiver, the target, and the situation that determines at any given moment of how people behave and whether a sex difference is observed.

Paid Worker Role and Family Role

A role is defined as a position in a society that is governed by norms and these norms are expectations for the behaviour. The roles have changed over the period of time. From a traditional family to modern family, the belief that it is better for men to earn money and women to take care of home and children has changed comparatively. Today, there are multiple roles for an individual which have the potential for role conflict also. Men and women have both the roles of paid worker along with the family roles.

Gender roles have existed through prehistoric cultures. Employment being equated with monetary benefits is a huge reason why the work of women at home is neglected and taken for granted. Paid employment has a positive effect on both women and men's health. Without the involvement of money for tasks done, the work that home-makers do is more often than not neglected and shunned away. Household work is disregarded due to absence of remuneration and hardly ever is taken into consideration. Neglect towards the work and worker indulging in such tasks is extremely common. In such a scenario, the sense of worth or accomplishment which the other, often the woman gets is nullified or non-existent. The house-wife or house-maker gets the designation, a list of targets to be achieved every day, but no matter how tedious the work, it holds no significance. Comparison between such work and that of another member's work which is paid for is often laughed about and ignored again, due to the absence of monetary compensation.

The cost-benefit analysis of the scenario is only made in terms of monetary capital gains and not the development of human capital. While it is the latter which gives way to the former, the role of those who help in the emergence of this cycle is not given due importance which proves to be detrimental for the well-being of women. Fostering the attitude that house work needs to be done because of compliance to social norms, takes away the meaning, value, and effort that the home-maker puts in to accomplish those tasks. When we talk of values associated to tasks, we speak of it in terms of how accomplishing something meaningful adds to one's self-esteem and sense of self-worth. But when this value is taken away or neglected in the name of "norms", it leaves the individual with a sense of worthlessness. This in turn, is a major contributing factor to the rise of mental issues and health problems in those faced with the phenomenon. The working women are able to break this cycle and enter the work front where their work is given a sense of worth, but the house-wives often struggle to make meaning of which they truly are, or even their identity.

As young children we all seek worth from our significant others, often our parents who are our mirrors, and reflect back who we are, to us. As we grow up, we seek the same reflection from our friends, partners, and peers. But as a house-wife, who looks into her hypothetical mirrors and is reflected back with nothing but a sense of how her duties are her meaning of existing, how does she answer the question of who she truly is? "Behind every successful man is a woman". The quote answers the question here, by denoting how a house-wife's sense of worth and value is derived from the achievements of her husband or her children. She lives vicariously through the success and failures of her family, and this becomes her identity. It is thus, not hard to comprehend the adverse effects that such living conditions bring with them, and how inimical this is to one's mental health. It is a question of identity, of virtue, of value and of worth. How does one assess the emotional well-being in this case which by definition is an integral part of mental health? Rosenthal, Carroll-Scott, Earnshaw, Santilli, and Ickovics (2012) concluded on the basis of a national survey, that people who worked full-time had lower levels of stress and lower levels of depressive symptoms than those who worked part-time or were unemployed. Those who worked full-time also had better eating habits, were more physically active and were less likely to drink and smoke as compared to unemployed and part-time employed people. These findings were applicable to both men and women.

For a lot of women seeking entry into the work domain, appropriate jobs that match their interests or needs are not available. The trend of flexible work timings and work from home which is extremely prevalent in the developed countries, is only in its nascent stages in India. There is a certain level of misallocation of talent in the labour force. Women with high ability are often employed in low skilled occupations, which are a significant hindrance to growth (Wang & Hsieh, 2013). It is projected that a 10 per cent increase in the ratio of females to males of workers could increase the per capita net domestic product by almost 8 per cent (Esteve-Volart, 2004). Working women face immense discrimination in terms of wages, opportunities, and equal treatment. The glass ceiling is far more common than thought off, but despite these drawbacks, employment comes with a benefit of independence. The notion of freedom and independence lacks an egalitarian basis when compared with respect to gender. Women are confined to the household as a means to often curtail freedom by stressing on the vulnerability that comes with being a female. Many such tags are often used to create a boundary or modern day "Lakshman Rekha" which in the name of protection is in fact, creating limits for women.

Working woman's capability to stand equal to men is a disruption in the prevailing system, which threats not only the norms of societies but also the very discourse and developmental norms of masculinity. Threats to the alpha male status by the multitasking female often prove to shake grounds of the practices that bear the burden of what we call society.

A study by Sarkar *et al.* (2017) sheds light on the employment conditions in India with respect to the entry and exit rates of female employees. The trend that emerges was that women were more likely to quit work with a substantial increase in the income of other members of the society. Women having new born children are much prone to quitting work due to unavailability of either appropriate childcare leaves or due to the social pressure placed on them to raise the children as a "good" mother. Quitting from the workforce is maximum after childbirth, due to which many women prefer to not work at all rather than working for a brief while, only to return and be confined to child rearing. Only 27 per cent of adult women in India had a job in 2012 as compared to 79 per cent men. The labour force is not even close to exclusive in terms of equality despite the rising GDP.

The image of the "good" woman has to be upheld even more strongly by a lot of women venturing into the workplace in order to fulfil the societal norms that enslave them. The work hours outside the house are often compensated by greater commitment to household chores on return, which leaves little or no space for meeting one's own needs (Bose & Das, 2014a; Sudarshan, 2014; Sudarshan & Bhattacharya, 2009). This negligence is what kick starts the development of various obstacles to well-being that hold the potential to develop into full blown psychological disorders. Working women are often faced with the stress of being skilled workers vs. skilled home-makers. Women employees show a greater degree of work stress as compared to men (Swanson, 2000). The task of balancing between the two is tedious and could be detrimental to well-being. Jobs created through globalization and liberalization has created job opportunities along with fueling necessities. With the movement of women outside the house, there has been an increase in the burden of managing the dual identity and working double to manage the household as well as the workplace. Moreover, these added responsibilities are now becoming extremely normalized due to re-structuring of society which is continuing to place the burden of being efficient home-makers as well as efficient at workplace.

So, even though there is a new world that the working women are venturing into, they are being pushed back harder into the household domain, often by the guilt they bear for simply working! Guilt and shame are powerful tools that hold the potential to deeply impact mental health and well-being. The identity of a woman as a caregiver and home-maker are hanging like an albatross around the necks of many women who have internalized this 'duty' so ardently, that looking beyond these domains seem sinful. And for those who do, compensatory mechanisms are in place to ensure that the guilt is overridden by greater commitment to the house. Working women often prefer to be employed in professions that require lesser part of the day so as to be able to spend adequate time with their children. Many of them join work only after the child is old enough and going to school.

For the housewives on the other hand, the guilt factor seems to be lesser due to their indulgence with the family life. This not only helps them to focus on self-care in a more guilt free manner, but also contributes to greater well-being in the long run. Many of the house-wives indulge in productively channelizing their time and energy by venturing into learning new skills and activities. With a little push and support, those who excel in a particular skill emerge as small entrepreneurs eventually, even if it is by means of hosting skill-based classes or opening their own line of work. Passion for activities is immensely important when one speaks of mental health, since it helps the individual focus inwards, into what one really wants. Akin to introspection, skills evoke a sense of fulfilment which has deeper connotations than just being one's interest. It is about designating some time in doing what the individuals desires to do. In common parlance, it is focusing inwards on the needs and desires of the self, or self-care! Well-being cannot be talked about without understanding the importance of putting aside time for oneself, which is why solitary activities like reading, meditation, etc are so well encouraged. For the modern-day woman, this has gained optimum importance and is subliminally resulting in a much-improved level of mental health. For the working women, this poses to be one of the greatest challenges because it adds to the 'guilt' of taking away time to venture into one's selfish interests rather than catering to the needs of the household and family.

Mental health and well-being are largely influenced by the perceived power that one upholds. Working women get a sense of power from the workplace, from success and achievements at their work front which proves to make a huge difference. Working women tend to be autonomous with respect to their decision-making ability, which defies the gender conformation to the norms and may seem as very unacceptable, causing a great deal of rejection. Women in India are often, by virtue of gender norms, asked to prioritize housework which may be explicitly stated after marriage (Sudarshan & Bhattacharya, 2009). Although exceptions exist in terms of women who have surpassed the glass ceiling and reached the top, but the numbers are few. Prominent personalities like, Arundhati Bhattacharya (the former Chairman of the State Bank of India, and was acclaimed as the 25th most powerful woman by Forbes, 2016); Shikha Sharma, (former CEO of Axis Bank); Vanitha Narayanan (has played a leadership role in IBM's growth trajectory) remain either unheard or insignificant due to the undue focus on the success of their male counterparts.

For housewives however, the sense of power often comes from either dominating those beneath them by virtue of relations, or through the accomplishments of their family members. But this vicarious sense of power is in turn, not their own and sooner or later fades off. The women in the household often exert their influence, their need for power and superiority by dominating the other members of the family. It is akin to the working of the Prime Minister and the President, which men being the latter and women being the former. However, such influences are very subliminal and sometimes may not exist. In such a scenario, it seems hard to envision the life of a home bound woman in the 21st century and how they deal with the transitions that come across while keeping their well-being intact.

Being an employed, earning member of the family brings with it certain powers which the working women possess by virtue of their entry into the domain. These powers are not only outside, but also exerted within the family by the women, giving them an equal right, and a voice which is otherwise subdued. Rosenfield (1989) speaks about how married women experience greater anxiety and depressive symptoms than married men, but working women seem to experience a lesser degree of these as compared to housewives. She stresses the importance of power dynamics that come into play when an individual is employed, and the health benefits associated with it through this very power. But on the other hand, the results of many studies conducted with regard to the stress levels in working vs. non-working married women have had different results (Rosenfield, 1989; Lennon & Rosenfield, 1992). Some stress the importance of work as liberating and enhancing well-being, while others talk about the guilt associated with spending time away from one's 'duty' and how an over-compensation leaves the working women fatigued and mentally exhausted.

Emotional well-being is impacted by the needs of autonomy, competence and relatedness (Reis, Sheldon, Gable, Roscoe & Ryan, 2018).

The Self-Determination theory (Deci & Ryan, 1991) talks about how the well-being is associated with satisfaction of basic psychological needs. These needs are perhaps better fulfilled in working women, wherein the need for autonomy is met through being employed at one's will and desire; the need for competence is met through feeling of worth which rises out of accomplishments; and the need of relatedness is met through one's relation with significant others. But on the other hand, if one was to compare the fulfilment of these needs to that of a housewife's, one could see how the needs are still met but not directly, through the experiences of others. That is, the need for autonomy is met by being congruent with the self, beliefs and norms within which they function; the need for competence is brought about by the successful outcomes of the family members modulated by these women; and the need for relatedness is met through family interactions and time spent with friends. In lieu with the research then, it is not hard to see how the concept is complex and slightly haywire, bending in both directions equally. This is where the 'individualism' factor becomes significant. Mental health has a lot to do with how one perceives their situations. Two people having the same experiences may perceive the impact of those in contrasting ways. Similarly, when we talk about the well-being of women, we may see instances where housewives are actually happier and better off being in the domain of the household as compared to extremely good professionals who may experience guilt of not conforming to the gendered norms.

Pursuing personal strivings that are congruent to one's organismic needs have a healthier personality (Emmons, 1991). Panwar and Srivastava (2019) found out that working women tend to experience higher life satisfaction and lower mental stress as compared to housewives, along with lesser physiological complaints. Ahmad & Khan (2018) found out that although there were no differences between married working women and housewives, both groups differed on social and psychological factors. Non-working women were seen to have poorer mental health and lower self-esteem. They reported more depression due to a poor social life (Akbari, 2012). Socially, non-working women scored lower due to perhaps not being exposed to professional interpersonal relationships. This however, could be contradicted by the fact that many working women find it difficult to extend a social circle beyond the workplace due to added responsibility of managing the household. The housewives on the other hand, may be very adept at social gatherings and skills due to the time devoted for such activities willingly. Housewives on the other hand, are often very active members when it comes to socializing. The time they devote to such activities could make them extremely adept and efficient in social interactions, hence contributing to a significantly satisfactory social life.

Forming groups with other non-working women, indulging in educational and leisure activities could in fact, help these women to be adept socially. Some of these challenges are addressed if one closely examines the 'small spaces' women have created for themselves, knowingly or unknowingly. Socialization is an important component through which women are extending their feet into the outside world. One would often find small groups of women who would gather monthly to meet, or to discuss the latest trends in clothing or jewellery, or to simply share recipes of new dishes amongst each other. As a layman, one would interpret this as a fairly normal process which comes 'naturally' to women by virtue of their gender identity. But these small gatherings function as therapy groups where women get a chance to speak, and to be heard by other women who understand the experiences through the similarity that they hold.

Stigmatization of Man as the Home-maker

Social conditioning reinforces gender roles. The beginning of these can be traced to the hunter and gatherer era were men would hunt due to their built, which is a completely physiological difference, while women with their maternal instincts, would take care of the family and children. Switching to the modern-day scenario in a metropolitan city, we see that many of the jobs today are simply desk jobs which require mental capital rather than physical labour. However, this disparity is still extremely prevalent and does not cease. Researches through history have aimed to focus on the distinction between the genders and not the sexes, to the extent of gendering academic subjects as being more proficient by one gender as compared to the other. Men even in today's society are criticized for taking up humanities and social sciences, whereas women are doubted for their capacity to understand the sciences. These subtle processes that exist right from the birth of a child to adulthood subliminally mould individuals in a certain way, without even realizing. The process of gendering is not only to do with the capacities that men and women later deem fit to pursue, but also creates a mindset which becomes detrimental to growth and seeps into every area of functioning. The development of self-esteem and self-worth largely arise from our interaction with significant others who reinforce the idea of what we believe in, of our abilities, capacities and worth. But if only a certain kind of worth is highlighted from a woman's many areas of specializations, she goes on to developing that and only that further. A very simple example that one can think of is instincts. Maternal instincts are by far, extremely talked about when we talk of the process of gendering. Looking in a little deeper, there are other instincts too which Freud postulated as the basis of his theory, namely the life and the death instinct—*Eros* and *Thanatos*. But the expression of Eros by women, the desire to procreate, and the desire to indulge into a gratifying sexual relationship is shamed and looked down upon almost as a sin. One instinct, on which the society wants us to focus, is highly glorified whereas all the others are simple excluded very subtly. Similarly, the death instinct too is shamed if exemplified by a woman being too aggressive because the gendered identity does not permit dominance by a woman. It seeks submission, or rather demands submission by the 'good' woman, giving rise to the housewife who functions within these boundaries and the working woman who remains guilt ridden.

The concept of *stay-at-home dad* or *stay-at home father* is much prevalent in the developed countries, and especially in cosmopolitan cities like London, where it has become an acceptable practice for men to look after the family and for the women to be the breadwinners.

The breadwinner model talks about how one member of the family has the duty to support the family financially, while the non-earning members has to look after the functioning within the house. This has been extremely gendered in its approach wherein women are traditionally sought after as the home-makers while men are termed as the breadwinners in almost all societies. The model grew out of the increasing wages for work which would help suffice the needs of the entire family with only one earning members, thus forgoing the system of divided work contribution at home. Although the breadwinner ideology transitioned into removing children from waged labour, it pushed women back into the house.

Task at Hand

Although the number of women attending any educational institution in 1994-2010 doubled (Kapsos *et al.*, 2014), the rise in economic growth, the number of women in the labourforce is still very low. The government has realized the importance of the workforce being more inclusive as exemplified by the various programmes started to help women become more independent, like the 'Support to Training and Employment Programme for Women (STEP)' scheme, Women's Vocational Training Programme, and Start Up India initiative to empower women as job creators rather than seekers.

Women face 2-3 times more symptoms of depression and anxiety as compared to men (World Health Organization, 2001). Training programmes and educational policies need to account for including more women in inclusive programmes with more flexible schedules that are sensitive to their needs. Examining the connotations of mental health, along with frameworks for diagnosis and identification are important. It is quintessential to formulate policies and programmes to propagate mental health agendas to a wider array of the society and de-stigmatize it in order to make well-being modules available to the masses. Awareness, intervention and psycho-education are powerful tools to change the present scenario. These have to operate on a political and national level along with being propagated to individuals at the grassroot level as well, by spreading awareness about mental health and the connotations of its absence. The risk factors must be taken into account and rectified individually. Community settings in particular, must give importance to the socio-cultural, legal, infrastructural and economic restructuring that benefits women in the long run. Moreover, fostering women empowerment through posters and banners would not do any good unless the meaning is explained to the target groups along with the repercussions that follow when adequate steps are not taken to ensure well-being.

Conclusion

The decisive point that remains is that mental health for women is an extremely important issue which has been neglected for decades but has got public attention very recently. More than a debate about working vs. non-working women, the task at hand should be to educate women about the gendering process that has shaped us to be who we are. It is imperative to restructure the societal norms and expectations by first understanding them, and then trying to modify it according to the needs of the 21st century in a guilt-free manner. To be a housewife or to work is a personal choice which should not come with the baggage of feeling stuck or being overwhelmed. The limits of the human mind and physical capacity of the body to manage two extremely tedious areas must be considered and understood by the larger section of the society.

References

Ahmad, M. and Khan, A. (2018). Social Support and Marital Adjustment In:

Married Working Women. *Education, Sustainability and Society* (*ESS*), *1*(2), 5-7.

Akbari, A.J. (2012). Life satisfaction and stress among working and non-working women. *Indian Journal of Research. 1*(*9*), 174-176.

Bose, Nayana, and Shreyasee Das. 2015. "Women's Reservation and India's National Rural Employment Guarantee Scheme." Working Paper.

Chhabra, S. (2017). Stress among Working Women: Maintaining Balance as Housewives or Productive Employees. *International Journal in Applied Studies and Production Management*, *3*(3), 15.

Deaux, K., and Major, B. (1987). Putting gender into context: An interactive model of gender-related behaviour. *Psychological Review, 94,* 369-389.

Emmons, R.A. (1991). Personal strivings, daily life events, and psychological and physical well-being. *Journal of Personality*, *59*(3), 453-472.

Esteve-Volart, B. (2004). Gender discrimination and growth: Theory and evidence from India.

https://econpapers.repec.org/scripts/redir.pf?u=http%3A%2F%2Fsticerd.lse.ac.uk%2Fdps%2Fde%2Fdedps42.pdf;h=repec:cep:stidep:42 (accessed on 20.09.2019)

Helgeson, Vicki S. (2018). *Psychology of Gender.* Rutledge.

Kapsos, S., Bourmpoula, E., and Silberman, A. (2014). *Why is female labour force participation declining so sharply in India?* (No. 994949190702676). International Labour Organization.

Lennon, M.C., and Rosenfield, S. (1992). Women and mental health: The interaction of job and family conditions. *Journal of Health and Social Behaviour*, 316-327.

Panwar, N., and Srivastava, S. (2019). Job V/s. Home Demands: A Comparative Study between Life Satisfaction, Physical and Mental Stress in Indian Housewives and Employed Women. *Indian Journal of Physiotherapy and Occupational Therapy*, *13*(3).

Ram, U., Strohschein, L., and Gaur, K. (2014). Gender Socialization: Differences between Male and Female Youth in India and Associations with Mental Health. *International Journal of Population Research,* vol. 2014, Article ID 357145, 11 pages, 2014. https://doi.org/10.1155/2014/357145.

Sustainable Development Goals-United Nations.

https://www.un.org/sustainabledevelopment/sustainable-development-goals/ (accessed on 20.9.2019)

Reis, H.T., Sheldon, K.M., Gable, S.L., Roscoe, J., and Ryan, R.M. (2000). Daily well-being: The role of autonomy, competence, and relatedness. *Personality and Social Psychology Bulletin, 26, 419–435.*

Rosenfield, S. (1989). The effects of women's employment: Personal control and sex differences in mental health. *Journal of Health and Social Behaviour, 30,* 77-91.

Rosenthal, L., Carroll-Scott, A., Earnshaw, V.A., Santilli, A. and Ickovics, J.R. (2012). The importance of full-time work for urban adults' mental and physical health. *Social Science and Medicine, 75,* 1692-1696.

Ryan, R.M. and Deci, E.L. (1991). Self-Determination Theory and the Facilitation of Intrinsic Motivation, Social Development and Well-Being. https://selfdeterminationtheory.org/SDT/documents/2000_RyanDeci_SDT.pdf(accessed on 20.9.2019)

Sudarshan, R.M. (2014). Enabling Women's Work, ILO Asia-Pacific Working Paper Series, DWT for South Asia and Country Office for India, International Labour Organization,www.ilo.org/wcmsp5/groups/public/---asia/---ro-bangkok/---sronew_delhi/documents/publication/wcms_324624.pdf (accessed on 20.9.2019)

Sudarshan, R.M., and Bhattacharya, S. (2009). Through the Magnifying Glass: Women's Work and Labour Force Participation in Urban Delhi. *Economic and Political Weekly,* 44 (48), 59–66.

Swanson (2000). Working women and stress. *Journal of the American Medical Women's Association (1972)*, *55*(2), 76-79.

Wang, D.S. and Hsieh, C.C. (2013). The effect of authentic leadership on employee trust and employee engagement. *Social Behaviour and Personality: An International Journal*, *41*(4), 613-624.

9

Empty Nest Transition in Employed and Home-maker Mothers

An Exploratory Study

Parisha Jijina and *Aneri Shah*

Introduction

Normally, the Indian society is considered to have a very enduring, stable, and supportive family system. Until few decades ago, Indian society was dominated by the joint family system. Until recently this trend slowly gave way to nuclear families. Families split as a result of career opportunities. Youth from small cities and towns moved to bigger commercial cities in search of better job opportunities, further studies and to avail improved standard of living. While the parents, who stay emotionally, rooted to the place where they spent most of their life, choose to stay at the same place and accept with some sorrow their children starting out new life away from them (Chadda & Sinha, 2013).

As a convention, in India, parents were largely seen to reside in the home of their eldest son. However, across India, this trend is changing, and aging parents are going through their old age alone (Shapira, Barack & Gal, 2007). The phenomenon of the lonely elderly parent is becoming common across all levels of modern Indian society (Gentleman, 2006).

Empty Nest Transition

Carter & McGoldrick (1980) recognized six normal developmental stages of the family life cycle. These stages include: (1) Leaving Home: The Single Adult, (2) The Joining of Families through Marriage: The New Couple, (3) Families with Young Children, (4) Families with Adolescents, (5) Launching Children and Moving On, and (6) Families in Later Life.

Empty nest phase is usually identified as the post-parenthood phase. The empty nest period is defined as the phase of life when the children are grown but no longer live at home (Dinnerstein, Dudley & Guthrie, 2002). When a child leaves, it is an important experience for both parents and child. And even though many parents view it as a highly hopeful event, for others it is a difficult point, a stage of loving and letting go and a time when the daily parental role is diminished.

More intense and long lasting than the Empty Nest phase is the Empty Nest Syndrome which refers to feelings of depression, sadness, and/or grief experienced by parents and caregivers after children come of age and leave their childhood homes" (Sword, 2014). However, the validity of the Empty Nest Syndrome phenomenon is highly probed as it is predominantly not recognized as a clinical disorder or diagnosis in the psychiatric classification system followed worldwide but is rather viewed as a life transition that many people undergo (Moscucci, 1999).

Wu *et al.* (2010) has reported a cultural difference in the meaning attached to the empty nest. In predominantly individualistic cultures, nest leaving typically reflects the success of parents to raise their children into well-adjusted, independent adults. On the other hand, in cultures that are usually collective in nature, the empty nest reflects the failures of the parents of being unable to instil the family values in a child that keep the family bound together. Such negative conations of the Empty Nest are likely to have negative impact on the mother and father.

The Empty Nest may not always evoke negative emotions, but a series of mixed emotions with a relief towards the end of parental responsibilities and excitement towards much awaited freedom coupled with concern of the children's well-being as well as worry and anxiety over rejection by the children in the future (Mount & Moas, 2015). A recent study found that the women with their primary role as caretaker of children as say-at-home-mothers were looking forward to the departure of their child and were also preparing for the next stage in life such as seeking additional hobbies, etc. On the other hand, the fathers did not talk about their child's departure and were less prepared for the separation and later exhibited regrets over lost opportunities to play a greater role in their child's life before they left home (Mitchell & Lovegreen, 2009).

Research has revealed that working women are less likely to be negatively affected by the empty nest transition as compared to non-working women as they develop other aspects of their identity through work and other interests (Putz, 2012). Women who carry on with their work parallel through child rearing may be adequately engaging themselves in other roles that may reduce the impact of their children leaving home.

O'Connell (1976) explored the identity of women. He suggested two aspects of identity—a personal sense of identity occurs where she is considerate of her own ability, potential and needs and has the capacity to see herself as a separate individual, to occupy herself independently, and the other aspect of identity in which the woman's self-esteem and feelings of self-worth are the result of being associated with significant others. It was found that the sense of personal identity becomes a central issue after her role of wife and mother has been lessened and hence, they may feel the effects of empty nest more acutely.

Cessation of Active Parent Role in Mothers and Fathers

Role theory is one of the important theories of social aging. According to Role theory research, the idea of better health is often attached to the individual's feelings of control of life, social status and social control. Role loss is an important aspect in role theory. Role loss may be experienced by individuals as they grow older and they start losing their roles as a parent, employee or spouse. Their social network gets smaller as they are now in contact with less number of people (Tanner, 2010). Studies on the family life cycle have shown that empty nest phase may bring to parents this feeling of role loss. It has negative effects on emotional well-being and may lead to parental emotional trauma (Pinhey, 2004).

Much of the research related to the empty nest phase is done on women, as women are traditionally seen to be the primary caregiver to the child and they gain their identity from their role as a mother, while fathers are assumed to be more involved in bread earning activities and may gain their identity from their work role. The fathers who play a more traditional role of being more involved in working than spending time in raising the children, they may experience a loss and may wish that they had contributed more time and were more involved with their children (Putz, 2012).

Dennerstein, Dudley and Guthrie (2002) suggest that mothers who are over-involved in their children's lives and hold the traditional view of selflessly devoting themselves to their children's upbringing may perceive the loss of mother role as a major role loss.

Feelings of Loneliness, Depression and Anxiety due to Empty Nest Phase

Depression is observed to be a common condition in the middle age women due to the biological, psychological and social changes during this phase of life such as menopause, retirement etc. Changes such as empty nest phase, poor health, or loss of older parents taking shape within closed interval may accelerate the feelings of depression, anxiety and loneliness. Individuals going through empty nest syndrome may experience feelings of grief, sadness, irritability, change in their appetite or sleep disturbances. They may also have several somatic complains.

They may also feel anxious about being alone during the difficult situations like health problems faced by themselves or their children or any other complicated life situations. A comparative study revealed that empty nest group, had higher level of loneliness, lower physical and mental scores (Liu & Guo, 2007). In another study it was reported that when parents become alone, they find it difficult to identify any new activity that they can engage in to utilize their free time which in turn leads to experience of loneliness (Iman & Aghamari, 2011).

Effects on Marital Relations of Parents and Coping with the Empty Nest Transition

After launching their children, parents can attend to their individual needs as well as to their needs as a couple, how they return to their marital relationship, decides the quality of their marriage for remaining years (Putz, 2012). Researches in the west revealed that a large number of parents enjoy their freedom of being alone with their spouses and have a feeling of being reconnected with one another. In a study conducted by Clay (2003), the majority of parents enjoyed better independence, a reconnection with their partner and extra-opportunities to pursue their own goals and interests once their children go away. Parents stated that seeing a child on the path towards successful adulthood gave them a feeling of joy and pride.

It is found that if the children are more prepared for the transition in their life then it is more likely that the parents will also be well-prepared for the empty nest transition. On the contrary, it may happen that some parents during the child rearing process have forgotten how to be a couple. A couple who does not have a steady and a mutually satisfying relationship will have difficulties adjusting to the children leaving home and old age and are more likely to get divorced during this phase of life (Putz, 2012).

To cope with the empty nest, some parents become part of Parents Association of their child's university or visit their children during special occasions and find ways to continue their involvement in their children's lives. Empty nest transition for such parents is not a concern, because they still attach a parental role and responsibility to their children and do not sense the feeling of empty nest transition (Clay, 2003). Also, with the popularized use of internet and mobile phones, the number of ways of staying connected is more readily accessible with email, texting, Skype and more, which has helped the empty nesters to cope up and stay in touch with their children. The internet has also played a significant role by availing empty nesters with opportunities that include online therapy and counselling (Shapira, Barak, & Gal, 2007).

Rationale of Study in Indian Context

With the increasing number of nuclear families, and dispersion of joint families, members of the family are moving towards a situation where they are losing their support system that helped them keep themselves psychologically and physically resilient in many challenging life situations. Empty nest transition is one such challenging phase for mothers. Traditionally in India, boys would move out more of the house as compared to girls for further studies. But now even girls are leaving home for a better academic and professional future. Due to job opportunities and better living standards, families are shifting from their native cities and are becoming isolated islands. Women in mid-life are prone to be affected by Empty nest syndrome. There is a dearth of research in the Indian context. The needs of the empty nesters should be recognized thereby, this study is conducted so as to make a small contribution to the literature in the Indian context.

Method

Aim of the study: This study attempted to explore Empty nest transition in working and home-maker mothers and understand their experiences and coping.

Sample

Purposive Sampling and Snowball sampling technique was used for selecting participants of the study. The sample consisted of total ten participants: five working and five home-maker mothers, residing in Ahmadabad city, mean age of participants in the study was 50 years. The participants were selected according to the following Inclusion and Exclusion criteria:

Inclusion Criteria

(a) Last child should have left city for long-term commitment such as marriage, job, and academics and will return after minimum two years or may not return.
(b) Duration of time from the last child left home should be within three months to two years.
(c) Mothers staying in nuclear family or with in-laws.

Exclusion Criteria

(a) Mothers whose husband or either of the children has passed away.
(b) Mothers who are divorced/single mothers.
(c) Mothers who live in a joint family.

Participant characteristics: All the participants belonged to upper middle-class strata residing in Ahmedabad and were of similar age. The five working women belonged to various professions like, doctor, lecturer, and tuition teacher, administrative officer in government office and employed in a finance company.

Tool

Semi-structured interview schedule: For most purposes, exploratory research is conducted using qualitative approach. Among the various techniques available individual in-depth interview method has its own advantage in exploring individual experiences and perceptions. A semi-structured interview schedule was developed for this study based on the review of literature, discussions among the authors and keeping the present study's aim and objectives in mind. The interview schedule comprised of open-ended questions and probes. The semi-structured interview schedule was given for validation and feedback to two senior Psychology professors and changes were made in the interview schedule as per their suggestions. A pilot study with one participant was done. The feedback was taken from the participant and changes were made accordingly.

Procedure

After review of literature and discussion among the authors, the semi-structured interview schedule was developed based on the objectives of the study. It was sent to two experts for validation and a pilot study with one participant was done. The insights from the experts and pilot study were incorporated in the interview schedule.

Through purposive and snowball sampling the mothers were approached individually for participation. They were explained about the study and its objectives and their concerns and queries were addressed. Informed consent was taken and they were interviewed individually. Prior consent for audio recording was taken. General probing questions like "Could you elaborate? as well as techniques like summarizing, paraphrasing and clarification were used to deepen the interviewer's understanding about phenomena being discussed.

The average duration of the interview varied from sixty to ninety minutes and for the convenience of the participants, the interviews were conducted in their own homes. The interviews were conducted in the mother tongue of the participants (Hindi/Gujarati), were audio recorded and then transcribed for further analysis in study.

Analysis: Each participant's interview was read and re-read in entirety to get a holistic understanding of the participants' lived experiences and key phrases were highlighted. Braun & Clarke's (2006) Thematic Analysis method was employed.

Results and Discussion

The themes were collated under two super-ordinate themes: (1) lived experiences and feelings during the empty nest transition phase, (2) Dynamics of coping. Several sub-themes emerged.

Table 9.1: The super-ordinate themes with sub-themes

Super-ordinate themes	*Sub-themes*
Lived experiences and feelings during empty nest transition	i. Initial transition most difficult ii. Feelings of loneliness iii. Change in responsibilities iv. Preparation for launching child v. Pride in child's achievements vi. Perception of Change in communication with child vii. Perception of Change in relationship with spouse
Dynamics of Coping	i. Social media applications ii. Reassurance-Hope of better future for child iii. Keeping self-occupied iv. Cognitive distraction

Lived experiences and feelings during empty nest transition: The sub-themes are explained with specific illustrative quotations for working and home-maker mothers. The quotations provide deep insight into the feelings and perceptions of the mothers.

(i) Initial Transition Most Difficult

Three out of five working mothers reported that they found this transition very difficult initially, this is revealed in the following excerpt,

> "*It was difficult initially as we have stayed together for 17 years, we were much attached, and we were team of two as his father had been away for on and off, but I knew that I am going to miss him but I had prepared for it*".

When the home-maker mothers were asked about their feelings and thoughts about their children being away from home, four out of five mothers reported that they found this transition very difficult initially as they felt that their whole life was revolving around their children till the time they were staying with them. One mother reported,

> "*First you bring them up since their birth and then they go away. You would not even have thought that they would go away*".

The initial phase is reported to be difficult as changes such as empty nest phase may accelerate the feelings of depression, anxiety and loneliness (Pillay, 1998).

(ii) Feelings of Loneliness

Four out of five working mothers reported that their house had become empty without their children and they feel lonely after they come back from their work. It was reflected in the following excerpt,

> "*I had someone to talk to. At 4.30 when I get free from job I think that what I will do now going home....*"

Three of the home-maker mothers reported that they were very much attached and had become habituated to their child as they had stayed together with their children for so many years, groomed them with so much care and love and now they had to go away. They reported that their house had become empty without their children and they feel lonely staying at home. They also felt like crying many times. It was seen in the following excerpts,

> "*As I had seen him at home all the time, and now suddenly you don't see that person so it becomes very difficult right*".

> "*My house was full of people before when he was there. He has so many friends. At airport also all his friends had come to see off, they used to laugh and say that aunty we will come to meet you but none of them come, all are busy in their careers, now house looks all empty*".

One of the home-maker mother stated that she wanted her daughter to come back as she did not like staying without her. She also reported that she used to frequently tell her daughter to leave her job and come back.

> "*When she got her job I felt very happy for her, that she should focus on her career, she must not stay back for my emotions, but now I feel that it's enough and she should come back*".

The expression of feelings of loneliness and anxiety over adult child well-being is seen to be more in the home-maker mothers as compared to the working mothers. Three of the five home-maker mothers were found to get crying spells frequently when they remembered or missed their child at different occasions like when they visited their room, had made his favourite food or went out to dine.

Lal (2002) conducted a study, which revealed that women experiencing the empty nest experience come across intense feelings like feeling sad, intensely missing their children, and coping with anxieties and denial. It was thus proposed that counselling should be done based on situational determinants for each woman. Putz (2012) reports that many mothers who are over-involved in raising kids and hold the traditional view of selflessly devoting themselves to their children' upbringing may perceive the loss of mother's role as a major role loss.

(iii) Change in Responsibilities

Three out of five working mothers said that now they did not have to spend their time in cooking and keeping things ready for their child as per their timings and hence their responsibilities had decreased. However, one mother felt that her responsibilities had increased as now she does not have her child at home who was her helping hand.

Three out of five home-maker mothers reported that now they did not have to spend their time in cooking and keeping things ready for their child as per their timings. One of the mothers stated with great sadness that, she wants her daughter to be with her so that she can cook for her and be with her. As seen in the following excerpt,

> *"I tell her that now at Pune you work for two to four months and then we will find a job for you here in Ahmedabad, I will make food for you and you go for your job...".*

All the home-maker mothers reported that their child would help them in getting things from outside but that now they have got habituated to getting things by themselves, or ask their spouse to get it. As reflected in the following excerpt,

> *So during initial two months, I had become very busy. All small work that she used to do, I had to do them now. I would prefer buying things from nearby now. Else uncle would call in the evening before coming back from work to ask if anything is to be brought.*

It was evident more with the home-maker mothers that their responsibility of preparing food and keeping up with their child's time was no longer there. This added on to their feelings of maternal role loss. Previous research revealed that role loss may be experienced by individuals as they grow older and they start losing their roles as a parent, employees or as a spouse (Tanner, 2010). Children of working women are seen as more prepared and trained by parents to go away from their parental home. But home-maker mothers stated that their children learned more and worked more once they were away from their parent's home. This sensitivity of parents regarding their child's help in their day to day living gave them a sense of missing them and their company.

(iv) Preparation for Launching Child

Four out of five working mothers stated that they were prepared as they had always thought that their child will go away for further studies. They were aware that they will have to engage in a new routine. One mother who had not thought of sending her child away for further studies until her child was in the last year of college stated that she gradually prepared herself in the 6 months time period when the application procedures were going on.

Three out of five home-maker mothers stated that they were not prepared as they had always thought that their child will not go so away for further studies. But they said that gradually they managed to get into a new routine. Amongst them, one stated that she was not emotionally prepared for this transition. She used to often feel sad and would cry a lot,

> "*Today doctor told me that I should start with anti-depressants, so I told him that I will take three four days and see if I can get better without medicine, still if I feel the same way sad, then I will take medicine. He said that due to imbalance in the body due to constant thought processes it happens. Today I am feeling good. So I am trying.*"

It was seen that, four out of five working women had a tendency to perceive their children going away to pursue their careers as a mutual decision. They seemed to be more prepared to send away their child. But three out of five non-working women felt that it was sudden and unexpected for them and hence they did not prepare themselves to go through this phase.

(v) Pride in Child's Independence

All the mothers expressed that they were proud that their children were on their own feet now. Two home-maker mothers said with a feeling of pride that they were very happy that their children had now become independent and could take proper care of themselves as seen in the following excerpt.

> "*I can say with pleasure that my child has become self-dependent now*".
>
> "*Earlier she was dependent on me. We always had a helper and a cook at home, so certain things she would not do, but now she is very well-trained and I can say that she can go anywhere in the world alone. She was an average student during her school and college years here, but now she has progressed a lot*".

As seen in the responses given during the interview, all the participants felt that when their child was well settled or was doing well in life away from home, they gained the sense of pride, this in turn also helped them go through the transition more smoothly, they felt more prepared and gained better meaning in their lives, that they have groomed their child so well that now their child is making good progress in life and they have the feeling of peace and tranquillity of having carried out their duties.

(vi) Perception of Change in Communication with Child

Three of the working mothers stated that they feel that their communication and sharing with their child has in fact increased as when they were at home they used to be busy with their friends and college. As reflected in one of the excerpts,

> *"No in fact may be it has increased. Many times he would come home and would be so tired that he would go to sleep after dinner. In the morning, he would have to go to college, so we would not get to talk only. In fact we would hardly speak on the phone when he was here".*

Two of the five home-maker mothers stated that they felt that their child has become more close to them and shared more. They also feel that their children's value for family has increased. As reflected in one of the excerpts,

> *"Yes it has in fact increased since she has gone away. She has become more attached to me. Before she used to spend more time with her friend here, now she understands what family is".*

We see that previous research done has also pointed out the same; some parents reported that their relationship with their child improved when they went away from home (Clay, 2003). This indeed helps parents in coping through the transition as they feel closer to their child.

(vii) Perception of Change in Relationship with Spouse

Four out of five working mothers felt that there was no change in their marital relation with their husband. As reflected in the excerpt,

> *"We both are the same. I don't think our child going away has changed our intimacy, what it was previously is there today".*

While one of the mothers felt that they take more care of each other now. As reflected in the following excerpt,

"Ya it happens, because now it's only two of us. So, both of us we take more care of each other. Before we used to talk more about our son all the time, now also we talk about him only. He calls both of us separately; we tell each other what we spoke to him".

While four of the home-maker mothers felt that they take more care of each other now as a couple. They feel that now it's only both of them. Their husbands give them more time as compared to before. As reflected in the following excerpt,

> *"He talks very less, but yes I do feel that we have become more close to each other now".*

It's interesting to note the effect of empty nest transition on marital relations of parents, as per the findings; four working mothers stated that they do not see any significant change in their marital relationship. However, four out of five home-maker mothers perceived a change in their relations with their husbands. They feel that their husbands are giving them more time as compared to before. They feel that now it's only both of them and they only have to take care of each other more.

Literature suggests that sometimes when children are the focus of the relationship couples stay together and when the children leave home, the issues that create tension in the marriage are heightened in the absence of children (Black, 1984). There is however contradictory evidence that suggests positive emotions upon the nest emptying such as increased marital satisfaction, greater intimacy, more freedom and improved financial conditions and the couple rediscovering each other (Wang & Zhao, 2012).

Dynamics of coping: The next super-ordinate theme was related to the dynamics of the coping processes during the empty nest transition. The sub-themes are explained with specific illustrative quotations for working and home-maker mothers which provide insight and depth into the coping process.

(i) Social Media Applications

All the 10 mothers in the study reported that they would use Viber, Skype, Facetime or WhatsApp to stay in touch with their child. Social media applications have made it easy to speak to their children once or sometimes twice in a day, most mothers reported doing video calling once or twice in a week. They mentioned that any time in the day if they felt like, they would chat through messages. They feel good when they talk to their child. When they use video calling, they perceived the distance as less as seen in the following excerpt,

> *"WhatsApp makes me feel like he is here only with me. Like I can imagine when he says that he is doing this or that. I would feel like everything is all right. We feel less lonely. It has helped to a great extent. I feel less distance".*

It is found that participants feel that using video calling application via internet and free calling services have played a very significant role in their worries related to their child going to a new environment. They feel less distance and less worried when they do video calling. As previously stated, the popularized use of internet, staying connected is more readily accessible this has helped the empty nesters to cope up with the empty nest transition (Putz, 2012). Digitalization has brought many families closer and because of the internet, children abroad can always stay in touch with parents who use digital media to communicate at least once a day (Badiani & DeSouza, 2016).

(ii) Reassurance-Hope of Better Future for Child

All the mothers had hopes of better and brighter future for their child which is an important cognitive coping strategy. As seen in the following excerpt.

> *"He has not fought or left home and gone, that is anything that is good for him that is what I want"*

They feel good that their children are settling nicely and are currently not facing any major problems. Thinking this way helps them to accept that their child is away. As seen in the excerpts,

> *"So one thing is there that now he is very well set there with his*

> *routine, all his studies are going good and he does not have any problem there so I would first ask him in the morning whether his health is good, if he is alright and wish him good morning. So we have accepted it, there is no other option than accepting it. If his life is getting better then we have to compromise a little". "Well I feel good, with times they are pursuing their careers, and they too will be settled".*

(iii & iv) Keeping Self-occupied and Cognitive Distraction

The working mothers engaged themselves in the activities of their own interest like exercising, yoga, meditation and reading, which they could not engage in regularly before. Two of the mothers stated that this was the time for them to sit back rejoice and explore their own interests and socialize. As seen in the excerpt,

> *"I would go to crossword 3-4 times a week, browse through books. Plus, I like trekking, I like travelling so I increased that, I had my friends circle through that. In fact, I realized that this is the time to explore myself".*

When they had the feeling of missing their child, they would divert their mind by engaging in some activity. One of the mothers stated that she would avoid thinking about her child; else she would feel like crying. Two of the five working mothers, one who was a doctor and the other who was a tuition teacher stated that they had increased their working hours now, which they could not do so when their children were at home. It can be seen in the following excerpt,

> *"In evenings I used to spend more time with them, but since they are not there, I go to my clinic earlier now".*

For the home-maker mothers, it was initially difficult for them to identify the activities to engage themselves in. Two of the mothers stated that God has given them time explore their own interests and socialize. As seen in the excerpt,

> *"See honestly I tell you. I have taken it in this way that God has given me two years to spend in my own way, that I can live my own life".*

> *"We all ladies get together in the morning and do Yogasan for one hour. We read Dongre Maharaj's Bhagwat together. We then go out for food or movies sometimes. We make different things at home. So all this I have increased".*

One home-maker mother had joined an NGO and the other who used to engage herself in match making for marriages has increased her work. As seen in the following excerpts,

> *"I have joined NGO. I give my two hours there. I also teach the children of the helper at my house".*

One of the mothers stated that it was very difficult for her to engage herself in any activity because of which she was prescribed anti-depressants by her doctor before a day the interview was conducted. As seen in the following excerpt,

> *"That only, I am not able to engage myself in spare time, that's why all this medicine and things have started".*

According to the findings, four out of five working women's interview reflected in them the sense of being able to satisfactorily and more actively get into the new routine more easily as compared to the two non-working women, who were able to get into a new routine but did tend to reflect the sense of fulfilment in spite of engaging themselves in other activities when their children are away from them. Coping in the working mothers seemed to be concentrating more on self-development, while coping in non-working mothers included more of social and group activity.

It is believed that one's ability to adapt and adjust to other roles plays a critical role in coping with the empty nest phase. Women who are socialized to fulfil mainly the role of a mother tend to be over involved in the lives of her children, to a point where her own needs have been subjugated for the needs of her children. Hence, when the children leave, these mothers face an identity crisis, wherein they have to identify new roles to fulfil, and the inability to adjust to the new roles, in turn causes the anxiety and depression (Harkins, 1978; Rubins, 1979).

Shakya (2013) elaborates on how the parents can have preparatory coping when their last child is about to leave home. Adequate awareness about empty nest syndrome is needed and information of available services and resources, stress management and coping skills; support network are some of the strategies that might help mitigate such problems of the parents especially the mothers who are going through this phase.

Personal Observations and Experiences: Reflexivity of the Researchers

Researchers reflections on their actions and observations in the field, their impressions, irritations, feelings, and so on, become data in their own right, forming part of the interpretation, and are documented in research diaries or context protocols (Flick, 2009). During the interview the researcher observed that five of the participants while sharing their experiences started weeping as they were feeling sad, it could be that they were going through the process of catharsis. Two of the participants had mentioned that they were sharing such an experience for the first time with someone. As they were sharing their thoughts and experiences, they seemed to be realizing that they had actually never reflected back so much on their own feelings ever before.

From the interview with the mothers, it was sensed that fathers too were experiencing this phase with some difficulty. But they seemed not to be expressing it with their family members probably due to the prevailing Indian cultural belief that males as supposed to be strong. How fathers go through and cope with this transition should be studied to have a more comprehensive understanding of the empty nest transition. In a study by Oliver (1977) it was found that men do experience disequilibrium during the Empty Nest transition, but may be unwilling or express their response in terms that are neutral or ambivalent.

The findings thus indicate that working mothers adapted more actively and meaningfully to the empty nest transition phase as compared to the home-makers. Healthy coping methods to adapt with the empty nest transition period are discussed below.

Recommendations for healthy coping during the Empty nest transition phase:

(a) Familiarize yourself with latest technology which will help you stay in touch with your child.
(b) Mothers should engage themselves in the new activities before the child has left the house so as to reduce the experience of negative transition effects.
(c) Utilize this time to bond with your spouse.
(d) Utilize this time as an opportunity to focus on your self-development, rediscovering your old hobbies.

(e) Support groups can be started to give mothers an opportunity to vent out their feelings.

(f) Find out if there are any Parent Associations to the university where your child is studying so that you can have a more active part in their academics.

Implications for Practice

Mental health professionals need to be spread awareness regarding the empty nest syndrome and how counselling can help deal with this phase. As most of the mothers stated this was the first time, they were talking about their feelings regarding their child leaving home; counsellors could also consider establishing support groups for mothers and fathers going through this phase especially in states such as Kerala or Gujarat where there is a large incidence of immigration. Badiani and DeSouza (2016) strongly recommend that is vital that clinicians view the Empty Nest Syndrome (ENS) as real and for mental health professionals to consider psychological preparation for the ENS and having a preventive module in place for the same.

Summary and Suggestions for Future Research

To summarize, the findings indicated that initial transition was the most difficult for the mothers and included feelings of loneliness and changes in active role as mother. There were perceived changes in communication with the child and in the dynamics of marital relationship. Mothers coped with the transition through the use of social media applications, and increasing their social and the self-development activities. Emotional coping was found in sustaining the hope of a bright future for their child, a sense of fulfilment of parental duties and pride in seeing their child doing well. Overall, it was found that working mothers adapted more actively to the empty nest transition phase.

With more fathers taking on role of active care-giving and parenting in the Indian context, further research could focus on empty nest transition experienced by fathers. With technology making it easier for parents to communicate with their children even at vast geographical distances, it would be interesting to study the moderating role of technology on Empty Nest Syndrome.

References

Badiani, F. and De Sousa, A. (2016). The Empty Nest Syndrome: Critical clinical considerations. *Indian Journal of Mental Health*, *3*(2), 135-142.

Black, S.M., and Hill, C.E. (1984). The Psychological Wellbeing of Women in Their Middle Years. *Psychology Women Quarterly*, *8*(3), 282-92.

Braun, V., and Clarke, V. (2006). Using thematic analysis in psychology. *Qualitative Research in Psychology*, *3*(2), 77-101.

Carter, E.A., and McGoldrick, M. (1980). *The Family Life Cycle: A Frame Work for Family Therapy.* New York: Gardner.

Chadda, R.K., and Deb, K.S. (2013). Indian family systems, collectivistic society and psychotherapy. *Indian Journal of Psychiatry*, *55* (Suppl 2), S299–S309. doi:10.4103/0019-5545.105555.

Clay, R. (2003). An empty nest can promote freedom, improved relationships. *Monitor on Psychology*, *34*(4), 40.

Dennerstein, L., Dudley, E., and Guthrie, J. (2002). Empty nest or revolving door? A prospective study of women's quality of life in midlife during the phase of children leaving and re-entering the home. *Psychological Medicine*, *32*(3), 545-550.

Flick, U. (2018). *An Introduction to Qualitative Research.* Sage Publications Limited.

Gentleman, A. (2006). Indian parents hit by empty-nest syndrome-Asia-Pacific-International Herald Tribune. Retrieved from http://www.nytimes.com/2006/10/30/world/asia/30iht-parents.3334401.html?pagewanted=all&_r=0.

Harkins, E.B. (1978). Effects of empty nest transition on self-report of psychological and physical well-being. *Journal of Marriage and Family*, (1) 549-56.

Iman, B.T., and Aghamiri, S.F. (2011). A path analysis of the social and psychological factors influencing the psychological wellbeing of empty nest mothers in Sari city, Iran. *Sociation Today*, *9*(2), 1-10.

Lai, H.L. (2002). Transition to the empty nest: a phenomenological study. *Tzu Chi Nursing Journal*, *1*(3), 88-94.

Liu, L.J., and Guo, Q. (2007). Loneliness and Health-related Quality of Life for the Empty Nest Elderly in the Rural Area of a Mountainous County in China. *Quality of Life Research*, *16*(8), 1275-1280.

Mitchell, B.A., and Lovegreen, L.D. (2009). The Empty Nest Syndrome in Midlife Families A Multimethod Exploration of Parental Gender Differences and Cultural Dynamics. *Journal of Family Issues, 30*(12): 1651-70.

Moscucci, O. (1999). Medicine, age and gender: The menopause in history. *British Menopause Society Journal*, *5*(4), 149-53.

Mount, S.D., and Moas S. (2015). Re-purposing the "Empty Nest". *Journal of Family Psychotherapy*, *26*(3), 247-52.

O'Connell, A.N. (1976). The relationship between life-style and identity synthesis and resynthesis in traditional, neotraditional, and nontraditional women. *Journal of Personality*, 44, 675-688.

Oliver, R. (1977). The empty nest syndrome as a focus of depression: A cognitive treatment model, based on rational emotive therapy. *Psychotherapy Theory Research Practice*, *14*(1), 87-110.

Pillay, A.L. (1998). Midlife depression and the empty nest syndrome in Indian women. *Psychological Report*, 69, 591-594.

Pinhey, T.K. (2004). Empty nests and parental well-being in an Asian-Pacific population: an exploratory test. *Pacific Studies*, 27, (112).

Putz, K. (2012). *Transitions: The Family Life Cycle and the Empty Nest*. Published Masters project at the Adler Graduate School. Retrieved from Alfredadler. edu? sites/default/files/putzMP2012.pdf

Rubin, L.B. (1979). *Women of a Certain Age: The Midlife Search for Self*, pp. 7-8. New York: Harper & Row.

Shakya, D.R. (2009). Empty Nest Syndrome: An Obstacle for Alcohol Abstinence. *Journal of Nepal Health Research Council*, *7*(2), 135-137.

Shapira, N., Barak, A., and Gal, I. (2007). Promoting older adults' well-being through Internet training and use. *Aging and Mental Health*, *11*(5), 477–484.

Sword, K.M., and Zimbardo, P. (2014). *Empty Nest, Bring It On*! Retrieved from http://www.psychologytoday.com/blog/the-time-cure/201408/empty-nest-bring-it.

Tanner, J. (2010). *Aging and Role Loss*. Retrieved from http://www. brainybchaviour.com/blog/2010/11/aging-and-role-loss/.

Wang, J., and Zhao, X. (2012). Empty nest syndrome in China. *International Journal of Social Psychiatry*, *58*(1), 110-9.

Wu, Z.Q., Sun, L., Sun, Y.H., Zhang, X.J., Tao, F.B., and Cui, G.H. (2010). Correlation between loneliness and social relationship among empty nest elderly in Anhui rural area, China. *Aging Mental Health*, *14*(1), 108-12.

10

Learned Helplessness in Women

A Developmental Analysis

Aradhana Shukla and *Pooja Suteri*

Introduction

Learned helplessness is behaviour which can be characterized by maladaptive responses like avoidance of challenges, negative affect and the collapse of problem-solving i.e. inability to face or confront existing problems.

During the last 10 years, the learned helplessness model formulated by Seligman and his colleagues (Seligman, 1975; Seligman, Maier and Solomon, 1971) has had a major impact on theoretical development in social and clinical psychology (Abramason, Metalsky and Alloy, 1989) and on research on reactions to uncontrollable outcomes and depression (Benson & Kennelly, 1976; Geeta, 2010, Hammen & Krantz, 1975). As Abramson, Seligman and Teasdale (1978) have pointed out; however, the learned helplessness model was originally formulated on the basis of controlled experiments with infrahuman species (Maier & Seligman, 1976). As investigators started to extend the paradigm to research with human subjects and applying the theoretical constructs to reactions to uncontrollable life events, a plethora of problems appeared in existence. Individuals concerned with reactions to uncontrollable outcomes raised the following questions about the original helplessness formulation:

- Is uncontrollability a sufficient cause of helplessness, or must the outcome in question being aversive and/or highly important?
- Does the attribution of causality that an individual makes for his or her inability to influence an outcome affect the subsequent cognitive, motivational, or affective components of helplessness?
- Under what conditions do helplessness effects generalize whether

> these deficits are short lived or persist over time? Researchers primarily interested in depression began raising a parallel set of questions about the learned helplessness model of depression: does exposure to no contingent outcomes produce depression if the outcomes are positive how does the model account for lowered self-esteem a symptom frequently associated with depression? If depression stems from a belief in response outcome independence why do depressed individuals characteristically make internal attributions for their failure how can variations in the generality chronicity and intensity of depression be explained?

Abramson *et al.* (1978, 1981) have proposed a reformulation of the original model and posed a reformulation of the original model that addresses the majority of these problems. According to the reformulated account the individual first learns that certain outcomes and responses are independent and then makes an attribution about the cause. This attribution determines the person's subsequent expectation in turn, determines both the kind of deficit and its generality and chronicity. Abramson *et al.* (*1978*) have also argued that people's attributions for their inability to control their outcomes can be classified along three orthogonal dimensions. Two of these dimensions (internal-external, stable–unstable) have frequently been used by attribution theorists. The third (*global specific*) is new but so many psychologists do not define the internal external dimensions, but it is generally used to differentiate between causes that emerge from the person versus those that stem from situation or environmental factors. Stable factors are short lived and intermittent. Global factors across situations, whereas specific factors are more unique to the situation in which helplessness was induced. Abramson *et al.* (1978) have predicted that attributions to external factors. Attributions to stable factors should produce deficits with greater chronicity than attributed to global factors are expected to generalize further than those attributed to specific factors.

The Effect of Gender

So far many researchers investigated the difference between males and females regarding the attribution style and tried to uncover whether males or females are more likely to make pessimistic attributions leading to helplessness. In one study (Kiefer, 1990) the women being subject to uncontrollable adverse conditions were found to make more pessimistic attributions internal universal and stable attributions for failure and show symptoms of helplessness more compared to men. Researchers (Lazarus & Deese, 1952; Lee, Demons & Sullivan, 2001; Lee, 2002) found that women dealing with unsolvable anagrams in the first phase of experiment were found to be less successful and motivated in the second phase compared to women dealing with solvable anagrams and not dealing with anagrams at all. Lack of motivation and performance decrement was not observed among male participants. It was also suggested that males were less vulnerable to helplessness with socialization process and more equipped to cope with frustrating situations because of the training they got from their parents. Unlike many researchers claiming that women are more prone to feel themselves helpless Baucom and Danker-Brown (1979, 1984) stated that the role attributed to male and females by the society. According to researchers people scoring high on either masculinity or femininity are more likely to become helpless as compared to people scoring on high either masculinity and femininity or more likely to become helpless as compared to people having both masculine and femininity tendencies. Some researchers (Radloff & Monroe, 1978) claimed that women show helplessness because they are more exposed to situations which involve failure, lack of control and punishment. According to Seligman (1990) women are more prone to feel themselves helpless because of their tendency to well on their thought and explain unfavourable events and situations with pessimistic attributional style. It is noteworthy to mention that some studies (Dweck & Llicht, 1980; Overton & Meehan, 1982) reported conflicting results concerning the effect of gender on helplessness. For example in one study female students were found to exhibit less helplessness symptoms as compared to male students. Similarly, Rozell Gunderson and Tersptra (1998) found no difference between male and female university students with respect to helplessness they felt. Baucom and Danker-Brown (1979) researchers claimed that people having only feminine or masculine tendencies were more likely feel helplessness as compared to people having androgen tendencies or gender neutral identity.

Considering the conflicting results it is hard to conclude that particular type of sex induces learned helplessness. Getting lower wages and salaries and having to deal with prejudgments gender discrimination and role conflicts could make women employees more vulnerable to helplessness. However support given by coworkers' managers and family could alleviate the effects of adverse work conditions and lack of controllability hence increase resilience of women employees.

On the basis of above discussion it can be said that learned helplessness is just like an iceberg which is entirely different in its internal and external covers. The concept has been studied widely in west but in India the attempts are nominal. Geeta (2010) studied learned helplessness but it was focused on professional/non-professional student. Therefore, it was thought studied Indian women and learned helplessness. It is the sheer life of women who is a 24×7 home warrior and sacrifices her whole life on households and work place platforms. In spite of knowing the white and grey shades of all events he makes a compromised with the life and performs all chores with complete attention and care. Therefore, there is need to study the pattern of learned helplessness in women as affected by chronological age, marital status, cultural variation and job status. The objectives and hypotheses were as follows:

1. The first objective of the study was to find out the impact of age on learned helplessness. It was contended that variation in age would cause variation in learned helplessness.
2. The second objective of this investigation was to find out the relative efficacy of marital status on learned helplessness. It was proposed that marital status would lay its impact on learned helplessness.
3. The third objective of this investigation was to find out the impact of cultural variation on learned helplessness it was proposed that cultural variation would lay its impact on learned helplessness.
4. The fourth objective of this investigation was to find out the impact of job status on learned helplessness. It was proposed that variation in job status would lay its impact on learned helplessness.

Keeping these views in consideration this study was planned in factorial perspective.

Method

Sample: Two hundred forty participants ranging between 30-35 years of age, will serve as participants and they were arranged according to the requirements for four way factorial design with 3 levels of age (30-35 years, 40-45 years and 50-55 years), 2 levels for marital status (husbanded and widows), 2 levels of cultural variation (rural, urban) and 2 job status (employed and unemployed) i.e. 10 participants per cell. The design is given in Table 10.1.

Table 10.1: The schematic presentation is of experimental design

	A1				A2				A3			
	B1	B	B2		B1	B	B2		B1	B	B2	
	C		C		C		C		C		C	
	C1	C2	C1	C2	C1	C2	C1	C2	C1	C2	C1	C2
D1	10	10	10	10	10	10	10	10	10	10	10	10
D2	10	10	10	10	10	10	10	10	10	10	10	10

Legends

A = Chronological Age
A1 = 30-35 years
A2 = 40-45 years
A3 = 50-55 years
D = Job Status
D = Job Status
D1 = Employed
D2 = Unemployed

B = Marital Status
B1 = Living with Husbands
B2 = Widows

C = Cultural Variation
C1 = Rural
C2 = Urban

Measure: In this study only one measure was used and it is described below:

1. Learned helplessness scale: This measure is developed by ***Shukla and Suteri (2014)*** and consist of 64 point items that deal with the situations in which women find herself helpless although it is known by her. Test-retest reliably of this test is 0.79 and interrater reliability is given in Table 10.2.

Table 10.2: Inter-rater reliability of the test

Rates	*A*	*B*	*C*	*D*
1. A	–	62	66	70
1. B	–	–	64	56
1. C	–	–	–	79
1. D	–	–	–	–

Procedure: Data collection was done individually/in group as per availability of the participants and best attempts were made to avoid external distractions.

Results

Obtained data were analyzed by four way analysis of variance and interpreted in terms of chronological age, marital status, cultural variation and job status as affectors of learned helplessness. Summary of analysis of variance is appeared in the Table 10.3.

Table 10.3: Summary table of analysis of variance showing the impact of chronological age, marital status, cultural variation and job status on learned helplessness

Sources of Variation	Ss	Df	MS	F
A	16.86	2	8.43	4.74
B	3.15	1	3.15	1.79
C	5.98	1	5.98	3.36
D	0.95	1	0.95	0.54
AB	26.76	2	13.38	7.52
AC	18.26	2	9.13	5.19
AD	28.23	2	14.11	8.02
BC	7.99	1	7.99	4.49
BD	9.24	1	9.24	5.19
CD	5.35	1	5.35	3.01
ABC	31.89	2	15.94	8.96
ABD	30.90	2	15.45	8.68
ACD	32.58	2	16.29	9.15
BCD	6.48	1	6.48	3.64
ABCD	34.72	2	17.72	9.96
Error Within	384.48	216	1.78	
		239		

Table reveals that the main effect of chronological age was significant (*F, 2,216=4.74 p<.05*) and it was found that variation in chronological age, caused variation in the magnitude of experiential learned helplessness. It was found that youngest age group was least helpless (*x=142.80*) as compared to middle age group (*x=172.75*) and the oldest age group (*x=191.63*) respectively. The next main effect of marital status was insignificant (*F, 1,216=1.79 p>.05*). It was found that widows (*x=1.66.16*) and women living with husbands (*x=171.92*) were more or less similar in relation to their scores on learned helplessness. The third main effect of cultural variation was significant (*F,1, 216=3.36 p<.05*) and it was found that rural (*x=162.50*) and urban (*x=175.58*) women were apparently different in relation to their scores on learned helplessness. Also, it was seen that urban women had more helplessness than rural women. The main effect of job status was insignificant (*F, 1,216=0.54 p>.05*). It was found that employed (*x=170.58*) and unemployed women (*x=167.58*) were more or less similar in relation to their scores on learned helplessness.

The two way interaction of chronological age and marital status was significant (*F, 2,216=7.52 p<.01*) and is reported in Figure 10.1.

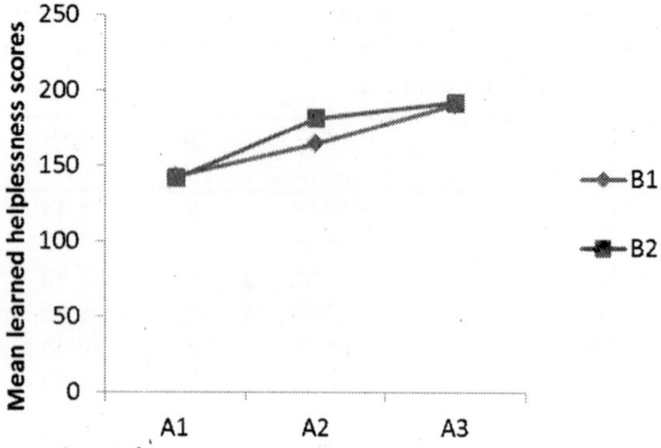

Legends

A=Chronological Age **_B=Marital Status_**

A1=30-35 years B1=Living with husbands

A2=40-45 years B2=Widows

A3=50-55 years

Fig. 10.1: Mean Values showing the Impact of Chronological Age and Marital Status on Learned Helplessness

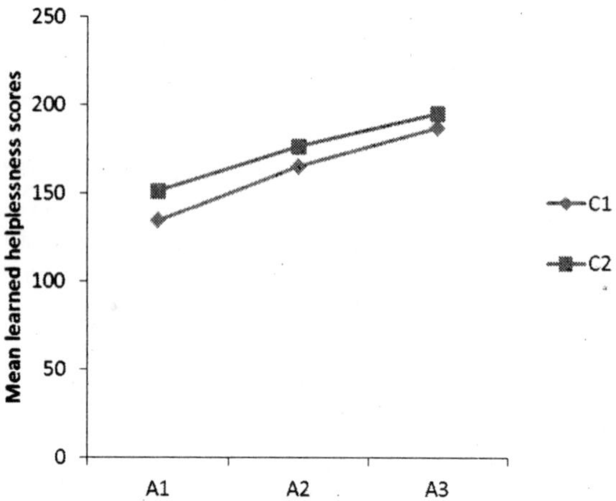

Legends

A=Chronological Age **_C=Cultural Variation_**

A1=30-35 years C1=Rural

A2=40-45 years C2=Urban

A3=50-55 years

Fig. 10.2: Mean Values showing the Impact of Chronological Age and Cultural Variation on Learned Helplessness

Above figure reveals that the discrepancy related to marital status was relatively higher in middle age group and the oldest and youngest participants were almost same. The chronological age and cultural variation interaction was significant (*F, 2,216=5.19 p<.01*). It is reported in Figure 10.2.

Figure show that this interaction was caused due to higher level of variation in learned helplessness scores at various cultural groups. Figure also manifests that highest level of discrepancy revealed at young age and with increase in age the gap narrowed down. Similarly, the chronological age, and job status interaction (*F, 2,216=8.02 p<.01*) was significant and it is reported in Figure 10.3.

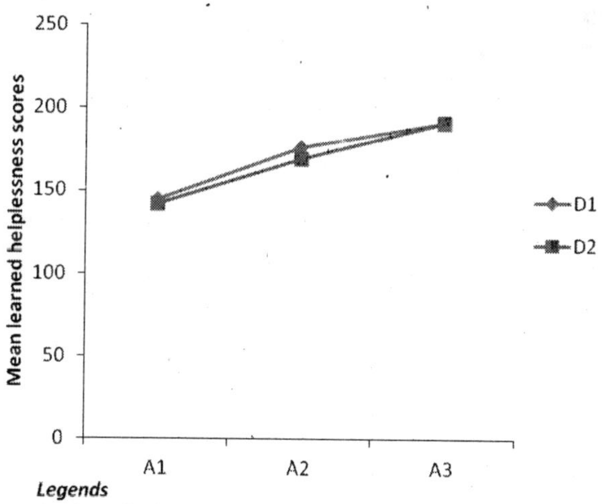

Legends

A=Chronological Age

A1=30-35 years

A2=40-45 years

A3=50-55 years

D=Job Status

D1=Employed

D2=Unemployed

Fig. 10.3: Mean Values showing the Impact of Chronological Age and Job Status on Learned Helplessness

Figure reveals a fine interaction and shows that the interaction occurred due to the discrepancy trend in middle age group youngest and oldest ones were almost equal. Marital status and cultural variation interaction was also significant (*F, 1,216=4.49 p<.05*) and it is appeared in Figure 10.4.

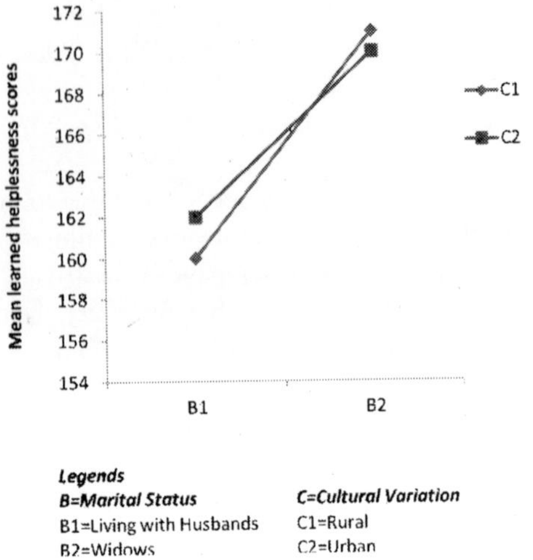

Fig. 10.4: Mean Values showing the Impact of Marital Status and Cultural Variation on Learned Helplessness

Figure reveals a good interaction. It was noted that although the trend of responses was quite similar, yet the magnitude of discrepancy was higher between the participants living with husbands. The marital status and employment status interaction was significant (*F, 1,216=5.19 p<.01*) and it is given in Figure 10.5.

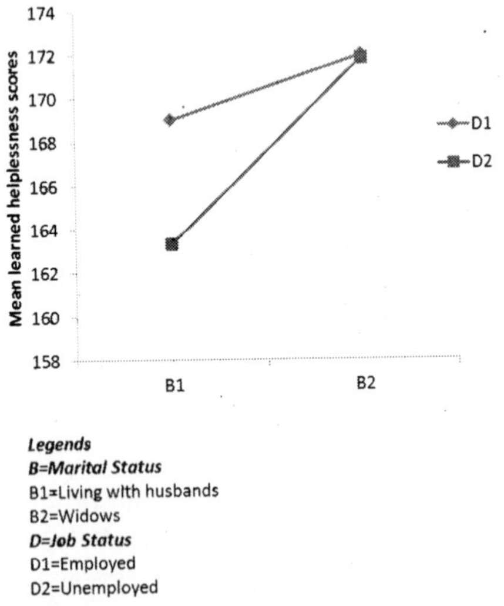

Fig. 10.5: Mean Values showing the Impact of Marital Status and Job Status on Learned Helplessness

Figure reveals a very good and notable interaction. A sharp increase in the scores was visited and it was shared by both participants i.e.; employed and unemployed women living with their husbands but the discrepancy disappeared in widows.

The cultural variation and employment status was significant (*F, 1,216=3.01 p<.05*) and it is given in Figure 10.6.

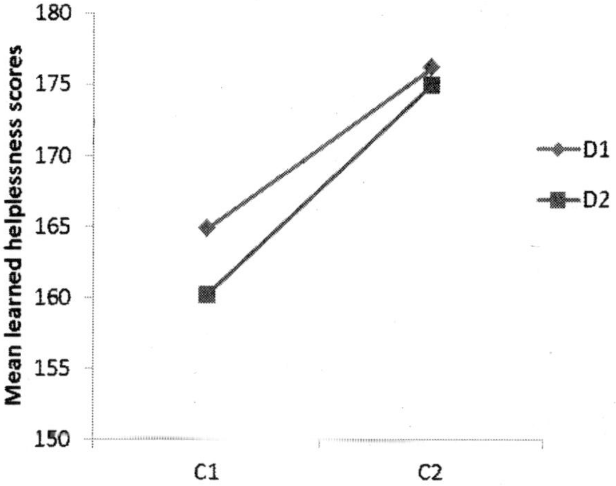

Legends
C=Cultural Variation
C1=Rural
C2=Urban
D=Job Status
D1=Employed
D2=Unemployed

Fig. 10.6: Mean Values Showing the Impact of Cultural Variation and Job Status on Learned Helplessness

Figure shows that rural employed participants were highly discriminant as compared to urban ones although the discrepancy excited. Also, the sharpness decreased in urban group.

The three way interaction of chronological age, marital status and cultural variation was significant (*F, 2,216=8.96 p<.01*) and it is given in Figure 10.7. A very beautiful and well-knitted interaction was seen and it was noticed that sharp difference between the scores was visited and the magnitude of discrepancy declined among widows of oldest age groups.

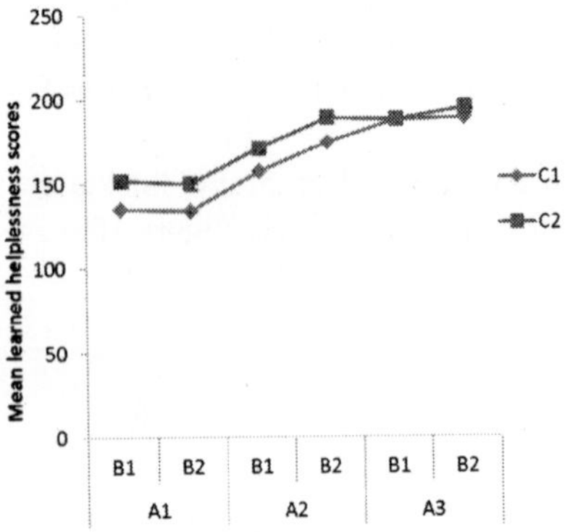

Legends
A=Chronological Age ***B=Marital Status*** ***C=Cultural Variation***
A1=30-35 years B1=Living with Husbands C1=Rural
A2=40-45 years B2=Widows C2=Urban
A3=50-55 years

Fig. 10.7: Mean Value showing the Impact of Chronological Age, Marital Status and Cultural Variation on Learned Helplessness

Figure reveals a good interaction. The chronological age, marital status and job status was also significant (*F, 2,216=8.68 p<.01*) and it is reported in Figure 10.8.

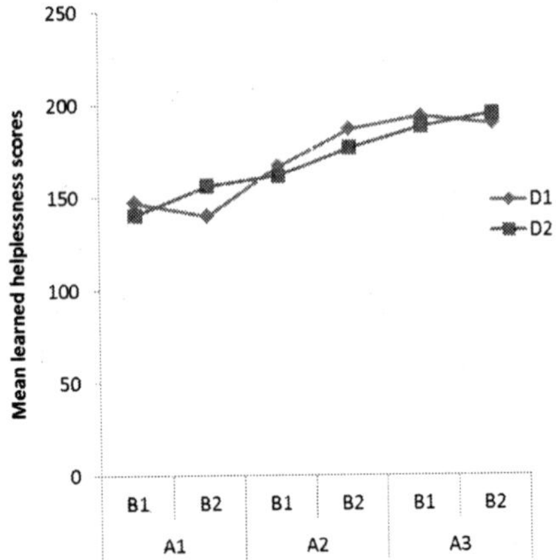

Legends
A=Chronological Age ***B=Marital Status***
A1=30-35 years B1=Living with husbands
A2=40-45 years B2=Widows
A3=50-55 years
D=Job Status
D1=Employed
D2=Unemployed

Fig. 10.8: Mean Values showing the Impact of Chronological Age, Marital Status and Job Status on Learned Helplessness

Figure tells a fine interaction. Totally diversification of scores was appeared here but the trends of responses of 30-35 years olds participants living with husbandry and 50-55 years participants living with husbands and widows were quite same. The chronological age, cultural variation and job status also significant (*F, 2,216=9.15 p<.01*) and reported in Figure 10.9.

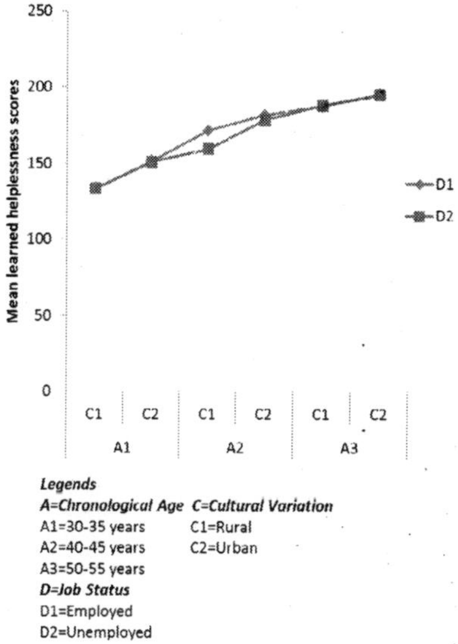

Fig. 10.9: Mean Values Showing the Impact of Chronological Age, Cultural Variation and Job Status on Learned Helplessness

Figure shows a sharp interaction in middle and rest of the place sheer similarly is visited. The marital status, cultural variation and job status interaction was also significant (F, 1,216=3.64 p<.01) and it is depicted in Figure 10.10.

It is an example of good interaction which is appeared here. The four way interaction of chronological age, marital status, cultural variation and job status was also significant (*F, 2,216=9.96 p<.01*) and it is appeared in Figure 10.11.

Figure shows that all variables laid their impact on learned helplessness.

Discussion

Obtained data were analyzed by four ways ANOVA and interpreted in terms of chronological age, marital status, cultural variation and job status

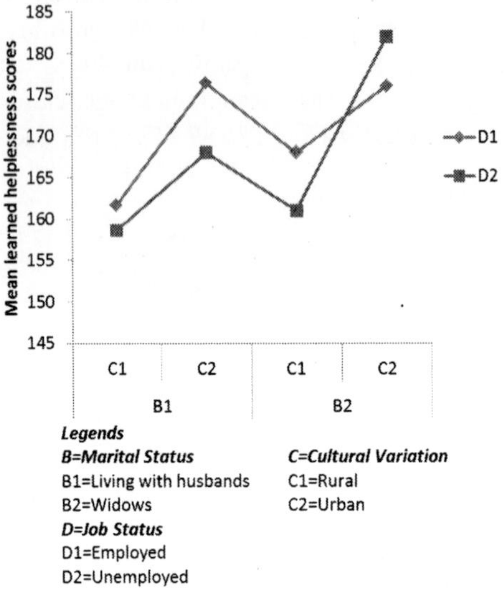

Fig. 10.10: Mean Values showing the Impact of Marital Status, Cultural Variation and Job Status on Learned Helplessness

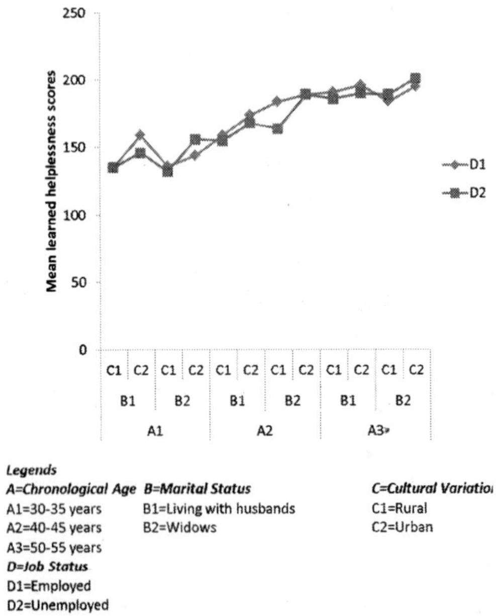

Fig. 10.11: Mean Values showing the Impact of Chronological Age, Marital Status, Cultural Variation and Job Status on Learned Helplessness

as affecters of **(*i*)** *learned helplessness* **(*ii*)** *depression and* **(*iii*)** *routine stress*. Moreover, a routine stress scale was also made. Prior to the inception of the work some hypotheses were formulated and the findings will be analyzed accordingly. There were thirteen objectives and hypotheses and they are clubbed in four consecutive hypotheses and they represented the pattern of *learned* helplessness. Findings are described below.

Our first notion was concerned with the pattern of learned helplessness in women. It was contended that women with various age, marital status, cultural variation and employment status would vary in relation to their scores on learned helplessness. When we see the results of the pattern of age-related change in women, it was found that systematic increase in the scores of learned helplessness was caused with increase in chronological age. It was resulted that the youngest participants (*aged 30-35 years*) were least in learned helplessness followed by middle aged participants (*40-45 years old*) and oldest participants (*50-55 years old*). The mean values were *142.80, 172.75* and *191.43;* respectively for youngest to oldest age and we have made a conclusion that the tendency of learned helplessness increases with increase in age. In this way we see that significant variation was seen between all age groups.

On the basis of this finding we come to know that chronological age is a significant factor and underlying determinant of learned helplessness in women. Increase in age enhances the magnitude of learned helplessness in women because as a woman grows older she finds her surrounded by many diseases that block her to do any work. Moreover, with increasing age she has to give up all her responsibilities to the younger ones like son, daughter or daughter-in-law. When they perform the work in an entire reversed way and pay less attention on her due to their job and other engagements she becomes completely helpless. Many participants stated "अब ये जैसा करें उसी में संतुष्ट रहना है हम तो बूढ़े हो गये राज तो इन्हीं का है" such words show their helplessness. One participant with tearful eyes stated "अब समझ में आ रहा है कि बागवान में अमिताभ हेमा ने क्या महसूस किया होगा". Such dialogue not only state the magnitude of learned helplessness in women but also they sketch the current scenario of Indian family system which is changing very fast. We see that with increase in age women feel a sense of mental deterioration and physical loss and many time related responsibilities like taking care of grand children or religiosity-based duties. Along with these duties she starts feeling the insane system and deficiency in her capacity. So, she leaves the attempts to do those deeds that were performed by her earlier and accepts the appearing result. This helplessness increases with advancing age. If we talk about the women of 30-35 years they are young and their psychophysical capabilities are far better than their older counterparts. In addition, they are young and they have to upbring their kids so they can be considered better than their seniors. Moreover, better and healthy psychophysical structure and awareness of rights (अधिकार बोध) reduces their helplessness. Many participants complained the less availability of time and the most important one that stroke the researcher was their complain regarding self-neglect (क्या करें सब खुद ही करना है....इतना भी टाइम नहीं मिलता कि अपने लिए कुछ सोचें) but they feel a sense of satisfaction and their self-esteem increases when they find them the *"Queen of home"* In addition, women at this age are supposed to be free and independent in nature and responsible for her work and duties. They are not dependent (*at least in domestic affairs*) but they are multitask master so there is no question to seek the amount of significant learned helpless in them.

So far as the matter of 40-45 years old participants was concerned they showed comparatively higher magnitude of learned helplessness because their dependency on others increases and this dependency increases their learned helplessness.

The magnitude of learned helplessness was found highest in the participants of 50-55 years. It was the oldest age group and it was seen that it is the age when a women find her physically weak and this weakness either occurs due to any decease or fairly due to menopause. This weaken also lays its impact on her behavioural mode. She dedicated her responsibilities on her daughter, daughter-in-law etc. and thus, her dependency over them starts and then increases day by day. On the ground of social reality, the young generation who is fit and fine in psycho-physical system in found ready to share the responsibilities. The multifaceted dependency produces a sense of dependency in them.

If we make a close perusal of the marital status of women and try to relate with their learned helplessness we noticed almost similarity in widow and the women with husbands in relation to their scores on learned helplessness. The mean values of women with husbands and widow were *166.16* and *171.92* and the main effect was insignificant. Although the difference was existed but it was very nominal so, we can say that widows are more learned helplessness as compared to women with husbands. Data analysis reveals that marital status, as an independent factor does not lay its direct impact on the magnitude of learned helplessness. Women, either single widow or with husband feels and passes through similar situations, and she possess similar tendencies so, it is quite sure that she is not influenced by marital status. Moreover, all participants were married. The difference may occur when they could be compared with unmarried.

When the data were analyzed on the ground of culture variation it was found this effect was significant and it can be stated that the magnitude of learned helplessness was influenced by cultural variation as revealed in the scores of rural and urban women. This F-ratio was significant. The mean values of rural and urban women were 162.50 and 175.58. It reveals the significant difference.

It is a well perceived fact that the climate structure of urban environment is comprised of more benevolent as compared to the rural environment. We see much experiential input that enriches the personality. The rural environment is based on patriarchal and has traditional values. The rural women are found more dependent on their husbands while in urban environment women have recognized their status and identity. In contrast, urban women found more conscious and aware about their social, economic, political and families rights and their socio-familial background is more benevolent than the rural ones. Perhaps, it has caused our findings that they felt less learned helplessness.

So far as the matter of the difference between employed and unemployed status was concerned, it was unable to yield its significant impact. It was found that the magnitude of discrepancy between employed (*X=170.00*) and unemployed women (*X=167.58*), in relation to their scores on learned helplessness was more or less equal. The hairline difference states that the unemployed women were less in learned helplessness as compared to employed women.

It is apparent from the analysis of scores that the main effect of employment status was failed to yield its impact on learned helplessness because women, in our society are found almost free from the economic liability of their families. Nowadays when women have proved them equal with men they share the financial responsibilities with their parents before marriage and with their husband after marriage. Moreover, in most middle and upper middle class society, if women are in service, male family members think to take the women's income as their insult or degradation in her eyes. She is supported to take and bear the responsibilities of home and she accepts it as the destiny. Our findings are in close consonance with Suteri (2015) and Geeta (2010) who in their studies traced the profile of learned helpless women in all walks of life.

Findings in sum several the university accepted phenomena of learned helplessness in women. Better attempts are required to understand the world and act accordingly so that the identity of women could not be spoiled and diminished in the darkness of life.

References

Abramson L.Y., Metalsky GI., and Alloy L.B. (1989). Hopelessness depression: A theory-based subtype of depression. *Psychological Review*, 96, 358-372.

Abramson, L.Y. Seligman M.E.P., and Teasdale, J. (1978). Learned helplessness in humans: critique and reformulation. *Journal of Abnormal Psychology,* 87, 49-74.

Abramson, L.Y. and Alloy L.B. (1981). Depression and the generation of complex hypotheses in the judgment of contingency. *Behaviour Research and Therapy*. 19, 35-45.

Baucom D.H. and Dankers-Brown, P. (1979). Influence of sex roles on the development of learned helplessness. *Journal of Consulting and Clinical Psychology, 47*(5) 928-936.

Berkman, L., Berkman, C., Kasi, S., *et al.* (1986). Depression symptoms in relation to physical health and functioning in the elderly. *American Journal of Epidemiology*; 124; 372-388.

Bibring, E. (1953). The mechanizing of depression. In: P. Greenare (Ed.), *Affective Disorders,* New York: International Universities Press.

Blazer, D., Hughes D. and George L. (1987). The epidemiology of depression in an elderly community population. *Gerontologist;* 27; 281-287.

Blazer D. (1989). Depression in the elderly, *N Engl J Med*; 320: 164-166.

Blazer D. Burchett B. Service, C. and George L. (1991). The association of age and depression among the elderly an epidemiologic exploration. *J Gerontol Med Sci:* 46 M210-M215.

Blazer, D. (2002). *Depression in late Life*, New York: Springer.

Dweck, C. and Llicht, B. (1980). Learned helplessness and intellectual achievement. In: J. Garber and M.E.P. Seligman *Human Helplessness*: *theory and application.* New York Academic Press.

Enns M.W., Cox B.J., Sareen J. and Freeman, P. (2001). Adaptive and maladaptive perfectionism in medical students. A longitudinal investment. *Medical Education 35*(11) 1034-1012.

Geeta (2010). Psychosocial Correlates of Learned Helplessness Among Professional and Non-Professional Students, Unpublished Ph.D. Thesis, Department of psychology, Kumaun University Campus, Almora.

Lazarus, Rechard S., Deese and Osler, S.F. (1952). The effect of psychological stress upon performance. *Psychological Bulletin,* 49: 293-317.

Lee, G.R., Demaris A., Bavin S. and Sullivian R. (2001). Gender Differences in the Depressive Effect of Widowhood in Later Life. *Journal of Gerontology: Social Science,* 56B: 556-561.

Lee, G.R. *Widowhood Encyclopedia of Aging* (2002). (Accessed on 18 March 2008). *Available at: http://www.agis.com/Document/363/windowhood.aspx*

Rozell E.J., Gunderson D.E. and Terpstra D.E. (1998). Gender differences in the factors affecting helpless behaviour and performances. *Journal of Social Behaviour and Personality, 13*(12) 265-280.

Seligman, M.E.P. (1975). *Helplessness.* Freeman, San Francisco, CA.

Seligman, M.E.P., Abramson, L.Y. Semmel, A. and Von Baeyer, C. (1979). Depressive attributional style. *Journal of Abnormal Psychology*, 88, 242-247.

Suteri, P. (2015). Social justice and learned helplessness. Paper presented in the National seminar on Justice System and Justice role for women in Society: Psychosocial impact and consequences, held at Saint Vinoba Post graduate College, Deoria, 27-28 Feb.

11

Motherhood and Mental Health

Postpartum Depression

Laxmi Vajpeyi

Introduction

Motherhood and womanhood stand in a complex and contradictory relationship with one another. Under patriarchy, mothers appear to have a mythological, mysterious and powerful status. Only women are granted this status, and it is one to which all women are expected to aspire. The reality of mothers' lives, however, often fails to match these aspirations. Motherhood is a challenge; although potentially enjoyable, it is also hard work and routinely stressful (Richardson, 1992). Becoming a mother often means economic dependence on another person or the state, and frequently reduces women's income. It affects relationships with men and other women, and changes occupational, domestic and sexual arrangements. Being a mother influences social and personal identity, and has implications for women's health (Nicolson, 1988).

Despite the prominence of motherhood as a social institution and the almost universal expectation that women will become mothers, the everyday reality of mothering is frequently invisible. For women caught up in the myths that accompany motherhood, failure to achieve that imaginary status is frequently a 'shock' (Antonis, 1981). Women who are not mothers are seen as failed and unfeminine women, and achievements and pleasures gained outside motherhood are condemned within patriarchy as substitutes for 'normal' femininity (Woollett, 1991).

Motherhood and Mental Health

WHO reports that worldwide about 10 per cent of pregnant women and 13 per cent of women who have just given birth experience a mental disorder, primarily depression. In developing countries this is even higher, i.e., 15.6 per cent during pregnancy and 19.8 per cent after child birth. In severe cases mothers' suffering might be so severe that they may even commit suicide. In addition, the affected mothers cannot function properly. As a result, the children's growth and development may be negatively affected as well. Maternal mental disorders are treatable. Effective interventions can be delivered even by well-trained non-specialist health providers.

Suicide is an important cause of death among pregnant and post-partum women. Psychosis is much less common but may also lead to suicide and in some cases even harming the newborn. Depression causes enormous suffering and disability and reduced response to child's need. Evidence indicates that treating the depression of mothers leads to improved growth and development of the newborn and reduces the likelihood of diarrhoea and malnutrition among them. Globally maternal mental health problems are considered as a major public health challenge. Though maternal mortality still lies at the heart of maternal health indicators; for the post-2015 agenda for development goals, WHO is considering Universal Health Coverage (UHC) and proposing Healthy Life Expectancy (HLE) related indicators as well. This implies stronger focus on mental health conditions in the integrated delivery of services for maternal and child health. The need is not just felt in high income countries. In fact, some academic and public health institutions in low and middle income countries have already initiated integrated maternal mental health programmes. These have been low cost interventions with the involvement of non-specialized or community health providers. Impact has been demonstrated not only on mothers but also on growth and development of children. Who is at risk of these disorders?

Virtually all women can develop mental disorders during pregnancy and in the first year after delivery, but poverty, migration, extreme stress, exposure to violence (domestic, sexual and gender-based), emergency and conflict situations, natural disasters, and low social support generally increase risks for specific disorders.

Effects of Maternal Mental Disorders after Birth on Mother and Infant

Prolonged or severe mental illness hampers the mother-infant attachment, breastfeeding and infant care. A specific kind of depression woman suffers called Postpartum Depression after deliver a baby. It affects woman's mental health as well. Postpartum period is a period which is very demanding and always specified by enormously the biological, physical, social, physical and emotional changes in the body of a woman. It is required and relevant individual and interpersonal adaptation. Pregnant women and their families have lots of aspirations and expectations from the postpartum period, which is coloured by the pleasant arrival of a new baby in the family. Woefully, a woman living in the postpartum period can be vulnerable to a range of many psychiatric disorders like postpartum blues, depression, and psychosis etc. Prenatal mental illness of a mother is not merely diagnosed and can have far-reaching aftermath for both the mother and the infant in the family. In the Early stage of screening, diagnosis, and management it is very important and must be considered as mandatory part of postpartum care of a mother.

Postpartum Disorders

Following labour, other may known as "baby blues", women may confront baby blues case that can influence their psychological well-being. The high hormonal changes and variances that happen in the body during and after labour could make mothers feel serious emotional episodes called "postnatal depression" which influences average 80 per cent of mothers. In the present case the side effects continue for in excess of two or three weeks, at that point it might be something revolutionarily serious, for example, a baby blues issue.

Identification according to Present Classification System

The current mental medical specialty has not ordered baby blues issues like a peculiar element. Specification of puerperal diseases like discrete nosological substances has been begging to be proven wrong for over 30 years. The best way of thinking see Postpartum issues as the baby blues initiation of a basic issue inside the bipolar range while others consider it absolutely as a particular medical specialty element.

Demonstrative and Statistical Manual of Mental Disorders, Fourth Edition, Text Revision (DSM-IV-TR) and the ICD-10 ranging of mental and demeanor concern: Clinical depiction and symptomatic rules, have cluster baby blues mental cases in an unforeseen course of action. DSM-IV-TR authorize Psychotherapist to utilize the "with baby blues beginning" specified to short and crazy case or to a present or latest significant and relevant burdensome, hyper, or blended scene in with maniacal high point in noteworthy burdensome topic or Bipolar Disorder, if starting happened inside about a month baby blues. In the ICD-10, decayed behaviours related with puerperium are converted by the introducing mental confusion; a consequent code (e.g., 099.3) indicates relationship with the puerperium. Now and again, the ICD-10 takes into consideration an exceptional code, F53 when there is inadequate data for labeling, or there are "remarkable extra highlights." F53 must be utilized if the turmoil happens inside about a month and a half of conveyance. DSM-V has supplanted the specified "with baby blues beginning" for burdensome and bipolar issues with the specified "with peripartum starting." The "with peripartum beginning" decides is utilized if the starting of mind-set side effects happens during pregnancy of women or inside the month following conveyance. Be that as it may, baby blues mental issues may show a long time past the first month or a month and a half after conveyance. Subsequently, the usefulness of DSM-V suggests and the ICD-10 remarkable code in the positioning of puerperal issues is constrained.

Clinical Features of Postpartum Disorders

Earlier postpartum disorders were classified as: (i) Postpartum blues (PBs), (ii) Postpartum depression (iii) Postpartum psychosis. This was an oversimplification. However, in addition to these, there are miscellaneous groups of anxiety and stress-related disorders occurring in the puerperium.

In contemporary times, postpartum disorders have been restricted into five considerable categories: (i) Postpartum Blues (PBs), (ii) Postpartum depression (PPD), (iii) Postpartum psychosis, (iv) postpartum post-traumatic stress disorder (PTSD), and (v) postpartum anxiety and obsessive compulsive disorder (OCD).

The characteristics of each postpartum disorder are described below.

Postpartum Blues

Postpartum blue is mainly known as "baby blues" or "maternity blues." It is a period of time of emotional responsibility in order to birth of a child, and its also characterized by very frequent crying episodes of infant, irritability of a mother, confusion, and anxiety of a mother. However, elation might also be perceived during the first few days of the following childbirth.

"Baby blues" are very common and experienced by most of the women to some extent. However, PB is more commonly seen in western countries because of the lack of strong familial support and bonding.

It is observed to be as high as 40–85 per cent. The symptoms make an appearance within the first ten days of child birth and the peak around of three to five days. Generally symptoms of Postpartum blues do not stand in the way of the social and occupational functioning of a mother. Postpartum blue is self-limiting and there is no requirement for agile intervention except social and family support and consolation from other family members also. Postpartum can be attributed to changes in hormonal levels of women, further compounded by the stress following delivery. However, PBs persisting for more than 2 weeks may make women vulnerable to a more severe form of mood disorders.

Postpartum Psychosis (PP)

Postpartum psychosis has an acute and abrupt onset, typically located inside the first two weeks following shipping or, at most, inside three months postpartum, and must be viewed as a psychiatric and obstetrical emergency. The presence of a psychotic sickness influences the prenatal and postpartum care adversely. Past records of psychosis with preceding pregnancies, records of bipolar disorder, household records of psychotic sickness (e.g., schizophrenia or bipolar disorder) are some of the important danger elements for the improvement of Postpartum psychosis.

Most typically signs and symptoms encompass elation, legal responsibility of mood, rambling speech, disorganized behaviour, and hallucinations or delusions. However, presentation and direction of PP may also be greater various and complex, with transient or alternating episodes of delusions of guilt, persecution, auditory hallucinations; delirium-like signs and confusion; and immoderate activity. At times, delusions revolve round the infant especially that the child is possessed, has exceptional powers, is divine, or is dead. Infanticide and suicide are located in 4 per cent and 5 per cent of the girls struggling from PP respectively. Enquiring about suicidal and infanticide ideas is indispensable at some stage in the evaluation of female struggling from Postpartum psychosis.

Postpartum Posttraumatic Stress Disorder (PTSD)

Bydlowski and Raoul-Duval (1978) did breakthrough work on postpartum PTSD is widely acknowledged. Many researchers have proven the incidence of postpartum PTSD to be round 5.6 per cent. It is typically characterized via tension, nightmares, flashbacks and autonomic hyper arousal that can proceed for some weeks or months, and may additionally recur towards the stop of the subsequent pregnancy. This can additionally end result in secondary tocophobia.

Anxiety Disorders Specific to the Puerperium

Many researchers have determined that postpartum anxiousness issues are under-diagnosed and are in truth extra-frequent than PPD. De Armond (1954) determined that concern of cot demise can attain up to a stage of pathological degree. The most frequent function is nocturnal vigilance specified by means of the mom mendacity wide awake listening to the infant's breathing, and normal checking ensuing in sleep deprivation. Many moms are excessively involved and preoccupied about the fitness and protection of their kids which is recognized as "maternity neurosis."

Obsessions of Child Harm

Women recognized with postpartum onset of main melancholy may additionally have repetitive, intrusive ideas associated to some happening to the child related with compulsive checking behaviour. Postpartum onset of OCD can show up for the duration of gestation or inside 6 weeks following delivery. The theme of the obsessions is regularly associated to thoughts/gruesome photographs of harming the baby.

Postpartum Depression (PPD)

Postpartum Depression is one of the most frequent psychiatric ailment discovered in the postpartum period. Postpartum despair is commonly hard to distinguish from despair going on at any different time in a mother's life. However, in Postpartum depression, the poor ideas are commonly associated to the newborn child. It is viewed in 10–15 per cent of postpartum females and, in addition to postpartum time specifies, the diagnostic standards is hard to differentiate from that of main depressive episode characterized by using pervasive depressed mood, disturbances of sleep and appetite, low energy, anxiety, and suicidal ideation. Additionally we can say that emotions of guilt or inadequacy about the new mother's capacity to care for the new born child, and a preoccupation with the child's overall well-being or protection are extreme ample to be regarded as obsession.

Arch (2003) observed that higher incidence of anxiety symptoms is observed in PPD than in non-PPD. Onset can range from few days to few weeks following delivery, generally in the first 2–3 months following childbirth. History of major depression increases the risk for PPD by 25 per cent, and past history of PPD increases the risk of recurrence to 50 per cent.

Many females experience a wide range of overwhelming emotions such as anticipation, excitement, happiness, fulfillment, as well as anxiety, frustration, confusion, or sadness/guilt during pregnancy and postpartum period. The postpartum period makes them highly vulnerable to various psychiatric disorders. Postpartum phenomenology is characterized by a range of emotions from transient mood liability, irritability, and weepiness, to marked agitation, delusions, confusion, and delirium.

Prenatal mental illness is largely under-diagnosed, and under-treated. Untreated postpartum psychiatric disorders can have far-reaching ramifications for a family. At times, the postpartum psychiatric condition can become so severe that it warrants hospitalization. Moreover, postpartum psychiatric disorders can adversely affect mother-infant interaction and attachment. Hence, early diagnosis and management of the postpartum psychiatric disorder is extremely crucial.

Postpartum depression is a type of mood disorder that can affect the mother after birth of a child. Mothers with postpartum depression may experience various feelings of extreme sadness, anxiety, and exhaustion and these feelings can make it difficult for mothers to complete daily care activities for themselves or for other members of the family. Postpartum depression (PPD) is a major form of depression and is less common than postpartum blues. PPD includes all the symptoms of depression but occurs only following childbirth. It can begin any time after delivery and can last up to a year. PPD is estimated to occur in approximately 10 to 20 per cent of new mothers.

How is Postpartum Depression Different from the "Baby Blues"?

"Postnatal depression" is a term widely used to depict the sentiments of stress, despondency, and weariness that numerous ladies experience in the wake of having a child. Children require a ton of care, so it is a typical for mothers to be stressed over, or tired from, giving that care. Postnatal depression, which influences up to 80 per cent of mothers, incorporates sentiments that are to some degree mellow, most recent up to 14 days, and disappear all alone. Mother's mood swings are the result of high hormonal fluctuations that occur during and immediately after childbirth. The onset of postpartum blues usually occurs three to five days after delivery, and should subside as hormone levels begin to stabilize. Symptoms generally do not last for more than a few weeks, and this condition is not considered a mental health disorder, however if a person continues to experience moods swings or feelings of depression for more than two weeks after childbirth, the problem may be more serious. With post-birth anxiety, sentiments of bitterness and tension can be outrageous and might meddle with a lady's capacity to think about herself or her family. In the light of seriousness of the indications, post-birth anxiety of mother as a rule requires treatment. The situation, which happens in almost 15 per cent of child births, may start in the blink of an eye previously or whenever after labour, yet regularly starts between a week and a month after conveyance.

What are the Factors that Contribute to PPD?

Postpartum depression does not have a single reason, but many similar results from a relevant combination of physical and emotional factors of a woman. Postpartum depression does not occur due to something that a mother does or does not do. After the birth of a child, the levels of hormones (estrogen and progesterone) in a mother's body rapidly drop. The causes of PPD are not quite clear but research suggests that the following factors may contribute to the onset of PPD:

- **Hormonal changes:** A woman experiences the greatest hormonal fluctuation levels after giving birth. Intense hormone fluctuations, such as decreased serotonin levels, occur after delivery and may play a role in the development of PPD.
- **Situational risks:** Childbirth itself is a major life change and transition, and big changes can cause a great deal of stress and result in depression. If a major event coincides with childbirth, a mother may be more susceptible than average to PPD.
- **Life stresses:** Ongoing stressful circumstances can compound the pressures of having a new baby and may trigger PPD. For example, excessive stress at the office added to the responsibilities of being a mother can cause emotional strain that could lead to PPD. The nature of the mother's relationship with the baby's father and any unresolved feelings about the pregnancy might also affect a mother's risk of getting PPD.

Do Mothers are more Credible to Occurrence Postpartum Depression?

Mothers are at more threat for growing postpartum despair because they need one or more danger elements, along with: signs of depression in the course of or after a previous pregnancy. Preceding revel in with despair or manic despair at once more in her existence. A loved one who has been diagnosed with depression or different mental disorder. A stressful lifestyles event during pregnancy or shortly after parturition, like job loss, death of a loved, violence, or non-public contamination. Scientific headaches all through childbirth, consisting of untimely transport or having a baby with clinical issues. The various emotions are related to the pregnancy of a woman, whether or not it had been deliberate or unplanned. As some examples like lack of robust emotional manual from her husband, partner, family, or friends, alcohol or other substance abuse troubles etc. Postpartum melancholy can have an effect on any female regardless of age, race, ethnicity, or financial status.

Diagnosis of Postpartum Depression

Postpartum melancholy has mostly been under-diagnosed, reiterating the truth that activities screening in the course of postpartum medical institution visits must structure a vital section of the assessment. Many time the use of a population-specific screening device such as the "Edinburgh Postnatal Depression Scale," and the "Mood Disorder Questionnaire", can enhance attention of healthcare companies and resource in the early prognosis of postpartum psychiatric disorders. Various studies using screening approaches have pronounced widespread will increase in prices of detection of postpartum psychiatric disorders. Laboratory investigations and thorough bodily examination ought to be performed to cut out natural etiology. Sometimes uncommon scientific conditions, such as front temporal dementia or frontal lobe tuberculoma, and Sheehan syndrome can mimic postpartum psychiatric disorders.

Remedy of Postpartum Psychiatric Depression

The therapy of PPDs is normally holistic and consists of reassurance, familial and social support, psycho-education, and in some cases, psychotherapy and/or pharmacologic treatment.

Pharmacology Therapy

In average to extreme despair and Postpartum, medicinal drug turns into necessary. Most psychotropic capsules are metabolized in the liver. During the first few weeks of a full-term infant's lifestyles potential for hepatic drug metabolism, is about one-third to one-fifth of the grownup capacity. The capability will increase step by step and by way of about three months it reaches to the degree of adult's capacity. In untimely kiddies or children with signs and symptoms of compromised hepatic metabolism breastfeeding need to be deferred if the mother is on psychotropic medication. Peak concentrations in breast milk are attained 6–8 hours after ingestion of medication. Therefore, breastfeeding can be restrained to instances when the breast milk drug attention is lowest, that is, simply earlier than or after taking medication.

Breastfeeding

Women with Postpartum depression have to be counseled towards breastfeeding their infants. Both breast feeding and nocturnal child care are essential motives of sleep loss, which in flip can lead to similarly temper instability mainly in girls with bipolar disorder. Additionally, owing to psychotic kingdom many girls are incapable of breastfeeding. However, for suppression of lactation, dopamine agonists need to be used cautiously as these capsules may additionally end result in psychosis in prone women. Women who select to breastfeed after enhancement have to be knowledgeable about the truth that all psychotropic pills are excreted in breast milk at various concentrations. The selection to breastfeed whilst taking medicinal drug needs to be made after cautious weighing the dangers and advantages to the mom as nicely as the infant.

Non Pharmacological Treatment

Individual psychotherapy is a vital section of treatment, in particular for females discovering it tough adjusting to motherhood and/or apprehensions about new responsibilities. Psycho-education and emotional assist for the accomplice and different household participants are important. Patient and the household participants ought to be concerned in the components of the remedy plan. Respite care offerings need to be encouraged in particular at night time to limit the patient's sleep disruption. In some cases, interpersonal remedy (IPT) would possibly be beneficial. IPT is proven to end result in increased discount in depressive signs and enhancement in social adjustment. In instances of PP, separation from the baby may be necessary. Reassurance and emotional aid towards the mom can improve the shallowness and self-assurance of the mother. Peer aid and psycho education about PP are essential interventions. Sometimes, crew psychotherapy may additionally be helpful.

Psychological Treatment of Postpartum Depression

There are some effectual remedies for the postpartum depression. A mother's health care provider can help her to choose the best psychological treatment, which may include:

Counseling/Talk Therapy: This therapy includes speaking one-on-one with an intellectual fitness expert (a counselor, therapist, psychologist, psychiatrist, or social worker). Here some sorts of counseling proven to be specifically advantageous in treating postpartum depression are:

Cognitive behavioural therapy (CBT): This therapy helps people to recognize and change their negative thoughts and behaviours; a person can modify his/her behaviour with the help of this type of therapy. CBT targets to assist the person to exchange the way they suppose (cognitive) and what they do (behaviour). Rather than searching at previous causes, it focuses on modern troubles and realistic options to assist the experience higher now. The way we assume about conditions influences the way we experience and behave. If we view a scenario negatively, we might also trip poor thoughts and emotions which lead us to behave in an unhelpful way. The therapist will assist the mother to become aware of and venture any poor questioning so she can deal with conditions higher and behave in a greater superb way. CBT is very useful technique for depression but this therapy can be also useful for anxiety, stress, phobias, obsessions, consuming problems and managing lengthy time period conditions. CBT is exceptional recognized for its efficacy in treating anxiousness such as OCD. CBT works with the appreciation that the way we assume influences the way that we feel, and so remedy is centred on supporting mom to have manipulate over her ideas so that she feels extra capable to trade them. A CBT therapist will work with a mother to perceive and renowned her automated thoughts, consider these ideas and end up conscious of when these ideas are now not helpful, discover and trade underlying beliefs, differentiate between practical and false threats, and advance new and extra-beneficial perspectives. CBT helps a mom to enhance coping techniques so that she feels higher outfitted to manipulate distress. CBT makes use of equipment such as homework, relaxation, publicity therapy, thinking stopping, intellectual imagery, and equipment for altering catastrophic ideas and irrational thinking. Mindfulness-Based Cognitive Therapy (MBCT) is a shape of CBT that additionally contains tremendous thing of mindfulness meditation.

- **Interpersonal therapy (IPT)**: This type of therapy helps people to understand and work through problematic personal relationships. Interpersonal remedy (IPT) is a structured, time-limited strategy centred on relationships. It can be beneficial for customers with melancholy and temper disorders, mainly round bereavement, battle and lifestyles changes. The IPT therapist will assist to perceive any patterns or issues in the relationships with different humans so it can work out techniques for coping with these. IPT is based on the premise that Postpartum depression is mainly rooted in four problem areas:

1. *Grief*: Acknowledging the losses that appear to experience of self, adjustments in relationships, or extra unique loss.
2. *Role Transitions*: Life stage transitions and social transitions which includes loss of independence and altering social networks.
3. *Interpersonal Disputes*: Oncs that regularly manifest after the start of a baby consisting of unmet expectations and intimacy struggles inside partnerships.
4. *Interpersonal Deficits*: Looking at struggles with attachment in different relationships that may additionally be inflicting distress.

- **Integrative Counseling:** Integrative counseling appears at the entire person, taking into account the mental, bodily and emotional needs. The therapist will use strategies and equipment from distinctive modalities to tailor a person method for client. An integrative counsellor target to build a trusting and non-judgmental relationship that helps to improve self-awareness. When a person apprehend the reasons of issues or triggers for the behaviour, can confidently set desires and boost new behaviours to enhance the delight with life.
- **Relationship Counseling:** This kind of counseling targets to assist human beings realizes and control variations and bad patterns inside their relationships. The therapist will discover the emotions and the communication process. The intention is to assist and discover methods to exchange and adapt for a greater superb future.
- **Dialectical Behavioural Therapy (DBT):** It is started out as a therapy for Borderline Personality Disorder, however is now

acknowledged to be tremendous in many situations the place misery is prominent. Like CBT, DBT makes use of exercise and homework as a section of its process. DBT teaches abilities in the following categories: mindfulness, misery tolerance, emotional regulation, and interpersonal effectiveness. DBT is regularly supported via each crew and man or woman remedy and follows a unique tenet for instructing capabilities to limit signs associated to distress.

- **Psychodynamic psychotherapy:** Psychodynamic psychotherapy is one of the earliest kinds of psychotherapy and focuses on unconscious and previous experiences in grasp present day behaviour. Psychodynamic psychotherapists trust that our earliest childhood experiences have a direct effect on our existing distress, and that when mothers are in a position to pick out and take delivery of these experiences as taking part in a position they are capable to start the manner of restoration and turning into much less entangled in the past. This kind of remedy appears into early experiences that play a position in forming beliefs about ourselves as adults, and identifies these beliefs that are no longer helpful. When working with a psychodynamic psychotherapist, a mother will be influenced to speak about relationships with dad and mom and different considerable humans in an effort to discover the unconscious content material of a mom's way of thinking. This technique reduces anxiety and distress. A psychodynamic strategy to cure is notion to be necessary due to the fact trade requires focus and appreciation to occur. Often in this kind of therapy, the "aha" moments permit for self-validation, empathy, and, ideally, freedom from self-judgment.
- **Eye Movement Desensitization and Reprocessing (EMDR):** EMDR is presently concept to be one of the nicest sorts of remedy when working through a hectic trip and is being used greater in the therapy of postpartum PTSD. This specialized kind of remedy requires precise education and credentialing. EMDR makes use of factors of each CBT and Psychodynamic remedy alongside with particular methods that are used to minimize the sensory affect of nerve-racking memories. Because worrying recollections are regularly saved in EITHER the proper (feeling-based and emotional) OR left (logical and intellectual) facet of the brain, EMDR makes use of a bilateral stimulation of the Genius (though eye movements, bilateral sound, or bilateral tactile stimulation) blended with beliefs, visualization, and interest to physique cognizance as a way to re-process reminiscences greater effectively. A considerable piece of EMDR includes supporting mother to get admission to ideas and emotions that are positive, grounding, and healing.

• **Solution-Focused Brief Psychotherapy:** Solution-Focused Brief Psychotherapy focuses on a particular trouble and works towards fantastic change. Unlike different healing procedures that perceive early experiences as taking part in a position in contemporary distress, solution-focused remedy stays away from previous issues and highlights, and instead, on a mom's strengths and skills. Much of this kind of remedy is about putting dreams and is solution-based alternatively than trouble solving. This very temporary remedy regularly requires various periods to be beneficial, alternatively many different kinds of clinicians might also experience that this kind of remedy does now not tackle the root reason of troubles correctly sufficient to create lasting change.

• **Group Therapy:** Group remedy makes use of the position of neighbourhood in support. A genuine crew remedy session is facilitated through one or greater educated psychotherapists and makes use of the dynamics that take place between individuals of the crew to assist discover trouble areas and interpersonal distress. A postpartum melancholy guide team regularly combines psycho-education (teaching about maternal intellectual illnesses, causes, therapy options, existence techniques for wellness, regular new mother stresses, etc.) with the essential function of validation from others in the group. The aim of a PPD guide crew is to assist construct community, supply house for a mother to be heard with the aid of others and to examine that she is no longer on my own in her struggles, and to speak about and share thoughts concerning stress management, coping, and early mothering.

• **Couples Therapy:** Couples Therapy gives a house for companions to be heard in the course of a time of crises. In a couples remedy setting, recurrent poor patterns inside the relationship will be addressed and couples will study conversation and listening techniques vital in working via these challenges. Often in postpartum work, couples remedy will tackle problems associated to PMADs, altering dynamics in a relationship, intimacy challenges, man or woman wishes that may additionally be interfering in connection, and person wishes that are vital in preserving the fitness of a couple relationship. When interviewing new therapists, it is actually splendid to ask him/her what type of remedy he/she practices. However in most instances you will locate that therapists use portions of many extraordinary sorts of remedy in their work. A therapist who has a precise education and therapeutic history might also permit for different sorts of remedy in his/her work when working with a mother struggling with a PMAD. Specialists in the remedy of PMADs will be pushed through what is recognized about vital factors in PMAD remedy (biological causes, symptom reduction, existence exchange management, expectation, infant-attachment support, etc.) and will both include therapeutic strategy into this work and wait to commence that section of cure till a mother's preliminary misery is managed. These treatment methods can be used alone or together.

Postpartum Depression and Marital Satisfaction

The relationship between childbirth and is often connected. Many earlier studies do indicate that in the postnatal period, mother and child are more vulnerable to mental and psychological dilemmas. Particularly we find in women baby blues and post-natal depression which hampers her handling of infant properly and as per cultural and social demands. Our problem of the research therefore focuses around the questions that whether life and marital satisfaction are related negatively to post-natal depression or not, and whether post-natal depression is more intensive in mothers of nuclear than joint family systems in Pakistani culture or it is of similar intensity. The Diagnostic and Statistical Manual of Mental Disorders (DSM-IV-TR, American Psychiatric Association, 2000) categorize this postnatal depression under Postpartum onset specifier and specify it as postpartum major depressive episodes if its onset occurs within the first four weeks of child birth. Investigators believe that these rapid changes in hormones may lead to depression. Priest (1983) considers postnatal depression as a common reaction, from which women may quickly recover. It appears from various researches that if empathy and support is provided to women during the postnatal period than their depression can become less and manageable. In spite of innumerable researches the only one contributing factor in the development of postpartum depression (PPD) is not yet clear. It is believed that various/few factors together may add to hormonal changes in the postnatal period of women resulting in depression. As cited in Mason, Risk factors, such as a lack of social support, marital discord, a history of depression, and socioeconomic hardship, are reported as contributing to PPD (Beck, 1996, 1998; Unterman *et al.*, 1990; Wood, Thomas, Droppleman, & Meagan), Life satisfaction is one of the significant factors influencing psychological wellbeing in the postnatal period and is usually connected with family and social support, financial position, marital satisfaction, family setup etc. The work of Aquino, Russell, Cutrona, and Altmaier (1996), shows that life satisfaction is significantly related to social support. Hence we can expect that if a woman finds social support during postnatal period then she can experience satisfaction with her life and may not feel depression with high intensity resulting from hormonal changes. Apart from life satisfaction another important variable is of marital satisfaction or marital quality and adjustment with attitude, love and attention during pregnancy and after delivery; verbal and nonverbal supporting communication reduces her dilemmas. Hara *et al.,* (1984), believe that uncomfortable relationship with husband and parents makes women susceptible for post-partum depression. In Pakistan if it is joint family then in post- and prenatal period women gets support from majority of family members, whereas in nuclear family there are few people to support each other. Mumford, Saeed, Ahmad, Latif and Mubbashar (1997) found remarkable relationship between depression and females residing in nuclear families. Similar findings can be seen in the work of Husain, Creed, and Tomenson (2000). Reference to depression in women after delivery Ahmad and Munaf (2006) concluded from their study that in their postnatal period women in nuclear family are more vulnerable to baby blues than those residing in joint families. Rahman, Iqbal, Harrington (2003) study on women living in southern Kahuta, Pakistan, found that 25 per cent and 28 per cent women experienced depression in their antenatal and post-natal period respectively. Hence it appears from the literature that together with hormonal changes other social factors do play important role in making women depress during their postnatal period. Thus, the purpose of research was to study the relationship of post-natal depression of women with their life and marital satisfaction. This study further investigated the difference in post-natal depression of women residing in two different family systems in city of Karachi, Pakistan.

Postpartum Depression and Social Support

However, depression could be linked to many other factors such as psychological, social, and financial, lifestyle stressors, or weight changes. These factors are beyond the scope of studies conducted earlier, and thus the findings could be related to such contributing factors. In addition, there may have been a communal allure bias at work, meaning that under pressure from their conventional culture, postpartum mother might have never reported depression in study. The family members might contradict the fact that women with newborn child can literally become depressed, especially given the fact they acknowledge the birth of a child as a social occasion. The members of family and friends may be the first to recognize symptoms of postpartum depression in a new mother. They can inspire her to talk with a health care provider, offer emotional and social support, and help with routine piece of work such as caring for the baby or the house. The reliance of postpartum mother can be nitrify by advising her husband and family members to provide her support throughout this experience. Health care providers should advise the mother prior to delivery to seek help postpartum whether from a family member, a friend, a health provider, or even religious scholars. The formation of postpartum social clubs under the kinship of health care institutions provides a great opportunity to counterbalance depression.

Mothers across all racial/ethnic groups identified fulfilling basic personal care needs, household chores, and getting sleep as the major challenges during the postpartum period. They discussed additional challenges with caring for other children and work-related stress. Researchers said that mothers mentioned physical symptoms such as post-delivery c-section pain or breastfeeding discomfort as obstacles to their postpartum recovery. Personal care needs such as bathing, eating, and sleeping were the most common needs mentioned and mothers also placed cleaning and cooking in the same category of importance. Fulfilling these basic needs was essential for women to feel they were more capable of dealing with the physical and emotional stressors inherent to the postpartum period. Lack of the instrumental support to help with these basic needs can be seen as the cause for depressive symptoms. Friends and other family members including fathers, godmothers and sisters-in-laws were also played a vital role to provide their support during the period of pregnancy. Today women speak about emotional support as being able to talk to someone about what they were going through, receiving words of encouragement, and pampering. Partners are identified as the primary resource for emotional support, but some women also sought cousins, godmothers, and other mothers from mother support groups to talk about their feelings and experiences.

Instrumental support postpartum is an important factor in the emotional and physical wellbeing of mothers and their newborns. The study (Rennie Negron *et al.,* Matern Child Health, May, 2013) gathered information on the techniques used to mobilize support and the barriers that hinder the mobilization of the support for a diverse sample of mothers. The results suggest that helping women identify their own needs and expectations surrounding support could impact their ability to mobilize support. Further, interventions aimed at strengthening mothers' ability to rally social support may not only reduce early postpartum depressive symptoms but may enhance a mother's postpartum recovery. The findings also highlighted the importance of continued examination of social support in the postpartum period and the differences and similarities existing among women from different racial/ethnic backgrounds.

Postpartum Depression and Well-being

Several researches demonstrated that postpartum depression (PPD) is a common problem. In a study, Kheirabadi and Maracy (2010) found that the rate of PPD during six to eight weeks after delivery was 20.1 per cent. In a review of studies from different countries Halbreich and Karkun (2006) established that incidence of postnatal depression has been reported between 0 per cent to nearly 60 per cent. The beginning of postpartum depression may be at the fourth week postpartum, although it is usually detected between sixth and twelfth weeks postpartum. The general symptoms of these women include depressed mood, weakness, disappointment, agitation, psychological distress, and sleep disorders. Number of changes is made during pregnancy and postpartum including organic, emotional, and societal alteration. Adjusting to these alterations may cause emotional problems in women after birth. The main predisposing factors for depression after delivery are history of mental disorders, depression during pregnancy, socio-economic insufficiency, and existence of other medical conditions. In addition, physical health problems after delivery are frequent and nearly 70 per cent of the mothers experience at least one problem in physical well-being due to birth. These problems are related to functional restrictions. Quality of life (QOL) after delivery is related to maternal social and demographic characteristics, birth factors, type of delivery, and social support. Postnatal depression has serious impact on mothers that manifests as lower quality of life and inability to care of themselves, their partner, and infants; moreover, occurrence of depression in these women is higher later in life. In a research, results showed there were significant correlation between postnatal depression and wellbeing condition. In another study, occurrence of the PPD was 15 per cent and mothers with PPD had lower quality of life scores based on World Health Organization Quality of Life-Bref (WHOQOL-BREF) scale. Other researchers indicated that all domains of SF-36 QOL scale were lower significantly in mothers with PPD compared to mother without PPD; however, worse physical health condition was not related to intensity of depression. A study was performed by Barbosa *et al.* in Portuguese revealed that some of SF-36 sub-scales are impaired in women with PPD. Boyce *et al.* found inverse correlation between PPD and five out of eight domains of SF-36 scale. Although undesirable effects of PPD are well-known, the influence of postnatal depression on quality of life or health status of mothers after birth has not been understood and few researches are done concerning this important issue.

Concluding Remarks

India is experiencing a consistent decline in maternal mortality, which skill that the centre of attention of care in the future will shift in the direction of decreasing maternal morbidity, such as intellectual fitness disorders. Despite the developing range of empirical research on postpartum melancholy in India, there is a lack of sturdy systematic proof that appears now not solely at the common burden of postpartum depression, however additionally its related danger factors. Despite the launch of India's countrywide intellectual fitness application in 1982, maternal intellectual fitness is nonetheless now not a outstanding factor of the programme. Dedicated maternal intellectual fitness offerings are generally poor in health-care facilities, and fitness people lack intellectual fitness training. The availability of intellectual fitness professionals is confined or non-existent in peripheral health-care facilities. Furthermore, there is presently no screening device specified for use in scientific exercise and no facts are mechanically accrued on the percentage of perinatal female with postpartum depression. Although facility-based deliveries are growing in many low-and middle-income countries, a excessive share of pregnant moms nonetheless supply at home. Beyond the lack of consciousness of postpartum despair via fitness professionals, there are troubles that may also be boundaries to instant consciousness and administration of the illness. In India, girls who supply at a fitness facility regularly remain for much less than forty eight hours after delivery. This leaves little possibility for fitness personnel to suggestions the mom and household individuals on the signs and symptoms and signs and symptoms of postpartum despair and when to are seeking for care. In low-and middle-income countries, the share of girls who go to the fitness facility for postpartum visits is typically low and subsequently intellectual problems regularly stay undetected and unmanaged, mainly for these handing over at home. Analysis of demographic and fitness survey statistics from seventy five countdown international locations confirmed that postnatal care visits for moms have low insurance among interventions on the continuum of maternal and infant care Postnatal traditions, such as the length of seclusion at domestic located in many cultures, can negatively have an effect on care-seeking conduct in the postpartum period. Furthermore, moms may also be reluctant to admit their struggling both due to the fact of social taboos related with despair or issues about being labeled as a mom who failed to supply the duties of toddler care. In the cutting-edge public health machine in most low- and middle-income countries, inclusive of India, primary-care people are supposed to be in normal contact with these days delivered mothers. However, at postnatal visits neighbourhood fitness people have a tendency to focal point on advertising integral toddler care practices, with decrease precedence given to the mother's health. These elements may additionally want to explain, to some extent, the lack of availability of reliable, movement's statistics on the burden of postpartum melancholy in low- and middle-income countries. There is a lack of research on prenatal intellectual fitness troubles from low- and middle-income nations and this hole in the proof hinders the procedure of organizing interventions to promote maternal psychosocial health. Gathering facts on prenatal intellectual fitness troubles will be fundamental in these countries, no longer solely to gauge the magnitude of the problem, however additionally to inform policy-makers. Such proof can stimulate governments to allocate assets for capacity-building in maternal intellectual fitness care, such as creating and enforcing tips and protocols for screening and treatment, and placing aims for decreasing the burden of postpartum despair on the Mother.

References

Baron, E.C., Hanlon, C., Mall, S., Honikman, S., Breuer, E., Kathree, T., *et al.* (2016). Maternal mental health in primary care in five low- and middle-income countries: A situational analysis. *BMC Health Service Research, 16*(1), 53.

Cheng, C.Y., and Pickler, R.H. (2009). Effects of stress and social support on postpartum health of Chinese mothers in the United States. *Research Nursing Health, 32*(6), 582–591.

Cutrona, C.E., and Troutman, B.R. (1986). Social support, infant temperament, and parenting self-efficacy: A meditational model of postpartum depression. *Child Development, 57*(6), 1507–1518.

Dennis, C.L., and Ross, L.E. (2006). Depressive symptomatology in the immediate postnatal period: Identifying maternal characteristics related to true- and false-positive screening scores. *Canadian Journal of Psychiatry, 51*(5), 265–73.

Dennis, C.L., and Stewart, D.E. (2004). Treatment of postpartum depression, part 1: A critical review of biological interventions. *Journal of Clinical Psychiatry, 65*(9), 1242–51.

Di Florio, A., Smith, S., and Jones, I. (2013). Postpartum psychosis. *The Obstetrician and Gynecologist, 15*(3), 145–50.

Field, T. (2010). Postpartum depression effects on early interactions, parenting, and safety practices: A review. *Infant Behaviour Development, 33*(1), 1–6.

Fisher, J., Cabral de Mello, M., Patel, V., Rahman, A., Tran, T., and Holton, S., *et al.* (2012). Prevalence and determinants of common prenatal mental disorders in women in low-and lower-middle-income countries: A systematic review. *Bull. World Health Organization, 90*(2), 139–49G.

Gjerdingen, D., Froberg, D., and Fontaine, P. (1991). The effects of social support on women's health during pregnancy, labour and delivery, and the postpartum period. *Family Medicine, 23*(5), 370.

Halbreich, U., and Karkun, S. (2006). Cross-cultural and social diversity of prevalence of postpartum depression and depressive symptoms. *Journal of Affect Disorders, 91*(2-3), 97–111.

Herzog, R., Álvarez-Pasquin, M.J., Díaz, C., Del Barrio, J.L., Estrada, J.M., and Gil, Á. (2013). Are healthcare workers' intentions to vaccinate related to their knowledge, beliefs and attitudes? A systematic review. *BMC Public Health, 13*(1), 154.

Higgins, J.P.T., and Green, S., editors. (2008). Cochrane handbook for systematic reviews of interventions. London: The Cochrane Collaboration.

Horowitz, J.A., Murphy, C.A., Gregory, K.E., and Wojcik, J. (2011). A community-based screening initiative to identify mothers at risk for postpartum depression. *Journal of Obstetrics and Gynaecology Neonatal Nursing, 40*(1), 52–61.

Howell, E.A., Mora, P., and Leventhal, H. (2006). Correlates of early postpartum depressive symptoms. *Maternal Child Health, 10*(2), 149–157.

Henshaw, C.A. (2003). Women's Mental Health. Review Mood disturbance in the early puerperium: a review. 6 Suppl 2, S33-42.

Kheirabadi, G.R., and Maracy, M.R. (2010). Prenatal depression in a cohort study on Iranian women. *Journal of Research in Medical Sciences, 15*(1), 41.

Kennedy, C.E., Hurley, K.M., and Black, M.M. (2011). Maternal depression and early childhood growth in developing countries: Systematic review and meta-analysis. *Bull. World Health Organization, 89*(8), 608–15D.

Kheirabadi, G.R., and Maracy, M.R. (2010). Perinatal depression in a cohort study on Iranian women. *Journal of Research Medical Science, 15*(1), 41–9.

Lee, D.T., Yip, A.S., Chan, S.S., Tsui, M.H., Wong, W.S., and Chung, T.K. (2003). Post-delivery screening for postpartum depression. *Psychosomatic Medicine, 65*(3), 357–61.

Logsdon, M.C., and Usui, W. (2001). Psychosocial predictors of postpartum depression in diverse groups of women. *West Journal of Nursing Research, 23*(6), 563–574.

McGarry, J., Kim, H., Sheng, X., Egger, M., and Baksh, L. (2009). Postpartum Depression and Help-Seeking Behaviour. *Journal of Midwife Women Health, 54*(1), 50–6.

O'Hara, M.W., Rehm, L.P., and Campbell, S.B. (1983). Postpartum depression: A role for social network and life stress variables. *Journal of Nerve Mental Disorder*, *171*(6), 336–341.

O'hara, M.W., and Swain, A.M. (1996). Rates and risk of postpartum depression—A meta-analysis. *International Review of Psychiatry*, *8*(1), 37–54.

Posmontier, B. (2008). Functional status outcomes in mothers with and without postpartum depression. *Journal of Midwifery Women's Health*, *53*(4), 310–8.

Rojas, G., Fritsch, R., Guajardo, V., Rojas, F., Barroilhet, S., and Jadresic, E. (2010). Characterization of depressed mothers in the postpartum. *Review of Medical Children, 138*(5), 536–42.

Saxena, S., Thornicroft, G., Knapp, M., and Whiteford, H. (2007). Resources for mental health: Scarcity, inequity, and inefficiency. *Lancet,* 8, *370*(9590), 878–89.

Shivalli, S., and Gururaj, N. (2015). Postnatal depression among rural women in South India: Do socio-demographic, obstetric and pregnancy outcome have a role to play? *PLoS One*, *10*(4), e0122079.

Shrestha, N., Hazrah, P., and Sagar, R. (2015). Incidence and prevalence of postpartum depression in a rural community of India. *Journal of Chitwan Medical College*, *5*(2), 11-9.

Sohr-Preston, S.L., and Scaramella, L.V. (2006). Implications of timing of maternal depressive symptoms for early cognitive and language development. *Clinical Child Family Psychology Review*, *9*(1), 65–83.

Stewart, D.E., Robertson, E., Dennis, C.L., Grace, S.L., and Wallington, T. (2003). Postpartum depression: Literature review of risk factors and interventions. Toronto: University Health Network Women's Health Programme.

Trends in Maternal Mortality: 1990 to 2015: estimates by WHO, UNICEF, UNFPA, World Bank Group and the United Nations Population Division. Geneva: World Health Organization.

Vander Kruik, R., Barreix, M., Chou, D., Allen, T., Say, L., and Cohen, L.S. (2017). Maternal Morbidity Working Group. The global prevalence of postpartum psychosis: A systematic review. *BMC Psychiatry*, 28, *17*(1), 272.

Verkuijl, N.E., Richter, L., Norris, S.A., Stein, A., Avan, B., and Ramchandani, P.G. (2014). Postnatal depressive symptoms and child psychological development at 10 years: A prospective study of longitudinal data from the South African Birth to Twenty Cohort. *Lancet Psychiatry*, *1*(6), 454–60.

Wells, G., Shea, B., O'Connell, D., Peterson, J., Welch, V., and Losos, M., *et al.* The Newcastle-Ottawa (NOS) for assessing the quality of nonrandomized studies in meta-analysis. Ottawa: Ottawa Hospital Research Institute.

12

Mental Health of Women having Polycystic Ovary Syndrome (PCOS)

Vibha Kriti and *Shobhna Joshi*

Introduction

Polycystic ovary syndrome (PCOS) is the most common and pervasive endocrine condition with multiple phenotypes found in reproductive age females all around the world and it is mainly characterized by hyperandrogenism (high level of androgen), menstrual disturbance, and infertility. In addition to this it is well recognized reproductive consequences (Rees *et al.*, 2016), PCOS is now established as a metabolic disorder underpinned by insulin resistance and leading to an increased risk of type 2 diabetes (Morgan *et al.*, 2012).

There are several features for characterizing PCOS, such as menstrual disturbances (amenorrhea and oligomenorrhea) and hyperadrogenism (hirsutism or acne, and very often obesity). Besides these, chronic anovulation and infertility are the prevalent consequences of PCOS (Podfigurna-Stopa *et al.*, 2015). Common physical symptoms include weight gain, excess facial hair, severe acne, and irregular menstruation. Biochemical symptoms include excess androgen and decreased progesterone (Chang & Katz, 1999).

The term PCOS is evolving over time with its conception and meaning that make the term curious one. Unfortunately there is no cure for PCOS and it can affect women of any age, race, ethnicity, or sexual orientation. The endocrinopathy begins at puberty and ends at menopause, which has adverse consequences based on clinical presentation and laboratory findings (Sayyah-Melli *et al.*, 2015). Thus, the syndrome has a lifelong duration and thus symptoms need to be monitored and managed from its onset until the end of a woman's life. Since PCOS is associated with a wide range of medical problems, it has gained remarkable attention over the last decade (Himelein *et al.,* 2006). Although PCOS is largely considered as a medical disorder hence its psychosocial aspects have been neglected or misunderstood by researchers and clinicians. According to Elsenbruch and colleagues (2003) almost all females diagnosed with PCOS go through experience of mental health problems, some may have less extent of sadness while other have severe depression or anxiety that may be because of enormous physical as well as endocrinology changes (Elsenbruch *et al.*, 2003; Zafari-Zangeneh *et al.,* 2012).

Thus, PCOS symptoms create psychological problems through which women suffer throughout life time and the lack of awareness about PCOS and its relationship with mental health issues has left many women struggling to find the support that they need from the mental health community (Castillo, 2008). The syndrome's complexity and a lack of knowledgeable specialists, PCOS can go undiagnosed and untreated for years (Richardson, 2003). There is no single test that can be used to diagnose PCOS; complex signs and symptoms, including both physical and biochemical markers, evolve over time (Azziz, 2008). However, a comprehensive and clear explanation for the pathogenesis of this disorder has remained questionable (Elsenbruch *et al.*, 2003; Sayyah-Melli *et al.*, 2016). The PCOS is complex endocrine condition, so for the deep understanding it is important to see its origin.

The two American doctors, Stein and Leventhal (1935), first discovered polycystic ovary syndrome. It was initially called as Stein-Leventhal Syndrome (Stein, 1958). They investigated seven women who had either lack of menstruation or abnormal menstrual cycles along with sterility and/or ovaries with multiple cysts and identified masculine traits in them. According to Stein & Cohen (1939) and Geist & Gaines (1942) the very first treatment for PCOS was ovarian surgical procedures such as surgical removing sections of the ovary. In addition Birnbaum (2003) called PCOS as a "total body endocrine disease" of which the abnormality of the ovary are outcome of the problem in endocrine system.

In medical literature the work by Stein and Leventhal on " polycystic ovaries" had begun appearing largely by the 1940s and 50s (Buxton & Van de Wiele, 1954; Leventhal & Cohen, 1951; Stein & Cohen, 1939) and it was referred as, Polycystic Ovarian Syndrome (Evans & Riley, 1958; Keettel, *et al.*, 1957) by the late 1950s. This clearly shows that the nomenclature of the syndrome was changed according to its morphological characteristics from time to time. Around the same time being PCOS symptomatic spectrum extended as more variety of symptoms is added alongside with cystic ovaries, hirsutism and body weight (Leventhal

& Cohen, 1951). Further in 1980s, it was found linked among insulin resistance, metabolism and PCOS (Plymate, *et al.*, 1981; Shoupe, *et al.*, 1983) as well as stress and PCOS (Lobo, *et al.*, 1983). Thus, Erhmann in 2006 stated that the discovery of PCOS has become well-recognized as it has major effects throughout on reproductive and metabolic area of women's life. In addition to the physical effects of PCOS, it has significant impact on women's mental health too.

The problem compounded as PCOS does not have a universal definition and its diagnostic criteria which ranging from very strict to more inclusive. The most recent criteria for PCOS require that a diagnosis should include both hyperandrogenism and ovarian dysfunction. While some clinicians and researchers argue that a more inclusive definition is important, Azziz (2008) encouraged the sub-categorization of PCOS for both research purposes and clinical applications.

The pathogenesis of PCOS is poorly understood (Goodarzi & Azziz, 2006; Ong, Theodoru & Ledger, 2006). Indeed, Franks, McCarthy and Hardy (2006) suggest that although the aetiology of PCOS remains uncertain, there is increasing evidence for a genetic basis: they proposed that the genesis of the syndrome may be during early development, perhaps in utero. However, De Melo *et al.* (2015) reported that whilst PCOS might have its origin in utero, interaction between genetic and environmental factors is crucial for its appearance.

The exact etiology for occurring to PCOS is not clear because of the complex nature of symptoms of PCOS. Polycystic Ovarian Syndrome, can include insulin resistance, obesity, acne, hair loss and infertility (Elsenbruch *et al.*, 2003). Specifically, women with PCOS may experience anovulatory infertility which is infertility due to lack of ovulation (Franks, Stark & Hardy, 2008). PCOS is the most common cause of anovulatory infertility in women (Balen & Rutherford, 2007; Gorry, Davima & Franks, 2006). In addition, women with PCOS can experience hirsutism, which can occur as a result of hyperandrogenism (excess levels of androgens; Oláh, 2004) and is defined in women as excessive facial and/or body hair in a male like distribution (Archer & Chang, 2004). Thus, hyperandrogenism, menstrual irregularity, and the presence of multiple follicles in ovaries are the most common physiological manifestations of PCOS (Norman, *et al.*, 2007) as shown in Table 12.1 but these symptoms may vary between individual especially when cultural context are considered, there experience of PCOS is quite subjective and distinct. For few PCOS people overweight and obesity may be main concern while for other it may be struggle for conceiving, or might be frequent shaving, and laser sessions, acne treatments or searching and trying out for new diet schedule are major problem. Thus, PCOS have different meaning for different people.

From the above paragraph it can be clearly said that the condition of PCOS is still very vague because of its definition, etiology as well as diagnostic criteria. Thus, it is important to work more carefully for the condition to make the term more understandable. Further long term outcome has been discussed.

Table 12.1: Features of Polycystic Ovary Syndrome

Clinical Features	*Metabolic Features*	*Psychological Features*
• Infertility • Hyperandrogenism • Hirsutism	• Insulin resistance • Impaired glucose tolerance • Type 2 diabetes mellitus • Cardiovascular risk	• Anxiety • Depression • Worsen quality of life

Polycystic Ovary Syndrome has enormous clinical and metabolic outcome, in which some have long-term consequences. Long-term illness was defined by De Ridder (2008), as a disorder which persists for longer period of time which is hard to cure. Moreover Forshaw (2002) suggest that long term illness is not something that can be easily cured but is a long lasting, and often permanent condition which becomes part of a person's life. In addition the DOH (2015) suggest that long term conditions can impact all aspects of an individual's life it curb their ability to work and disturbed their social relationship and these characteristics are embodied in PCOS, thus it can clearly said that PCOS is a long term condition. Long term outcome associated with PCOS like cardiovascular disease, type II diabetes mellitus and endometrial cancer (Navaratnarajan *et al.*, 2008; Chittenden, *et al.*, 2009; Fearnley *et al.*, 2010). Along with its physical health implications these symptoms have significant contribution in curbing their social, psychological and economical aspect of life (Azziz *et al.*, 2005).

PCOS conditions have long term consequences but to date there have been very less studies which explored PCOS from qualitative perspective (Amiri *et al.*, 2018; Crete & Adamshick, 2011)

There are currently three widely used PCOS diagnostic criteria. In the year of 1990, National Institute of Health (NIH) conference were held on PCOS in which the first formal diagnostic criteria was established which include the presence of chronic anovulation and clinical or biochemical signs of hyperandrogenissm and not polycystic ovaries and PCOS seen as disorder of androgen over-production (Azziz, 2006, p. 781). Later in 2003 this criteria was revised in Rotterdam conference (Fr & Tarlats, 2004) which included presence of any two symptoms from the following three symptoms and these are oligo and/or anovulation, clinical and/or biochemical signs of hyperandrogenism, polycystic ovaries in ultrasound. Moreover in year of 2009, NIH criteria has been accepted as it was suggested by Androgen Excess and PCOS Society, however it was a modification of two previous criteria and holds that women with oligomenorrhea and polycystic ovaries, but no hyperandrogenism should not be considered to have PCOS (Azziz *et al.*, 2006). Therefore, Rotterdam Criteria identified four phenotypes of PCOS (Norman *et al.*, 2007). First is severe PCOS (all diagnostic criteria met), second is mild PCOS (anovulation and polycystic ovaries), third is Ovulatory PCOS (polycystic ovaries and hyperandrogenism) and fourth is Hyperandrogonism and anovulation. Thus, the Rotterdam criteria are therefore more inclusive than the NIH or AES (Norman *et al.* 2007).

Table 12.2: Diagnostic Criteria for Polycystic Ovary Syndrome

National Institute of Health (NIH) Criteria (1990)	*Rotterdam Criteria (Revised) (2003)*	*Androgen Excess & PCOS Society Criteria (2006)*
Oligo-anovulation Hyperandrogenism both criteria required	Oligo or anovulation Hyperandrogenism Polycystic ovaries 2 out of 3 criteria required	Hyperandrogenism Ovarian dysfunction Both criteria required

Thus, from the above diagnostic criteria it can be concluded that the four key features of PCOS are hyperandrogenemia, clinical hyperandrogenism, oligoanovulation and polycystic ovaries (Azziz *et al.*, 2009). In addition Fauser *et al.*, 2012 demonstrated that these symptoms of PCOS may result in infertility, gestational diabetes and pre-eclampsia, as stage of life passes over time. Not only this PCOS has also been associated with increased risk of endometrial cancer (Barry *et al.*, 2014; Gottschau *et al.*, 2015), kidney, colon and brain cancers are more serious long-term consequences as mentioned above, but there exact association among them can't be drawn clearly, it may be genetic (Xita *et al.*, 2002) or environmental factor or the combination of both.

The nomenclature of the term "polycystic ovarian syndrome" has long past as the name of the syndrome was shifted according to its morphological characteristics. The name of PCOS is quite misleading because it is often confused as the term mainly focused on cystic ovaries but it is important to note that it is only one possible criteria but not necessary symptoms for the recognition of the disorder. In fact, ovarian cysts are neither necessary nor significant for the diagnosis of this syndrome. It is important to note that Polycystic Ovary also occurs in the women who display no other condition associated with syndrome. Moreover, the name PCOS neither reflects the hyperandrogenism which is essential for diagnosis of PCOS. Thus, PCOS is called as misleading label (Lam & Raine Fenning, 2009). Generally the term 'cyst' is used interchangeably with 'follicle', hence using poly-cystic as the central part of the syndrome is confusing in many ways as it is not proper representative of the ovarian morphology. Similarly, another confusion created when the term doesn't differentiate among women who have only polycystic ovaries and those who have the signs of hyperandrogenism, menstrual irregularities, and metabolic features that constitute the syndrome (Polson, *et al.*, 1988) and lastly it curtail syndrome's endocrine and metabolic aspects and escalate the role of the ovary (Khadilkar, 2016).

Teede and colleagues (2014) in Australia had conducted a study to see how the term PCOS name is perceived by doctors and PCOS women in Australia. They found that half of women with PCOS misinterpret cysts as the most remarkable feature of PCOS and both 74 per cent of doctors and 48 per cent of patients accept that the name PCOS deliver unclarity in its name as well as most of the doctors among them support to change the name of the syndrome (Teede, *et al.*, 2014). So it is simple to raise the question that if the finding of the polycystic morphology of ovaries is not essential for diagnosis of this syndrome, why to retain the name PCOS as Androgen Excess and PCOS Society (AES).

From the above paragraph, it can easily be inferred that the 'PCOS' has long past in its emergence and nomenclature. Further controversy carried out among clinicians in the process of naming of PCOS but a suitable new option has not yet been established.

Despite constant debate on the nomenclature, there was also discrepancy in prevalence rate which is affected by chosen diagnostic criteria. According to Azziz (2008) the prevalence rate of PCOS was approximately 6.5 in the year of 1990 and it become twice in the year of 2003 when Rotterdam criteria were established. This rate of increasing continuously in the case of PCOS condition in present scenario, it is not far to becoming an epidemic. So it is important to have a glance on its prevalence rate in today's world. Calculation of prevalence varies according to population studies and ethnicity as well as depends on the choice of diagnostic criteria (2–26%). As the syndrome is not defined precisely, its exact prevalence is not known. PCOS does not have a universal definition with its diagnostic criteria ranging from very strict to more inclusive. World Health Organization (WHO) estimates that it affected 116 million women worldwide in 2012 (3.4% of women). Globally, prevalence estimates of PCOS are highly variable ranging from 2.2 per cent to as high as 26 per cent, even the symptoms of PCOS vary from women to women in terms of even the severity with which they manifest. Joshi, B. and colleagues in 2014 found that the prevalence of PCOS was 22.5 per cent by Rotterdam and 10.7 per cent by Androgen Excess Society criteria. The prevalence rate of PCOS is also varies according to regions.

In European region, women labelled with PCOS when polycystic ovaries were observed on ultrasound co-exist with at least one of these following symptoms, irregular periods, elevated androgens, elevated luteinizing hormone, or obesity while in North American women labelled with PCOS when women had irregular menstrual cycles combined with increased androgen levels, and ovaries was not necessary condition for the diagnosis of PCOS (Hart, *et al.*, 2004). These differences in diagnosis also reflected that it is difficult to conclude the exact estimate for the prevalence of PCOS across populations. A study by March and colleagues (2009) on same group of women to assess the prevalence according to 3 diagnostic criteria of PCOS these are NIH, Rotterdam, and the AE-PCOS Society diagnostic criteria (March, *et al.*, 2009). They found different prevalence rates of PCOS from different diagnostic criteria within the same population. Similarly, Yildiz *et al.*, (2012) carried out a study on homogenous population in Turkey, he also find the same outcome as the three different diagnostic measures resulted to different prevalence rates. This clearly shows that PCOS prevalence rates will affect according to the criteria used so far. Not only has this, recently according to Hillman (2018) the prevalence of PCOS can't be estimated correctly as many women become remained undiagnosed from the condition (Hillman, 2018; March, *et al.*, 2009). Whilst there are conflicting views and explanations on the distribution of PCOS across different populations, although clustering different findings, the most frequent and prevalent endocrine condition found in women is PCOS all over (Knochenhauer, *et al.*, 1998).

PCOS is a heterogeneous health conditions, therefore it has unclear etiology and pathogenesis. Some studies have pointed that genetic factors also contribute to the development of PCOS. If someone in the family has it, they might be more likely to develop it as a women have more vulnerability for PCOS as her mother and sister have the syndrome

(Kahsar-Miller, *et al.*, 2001) or higher androgen levels (Legro, *et al.*, 1998) but the link cannot be drawn clearly as lack of universally accept diagnostic criteria. Another review study of Azziz (2008) reported that PCOS women have also impact on their male relatives like they manifest metabolic and androgenic outline similar to PCOS women (Azziz, 2008), it suggests two important things. Firstly, it lends weight to genetics as a predisposing factor for PCOS and secondly, that metabolic and endocrine factors beyond the female reproductive system underpin PCOS. The closest we come to understand the specific genetic pathways of PCOS to identify the cluster of genes that play an important role in the development of the condition (Chen *et al.*, 2011). Although it is well known that genetics play a role but the extent and degree of that role is still not certain (Diamanti-Kandarakis, *et al.*, 2006). Along with genetics, lifestyle is a highly significant factor in the development of PCOS. The etiology of PCOS looks at genetic and lifestyle factors hand in hand. Franks and colleagues (2006) hypothesis seems particularly relevant, propositioning that PCOS is rooted in genetic factors, but how it is manifested is also affected and varies by environmental and lifestyle factors, such as diet and nutrition. Metabolic disturbances e.g., insulin resistance have emerged as pivotal factors in the pathogenesis of PCOS (De Leo, *et al.*, 2016). An interaction of genetic, lifestyle, and environmental factors is the most comprehensive understanding of PCOS etiology that can be gleaned so far (Dumesic, *et al.*, 2015). As such, there remains a lack of consistency in diagnostic criteria utilized in practice, and reported in research (Lujan *et al.*, 2013). Thus, PCOS was observed and verified as a disease, a disorder, an abnormality, and a problem, that can be understood through multidimensional approach. This perspective sees PCOS as a sum of its symptomatic parts and correlates the syndrome and its symptoms (such as obesity, hirsutism, or infertility) with other co-morbidity such as sexual health, depression, anxiety, or quality of life.

From thorough review to literature related to PCOS, it can be said that despite the clinical and metabolic features there are number of psychological problems like depression, anxiety, bipolar disorder, borderline personality disorder and many more are related to the condition which adversely affect the mental health profile of PCOS women. To understand the mental health of PCOS women, it is firstly important to understand the term 'mental health'.

Mental health includes emotional, psychological and social well-being. Mental health can be influenced by a variety of factors, which effects in the way of thinking, feeling and acting for day to day life events. Mental health is also the key to relationships, personal and emotional well-being.

World Health Organization define mental health as a state of well-being in which the individual realizes his or her own abilities, can cope with the normal stresses of life, can work productively and fruitfully, and is able to make a contribution to his or her community (WHO, 2004). Mental health is considerable to PCOS disorder as the disorder is associated with many psychological problems.

Generally all females diagnosed with PCOS to have negative emotions of frustration, anxiety, and sadness to a lesser extent (Elsenbruch *et al.*, 2003; Zafari-Zangeneh *et al.*, 2012). However, several disorders such as changes in appearance, irregular or absent menstrual periods, and possibly disturbances in sexual attitudes and behaviour (Elsenbruch *et al.*, 2003) can lead to psychological distress and impaired emotional well-being (Silva *et al.*, 2010; Sayyah-Melli *et al.,* 2015). These can impact the patients' feminine identity and create psychological problems, such as anxiety, depression, as well as marital and social maladjustment (Podfigurna-Stopa *et al.*, 2015; Shakerardekani *et al.*, 2011). Almost all of the females diagnosed with PCOS had experienced significant levels of psychological disorders in all dimensions of their life compared to the general population (Jedel *et al.*, 2010; Rahiminejad *et al.*, 2014), with anxiety and depression, social interaction, body image and body weight, eating problems, hirsutism, fertility, and decreased Quality of Life (QOL) being the main consequences of psychosocial problems in PCOS (Lee, 2015; Krepula *et al.*, 2012). The majority of females with PCOS reported problems such as somatization, obsessive-compulsiveness, interpersonal sensitivity, and hostility (McCook *et al.*, 2015). Several other disorders have been reported by females with PCOS, including lower self-esteem, more negative body-image, decreased psychological wellbeing, impaired social and marital relationships, poor sexual performance (Janssen *et al.*, 2006; Kosari Moghadam *et al.*, 2015), and psychological morbidity (Hollinrake *et al.*, 2007, Sharma, 2015, Zafari-Zangeneh *et al.*, 2012). This further indicates the importance of emotional distress and psychiatric disorders in reducing psychosocial aspects of quality of life in such women. Thus, such studies which are related to mental health of PCOS women shows that such women experiences psychiatric problem such as depression, anxiety, bipolar disorder, borderline personality disorder and eating disorder and these severe problems have must underpinned by psychosocial issues which includes body image dissatisfaction and sexual functioning etc. Hence the psychological problem associated with PCOS has been categorized under two groups, first is psychiatric disorder and second is psychosocial problems. PCOS is accompanied by the array of symptoms such as obesity, acne, hair thinning, menstrual irregularity and infertility, these symptoms can also contributes to psychological impairment. Depression and anxiety are more likely to occur in such women.

Depression is a mood disorder that involves persistent feeling of sadness and loss of interest inactivates once enjoyed and these symptoms persist for at least two week. Simultaneously anxiety may also occur which is characterized by felling of worry, fear that are enough strong to interfere with one's daily activities. Another mood disorder that is found in such population is bipolar disorder which is associates with episodes of mood swing ranging from depressive lows to manic highs, means sometime such women might feel very energetic and low at the same time. Such severe problems might lead to chances for the occurrence of personality disorder like borderline personality disorder. Borderline personality disorder characterized by unstable moods, behaviour and rapid changes in self-identity that casing problems functioning in everyday life. The rapid changes in self-identity may create more concern for the eating pattern in PCOS women those results to eating disorder. Eating disorder is abnormal changes in food taking pattern. These problems have greater impact on the psychosocial aspect of PCOS women. One of the psychosocial aspects which curbs badly in PCOS women is their body image. It is known fact that eating disorder has direct impact on body image. Body image refers to perception that a person has of their physical self. In addition Poorandokht Afshari and colleagues (2016) study reported that body image is associated with sexual health. So it is very obvious that body image effects the sexual functioning in PCOS women. PCOS patient women markedly suffer from sexual dysfunction as they are less satisfied with their sex life. These above mentioned disorders can effect on the mental health of PCOS women. To understand the mental health profile of women with PCOS, firstly it is important to explicitly understand the construct.

On the basics of above studies it can be said that there are considerable number of mental health issues associated with PCOS with varied symptoms, so it is tough to explain each and every mental health problems in detail. Here some serious issues have been discussed in detail. Moreover Dr. Stener-Victorin (2011) notes that at least one mental health problem found in approximately 60 per cent of women having PCOS.

One of the most prominent mental health problem found in PCOS women is depression. Depression is common but serious mood disorder characterized by low mood, a feeling of sadness, loss of interest in daily activities. The prevalence of depression in PCOS is high (Trent *et al.*, 2002) but the risk of depression is yet unclear in females with PCOS (Hollinrake *et al.*, 2007). Nonetheless, studies that have investigated psychological causes of PCOS have found a relationship between depression and PCOS (Himelein & Thatcher, 2006). The symptoms of depression have been examined by a large number of behavioural scientists (Himelein & Thatcher, 2006).

Depressive disorders include major depressive disorder, dysthymic disorder and depressive disorder which are observable in PCOS patients (Himelein & Thatcher, 2006; Hollinrake *et al.*, 2007). Prior studies have found that depression increases cortisol levels while it decreases serotonin levels in the central nervous system (Zafari-Zangeneh *et al.*, 2012). According to the findings of several studies in this area, 28 per cent to 64 per cent of patients with PCOS had depression (Scaruffi *et al.*, 2014).

There are several efforts have been made to identify about the causes of depression in patients with PCOS but mixed results have been found. According to Rasgon & colleagues (2005), among PCOS women, there were no significant correlation found between depression and higher level of androgen as well as with between depression and hirsutism. A study by Weiner *et al.*, 2004 found positive mood state were associated with higher free testosterone levels (Weiner *et al.*, 2004). Some studies show symptoms of PCOS is associated with hyperandrogenism but there is lack of clear explanation for the relationship between clinical characteristics of PCOS and mental health aspect (Krepula *et al.*, 2012). One of the most critical causes of depression in patients with PCOS is increased body mass index, which is accompanied by negative perception towards their body (Gambineri *et al.*, 2002). Approximately, two-thirds of females with PCOS are overweight or obese (Azziz *et al.*, 2004). One of the main causes of depression in females of the general population is obesity. However, there are inconsistent findings regarding the relationship between obesity and depression in females with PCOS. Keegn and colleagues (2003) found incidence of depression in normal weight PCOS women as they not include women with body mass greater than 25 kg/m^2. Similarly, Weiner and colleagues (2004) reported that comparative to weight-matched control group there was greater depression in women with PCOS. Contrary, Benson in 2008 revealed that there was no association between depression and obesity in patients with PCOS (Benson *et al.*, 2008).

On the basis of above review it was observed that the condition of PCOS has potential vulnerability for the depression but actual reason for it still not clear.

Another common disturbance with prevalence rate of 34 per cent to 57 per cent that causes difficulty for females with PCOS is anxiety (Podfigurna-Stopa *et al.*, 2015). Anxiety is a mental health disorder characterized by feeling of intense, excessive and persistent worry and fear about everyday situations. In particular, women with PCOS have been found to be at an increased risk of social phobia and suicide attempts (Mansson *et al.*, 2008). According to Hussain and colleagues, one of the main reasons for anxiety is persistent fears regarding loss of sexuality, loss of fertility, and inability to have children (Hussain *et al.*, 2015). There are other PCOS symptoms such as hirsutism, acne (Harmanci *et al.*, 2013), obesity, and menstrual irregularities that might cause anxiety in PCOS patients (Michelmore *et al.*, 2001). Moreover, increasing level of androgen results to masculine body features in PCOS women that may experience higher level of anxiety and also awareness regarding possible chronic disorders (Harmanci *et al.*, 2013).

Negative reactions might trigger social phobia because of people attitude towards obesity and hirsutism (Hussain *et al.*, 2015). The underlying reason for development of depressive disorders is anxiety. Based on earlier findings, anxiety disorders are more prevalent than depression in patients with PCOS (Benson *et al.*, 2009; Harmanci *et al.*, 2013). Anxiety, as a strong predictor of functional impairment, has major effects on the role of function and quality of life in patients with PCOS (Hussain *et al.*, 2015). Overall, there is limited research regarding the link between anxiety and PCOS (Deeks *et al.*, 2011). As indicated by the literature, patients with PCOS have social phobia, specific phobia, and panic disorder (Harmanci *et al.*, 2013) anxiety in females with PCOS could be a byproduct of overall negative effects rather than independent problems (Harmanci *et al.*, 2013). Barry and his colleagues (2011) showed that PCOS patients were significantly more neurotic (had difficulty coping with stress), anxious and depressed than controls (Deurenberg *et al.*, 2002).

Above the two most frequent mental health problems are seen in detail but the counting are not limited to these only, other mental health issues are associated with PCOS condition. One of them is stress which is explained below in detailed.

The condition of PCOS is not only triggered depression and anxiety but it eventually leads to feeling of stress among such women. Stress is the experience of a perceived threat, resulting from a series of physiological responses and pathways (Canavatchel, 2014). Women with PCOS reported a significantly increased physiological reaction to stress compared with controls (Benson *et al.*, 2009; Farrell & Antoni, 2010). According to Lobo and colleagues (1983) the level of physiological stress hormone was high in PCOS patients. Moreover, patient with PCOS had higher felling of helplessness, self-blaming compared to healthy control but there is a paucity of studies investigating the relationship of stress with psychological health in PCOS (Guidi *et al.*, 2017). The persistence state of stress can affect the mood of the individual and leads of other mood disorder.

Another psychological disorder associated with episodes of mood swing ranging from depressive lows to manic highs that can significantly change mood, behaviour, thoughts, and energy level is bipolar disorder. There are three types of bipolar disorder, namely bipolar disorder I (mania and major depression), bipolar disorder II (hypomania and episodes of major depression), and unspecified bipolar disorder (not meeting the criteria of I or II). The incidence of bipolar disorder is 1 per cent (Krepula *et al.,* 2012). The relationship between bipolar disorder and PCOS has not yet been supported in the literature and there is little evidence in this regard. There are also contradictory and inconsistent opinions regarding such relationship. According to Himelein & Thatcher, 2006 research, valproic acid (VPA), which is used for treating bipolar disorder, highly influences development of PCOS (Himelein & Thatcher, 2006). Other studies state that these 2 disorders are directly linked. Specifically, hypothalamic-pituitary-ovary (HPO) level and likeness of metabolic abnormalities are common disturbances in both PCOS and bipolar disorder (Krepula *et al.*, 2012). Prior studies have demonstrated the existence of several PCOS disturbances such as menstrual irregularities, hyperandrogenism, and anatomic or hormonal evidences in bipolar females (Davari-Tanha *et al.*, 2014). Findings of a study revealed that bipolar females treated with valproate had a higher level of menstrual irregularities, hyperandrogenism, and metabolic syndrome than females without treatment (McIntyre *et al.*, 2003). This is mainly due to the medications used for treating bipolar disorder that could influence the hypothalamic-pituitary gonadal (HPG) axis and the reproductive system (Rassi *et al.*, 2010). This is a potential mechanism, by which valproate could induce PCOS symptoms (Himelein & Thatcher, 2006).

The condition of PCOS not only changes the mood badly but can also results to personality disorder. Among the mental health problem related to PCOS, Borderline personality disorder is emerging concern which needs to be investigated.

The most common personality disorder in clinical population is Borderline personality disorder (BPD) (Leichsenring *et al.*, 2011). BPD is a serious psychiatric disorder characterized by emotional dysregulation, interpersonal distress, stress related dissociation and suicidality (American Psychiatric Association, 2013). They become volatile when symptoms of BPD fluctuate rapidly and are severe (e.g. rage and self-injurious behaviour). Studies shows that approximately 75 per cent of BPD diagnosed individuals have attempted suicide at least once, and 10 per cent of them complete suicide (Black *et al.*, 2004).

Approximately half of BPD patients report experience of major depressive disorder (MDD) because interleukin (IL)-6 is associated with MDD as well as it is possible biomarker of BPD. Several studies reveal that PCOS has an association with personality including BPD (Azziz & Elyasi, 2017).

Women with PCOS are significantly more likely to develop metabolic complications such as obesity and type-2 diabetes, and cardiovascular disease (Fauser *et al.*, 2012). Similarly Moran and colleague in 2010 found double rates of metabolic disturbance in PCOS women comparatively to women without PCOS (Moran *et al.*, 2010). Likewise, emerging literature has shown that BPD is also associated with obesity, type 2 diabetes and cardiovascular disease (Dixon-Gordon *et al.*, 2015; Frankenburg & Zanarini, 2011; Kahl *et al.*, 2013). Recently Kahl and colleagues in 2013 reported that compared to other adults in primary care, BPD adults have twice rate of metabolic syndrome (Kahl *et al.*, 2013). However psychological consequences have strongly associated with both BPD and PCOS (Scaruffi *et al.*, 2014; Tomko *et al.*, 2014) but there is no clear explanation regarding there association.

Along with these severe mental health problem PCOS women have also face the challenges for food taking pattern that leads to eating disorder in such women.

PCOS is widely accepted that it include important causal role of eating disorders specifically bulimia (Polivy & Herman, 2002). There are eight types of eating disorders according to diagnostic and statistical manual V (DSM-V) that include Pica, Rumination, Restrictive Food Intake Disorder, anorexia nervosa, bulimia nervosa, and binge-eating disorder, Other Specified Feeding or Eating Disorder and Unspecified Feeding or Eating Disorder. It has been reported that the rate of eating disorders and suicidal behaviour among females with PCOS is increasing (Sayyah-Melli *et al.*, 2015). Females with bulimia nervosa are generally ashamed of their eating habits and behave secretly about their eating problem and weight control. Pica refers as persistence eating of non-nutritive substances for a period of at least one month while being eating refers to eating in a discrete period of time or lack of control over eating. Rumination disorder includes repeated regurgitation of food for a period of at least one month. This has caused females with eating disorders to be reluctant in exposing and discussing their eating habits (Michelmore *et al.*, 2001). It has been stated in several earlier studies that there is a relationship between PCOS and eating disorders. However, the etiology of such relationship has never been satisfactorily clarified (Hollinrake *et al.*, 2007; Davari-Tanha *et al.*, 2014). Several theories have been proposed that can explain the association between PCOS and bulimia nervosa (Michelmore *et al.*, 2001). One of the possibilities is emotional distress that brings about adverse symptoms of PCOS such as hirsutism, acne, menstrual irregularity, and obesity. These symptoms might develop eating disorders (Lee, 2015, Michelmore *et al.*, 2001). As revealed in an early study, being overweight or obese may lead to unhealthy eating habits such as binge eating purging, vomiting, dieting, and use of diuretics or laxatives to lose weight. As such, dissatisfaction with self-appearance in some adolescents with PCOS might cause them to think that their attempt for losing weight is not as successful as that of their peers without PCOS (Lee, 2015). Moreover, bulimia nervosa, by creating a hormonal environment, predisposes polycystic ovarian changes. One of the potential mechanisms is altered insulin secretion and insulin resistance in females with bulimia, however, the views regarding this mechanism varies in the literature (Michelmore *et al.*, 2001). Hence, it is of uttermost importance to clinically screen females with PCOS for their abnormal eating behaviour prior to suggesting any diet.

The above paragraph revealed that somewhere PCOS and eating disorder is associated with each other but which affect to whom is tough to answer, either PCOS may lead to bulimia or vice versa. Along with eating disorder other mental health problem are also found frequent in PCOS women, it is obvious that it affects body image among PCOS women.

Body image refers to the mental picture of someone's body, an attitude about physical self-appearance, wholeness, normal function, and sexuality. For females, body image has the elements of feminine and attractiveness that can be a symbol of social demonstration (Bazarganipour *et al.*, 2013). Therefore, negative perception among PCOS patients regarding their body image leads to a feeling of dissatisfied, and less self-consciousness with their appearance, loss of femininity, feeling less sexually attractive, and being unable to adapt to the normal society (Bazarganipour *et al.*, 2013,). Body dissatisfaction can have devastating impact on psychological functioning because symptoms such as hirsutism, obesity, acne, and infertility (Lee *et al.*, 2015) are painful, uncomfortable, and unpredictable for many PCOS patients because these symptoms are culturally defined as unfeminine and undesirable (Michelmore *et al.*, 2001, Tan *et al.*, 2008). Perhaps, losing femininity in females with PCOS can result in feelings of stigmatized and mood disorders such as depression, limited sense of well-being, and dissatisfaction with life (Kosari Moghadam *et al.*, 2015). Additionally, one of the reasons causing eating disorder is body dissatisfaction. This is because self-esteem, as an important element for a female's social function and interpersonal relationships, is exclusively based on their body image (Bazarganipour *et al.,* 2013). Another factor that affects the body image of females with PCOS is their weight. This could be rooted in cultural preferences that consider android fat pattern as unattractive (Deurenberg *et al.*, 2002). Obesity or weight gain might lead to a loss of self-esteem as well as poor body image and body satisfaction. This can ultimately reduce their quality of life while increasing their psychological disorders (Lee *et al.*, 2015). Therefore, is it paramount to carefully identify the patients' emotional well-being, which is particularly related to low self-esteem, poor body image and weight challenges, menstrual abnormalities, and hirsutism (Bazarganipour *et al.*, 2013).

The above studies show that body image disturbance is prominently found in PCOS women that eventually affect sexual functioning of such women. Further sexual functioning is explained.

Patients with PCOS experience multiple changes that may negatively influence their sexual functioning (Silva, 2010; Tan, 2008; Himelein & Thatcher, 2006). There are a very limited number of studies on the PCOS of patients' sexual functioning (Eftekhar, 2014). Elsenbruch and colleagues (2003) reported that speculation and frequency for intimacy, there is no difference between PCOS women and healthy women, although POCS women feel sexually less attractive and were downhearted with their sex life. Several factors, such as changes in body appearance, especially obesity and excessive body hair have been found to negatively impact quality of life, sexual dissatisfaction, and self-worth (Janssen *et al.*, 2006). Furthermore, another stressor for patients with PCOS is infertility that can negatively influence the couples' life, their marital relationships, and sexual performance (Kosari Moghadam *et al.*, 2015). Moreover another study by Eftekhar (2014) shows body mass and hirsutism is important contributor of women's negative perceptions of sexual attractiveness but acne is not one of it. Some other factors that can be related to sexual dysfunction are depression, anxiety, low self-esteem, and negative self-image (Eftekhar, 2014). Moreover, females with PCOS experienced lower levels of sexual thoughts and desires than the general healthy population (Bazarganipour *et al.,* 2013; Himelein & Thatcher, 2006, Bazarganipour *et al.*, 2014). Overall, in females with PCOS, the syndrome does not cause sexual initiation (forms of expressing sexuality), intimate communication with partners, and sexual satisfaction (Silva *et al.*, 2010). Although it is hypothesized that female libido increases with elevated androgen levels in PCOS, females with PCOS reported a decrease in libido and satisfaction (Bazarganipour *et al.*, 2014). Hence, no significant relationship has been established between androgen levels and sexual functioning. In summary, sexual functioning is very much dependent on psychological factors and the relationship between partners. Similarly, a study of married Iranian females with polycystic ovary syndrome indicated that the most common sexual dysfunction was related to hypoactive desire disorder and arousal disorder (Himelein & Thatcher, 2006).

Overall, studies of sexual functioning suggest that there is feeling of sexual discomfort and sexually unattractiveness has been found in women with PCOS but their clear causal factor cannot be drawn.

The literature regarding psychological problem of women with PCOS shows that mental health issues curbed their quality of life badly. So it is important to look after to the cause behind it. For this understanding the concept is firstly important.

The World Health Organization (WHO) define quality of life as "an individual's perception of their position in life in the context of the culture and value systems in which they live, and in relation to their goals, expectations, standards and concerns. It is a broad ranging concept as it includes person's physical health, psychological state, independence level, social relationships, their harmony with their environment and their spiritual, religious and personal beliefs" (WHOQOL Group, 1994, p. 1). Health-related quality of life has been proposed as a related construct and sub-domain of quality of life (Learmonth, Alwick, McAuley & Motl, 2015). Power *et al.* (1999) propose that the concept of health-related quality of life is a patient-perceived multidimensional construct. Moreover, Muldoon, Barger, Flory and Manuck (1998) suggest that health-related quality of life moves beyond manifestations of a condition to the impact of the condition on everyday life. Indeed, Bowling (1995, 2001) suggests that health is one of the most important areas of quality of life nominated by individuals and therefore, health-related quality of life should be included as a dimension within quality of life. However, Bowling (2001) reports that quality of life is often referred to as health-related quality of life in research.

Health-related quality of life is defined by Testa and Simonson (1996) as the physical, psychological and social domains of health that are influenced by a person's experiences, beliefs, expectations and perceptions. Moreover, Carr, Gibson and Robinson (2001, p. 1240) defined health-related quality of life as "those aspects of an individual's subjective experience that relate both directly and indirectly to health, disease, disability and impairment". Moreover, they suggest that quality of life is a broad concept concerned with whether disease or impairment limits a person's ability to fulfil a normal role. Quality of life, therefore, appears to be an assortment of interactive and subjective domains (Lawton, 1991). As such, whilst there are many differing definitions of quality of life there are arguably similarities within the underlying constructs, including; the individual's perspective, their goals and expectations, their psychological health, and physical and social domains of quality of life.

Barnard *et al.* (2007), Ching, Burke and Stuckey (2007) and Jones *et al.* (2010) all reported that women with PCOS have an impaired quality of life in comparison to control groups and/or normative data. McCook *et al.* (2015) identified that the symptom of weight was the highest health-related quality of life concern for women with PCOS, with hirsutism symptoms being the lowest related concern. Hahn *et al.* (2006) also found that obesity was significantly correlated with quality of life and, they reported that the symptom of hirsutism reduced quality of life. Recently, Benetti-Pinto Ferreira and his colleagues, (2015) reported that the domain of body weight, as measured by the PCOSQ, was correlated to worse quality of life in women with PCOS in Brazil, followed by infertility. However, women with PCOS often experience one or more co-morbid conditions including; type 2 diabetes and impaired glucose tolerance (Legro *et al.*, 2009) and thyroid disorders (Janssen *et al.*, 2004; Kachue *et al.*, 2012; Nisar *et al.*, 2012; Sinha *et al.*, 2013). Women with PCOS also experience higher risk factors for developing cardiovascular disease compared to matched controls (De Groo *et al.*, 2011; Milman *et al.*, 2016; Talbott *et al.*, 1995). Research also suggests that women with PCOS are also vulnerable for developing endometrial cancer (Gottschau *et al.*, 2015; Milman *et al.*, 2016; Haoula, Salman & Atiomo, 2012; Shafiee *et al.*, 2014).

The aforesaid thorough review of studies concern to mental health of women with PCOS, it could be stated that in addition to physical co-morbidities, women with PCOS likely to experience more psychological co-morbidities, including anxiety and depression (Deeks, Gibson-Helm & Teede, 2010; Lewis *et al.*, 2007; Månsson *et al.*, 2008; Rasgon *et al.*, 2005; Rassi *et al.*, 2010), body image disturbance, bipolar disorder, obesity, and many more. Lipton and colleagues (2006) also found that in a sample of women with PCOS over 74 per cent had clinical levels of anxiety, over

30 per cent had clinical levels of depression and just over 29 per cent of women had clinical levels of both depression and anxiety. It is clear that women with PCOS are more likely to experience co-morbid conditions, both physical and psychological that leads to occurrence of wide range of mental health difficulties.

Conclusion

In summary, this chapter reveals that polycystic ovary syndrome has numerous psychological impacts like depression, stress, anxiety, eating disorder and more leads to impaired physiological, behavioural, and social outcomes. The findings also revealed that patients with PCOS experience a great deal of stressful life events that can lead to psychological difficulties but the reason for such vulnerability of PCOS patients to mental health problems still remain unclear. Moreover mental health-related issues should be part of the initial screening and evaluation (Hussain *et al.*, 2015). Despite a justification for considering psychological side of PCOS women, there are very few studies available regarding it. Thus, more studies are now needed to understand the mechanism underlying for mental health problems in women with PCOS. PCOS is not curable so it is necessarily managed by facilitating a strong multidisciplinary taskforce together. Although a medical condition, PCOS required a holistic treatment approach. This approach is better than medication alone. Thus, gynecologist must be aware towards the significant psychological issue and specific interventions for required specific psychological problem that improve the mental health status of women with PCOS.

References

Afshari, P., Houshyar, Z., Jeevadifar, N., Pourmotahari, F., and Jorti, M. (2016). The relationship between Body Image and Sexual function in Middle-Aged Women. *Electronic Physician, 8*(11), 3302-3308.

American Psychiatric Association (2013). *Diagnostic and Statistical Manual of Mental Disorders*, 5th Edition. Arlington, VA: American Psychiatric Association.

Amiri, M., Kabir, A., Nahidi, F., Shekofteh, M., and Ramezani Tehrani, F. (2018). Effects of combined oral contraceptives on the clinical and biochemical parameters of hyperandrogenism in patients with polycystic ovary syndrome: A systematic review and meta-analysis. *The European Journal of Contraception and Reproductive Health Care, 23*(1), 64-77.

Archer, J.S., and Chang, R.J. (2004). Hirsutism and acne in polycystic ovary syndrome. *Best Practice and Research Clinical Obstetrics and Gynaecology, 18*(5), 737-754.

Azziz, R. *et al.*, (2004). The prevalence and features of the polycystic ovary syndrome in an unselected population. *The Journal of Clinical Endocrinology and Metabolism, 89*(6), 2745-2749.

Azziz, R., (2005). Diagnostic criteria for polycystic ovary syndrome: A reappraisal. *Fertility and Sterility, 83*(5), 1343-1346.

Azziz, R. *et al.*, (2006). Criteria for defining polycystic ovary syndrome as a predominantly hyperandrogenic syndrome: An androgen excess society guideline. *The Journal of Clinical Endocrinology and Metabolism, 91*(11), 4237-4245.

Azziz, R., (2008). Polycystic Ovary Syndrome Is a Family Affair. *The Journal of Clinical Endocrinology and Metabolism, 93*(5), 1579–1581.

Azziz, R. *et al.*, (2009). The Androgen Excess and PCOS Society criteria for the polycystic ovary syndrome: the complete task force report. *Fertility and Sterility, 91*(2), 456-488.

Azziz, R., Dumesic, D. and Goodarzi, M. (2011). Polycystic ovary syndrome: An ancient disorder?. *Fertility and Sterility, 95*(5), 1544-1548.

Azziz, R. *et al.*, (2016). Polycystic ovary syndrome. *Nature Reviews Disease Primers 2,* p. 16057.

Azizi, M., and Elyasi, F. (2017). Psychosomatic Aspects of Polycystic Ovarian Syndrome: A Review. *Iranian Journal of Psychiatry and Behavioural Sciences, 11*(2).

Balen, A.H. and Rutherford, A.J. (2007). Managing an ovulatory infertility and polycystic ovary syndrome, *BMJ Publishing group, 335*(7621), 663-666.

Barnard, L., Balen, A.H., Ferriday, D., Tiplady, B., and Dye, L. (2007). Cognitive functioning in polycystic ovary syndrome. *Psychoneuroendocrinology, 32*(8-10), 906-914.

Barry, J.A., Hardiman, P.J., Saxby, B.K., Kuczmierczyk, A. (2011). Testosterone and mood dysfunction in women with polycystic ovarian syndrome compared to subfertile controls. *Journal of Psychosomatic Obstetrics Gynecology, 32,* 104–111.

Barry, J.A., Kuczmierczyk, A.R., and Hardiman, P.J. (2011). Anxiety and depression in polycystic ovary syndrome: A systematic review and meta-analysis. *Hum Reprod*, 26, 2442–2451.

Barry, J.A., Kuczmierczyk, A.R., and Hardiman, P.J. (2014). Reporting the rates of depression in polycystic ovary syndrome (PCOS). *The Journal of Sexual Medicine, 11*(7), 1882-1883.

Bazarganipour, F., Ziaei, S,, Montazeri, A., Foroozanfard, F., Kazemnejad, A., Faghihzadeh, S. (2013). Body image satisfaction and self-esteem status among the patients with polycystic ovary syndrome. *Iran Journal of Reproductive Medicine, 11*(10), 829–36.

Benetti-Pinto, C.L., Ferreira, S.R., Antunes, A., and Yela, D.A. (2015). The influence of body weight on sexual function and quality of life in women with polycystic ovary syndrome. *Archives of Gynecology and Obstetrics, 291*(2), 451-455.

Benson, S., Janssen, O.E., Hahn, S., Tan, S., Dietz, T., Mann, K., Pleger, K., Schedlowski, M., Arck, P.C., and Elsenbruch, S. (2008). Obesity, depression, and chronic low-grade inflammation in women with polycystic ovary syndrome. *Brain Behaviour Immunity, 22*, 177–184.

Benson, S., Hahn, S., Tan, S., Mann, K., Janssen, O.E., Schedlowski, M., and Elsenbruch, S. (2009). Prevalence and implications of anxiety in polycystic ovary syndrome: Results of an internet-based survey in Germany. *Human Reproduction, 24*(6), 1446-1451.

Black, D.W., Blum, N., Pfohl, B., and Hale, N. (2004). Suicidal behaviour in borderline personality disorder: prevalence, risk factors, prediction, and prevention. *Journal of Personality Disorders, 18*(3), 226-239.

Bowling, A. (1995). Measuring disease: A review of disease-specific quality of life measurement scales.

Bowling, A. (2001). Measuring disease: A review of disease-specific quality of life measurement scales. *Philadelphia: Open University Press.*

Buxton, C. and Van de Wiele, R. (1954). Wedge resection for polycystic ovaries: A critical analysis of 40 operations. *New England Journal of Medicine, 251*(8), 293-297.

Canavatchel A. (2014). The experience of stress in women diagnosed with polycystic ovary syndrome. Syracuse University Honours Programme Capstone Projects: Springer, 1-55.

Carr, A.J., Gibson, B., and Robinson, P.G. (2001). Is quality of life determined by expectations or experience? *British Medical Journal, 322* (7296), 1240.

Castillo, Y. (2008). Understanding the social and emotional experiences of females with polycystic ovary syndrome (PCOS). *International Journal Humanities Social Science, 69*, 2154.

Chang, R.J. and Katz, E.S. (1999). Diagnosis of polycystic ovary syndrome. *Endocrinology and Metabolic Clinics of North America, 28*(2), 397-408.

Chen, Z.Z. *et al.*, (2011). Genome-wide association study identifies susceptibility loci for polycystic ovary syndrome on chromosome 2p16. 3, 2p21 and 9q33. 3. *Nature Genetics, 43*(1), 55.

Ching, H.L., Burke, V., and Stuckey, B.G.A. (2007). Quality of life and psychological morbidity in women with polycystic ovary syndrome: Body mass index, age and the provision of patient information are significant modifiers. *Clinical Endocrinology, 66*(3), 373-379.

Chittenden, B.G., Fullerton, G., Maheshwari, A., and Bhattacharya, S. (2009). Polycystic ovary syndrome and the risk of gynaecological cancer: A systematic review. *Reproductive Biomedicine Online, 19*(3), 398-405.

Crete, J., and Adamshick, P. (2011). Managing polycystic ovary syndrome: What our patients are telling us. *Journal of Holistic Nursing, 29*(4), 256-266.

Davari-Tanha, F., Hosseini, Rashidi B., Ghajarzadeh, M., Noorbala, A.A. (2014). Bipolar disorder in women with polycystic ovarian syndrome (PCO). *Acta Med Iran, 52*(1), 46–8.

De Ridder, D., Geenen, R., Kuijer, R., and van Middendorp, H. (2008). Psychological adjustment to chronic disease. *The Lancet, 372*(9634), 246-255.

Deeks, A.A., Gibson-Helm, M.E., Paul, E., Teede, H.J. (2011). Is having polycystic ovary syndrome a predictor of poor psychological function including anxiety and depression? *Hum Reprod, 26*(6), 1399–407.

De Groot, P.C.M., Dekkers, O.M., Romijn, J.A., Dieben, S.W.M., and Helmerhorst, F.M. (2011). PCOS, coronary heart disease, stroke and the influence of obesity: A systematic review and meta-analysis. *Human reproduction update, 17*(4), 495-500.

De Leo, V. *et al.*, 2016. Genetic, hormonal and metabolic aspects of PCOS: An update. *Reproductive Biology and Endocrinology, 14*(1), p. 38.

Deurenberg, P., Deurenberg-Yap, M., Guricci, S. (2002). Asians are different from Caucasians and from each other in their body mass index/body fat per cent relationship. *Obes Rev, 3*(3), 141–6.

Diamanti-Kandarakis, E., Kandarakis, H. and Legro, R., (2006). The role of genes and environment in the etiology of PCOS. *Endocrine, 30*(19), 19-26.

Dixon-Gordon KL, Whalen DJ, Layden BK, *et al.* (2015). A systematic review of personality disorders and health outcomes. *Canadian Psychology (Psychologie Canadienne)*, 56, 168–190.

Dokras, A., Sarwer, D.B., Allison, K.C., Milman, L., Kris-Etherton, P.M., Kunselman, A.R., and Fleming, J. (2016). Weight loss and lowering androgens predict improvements in health-related quality of life in women with PCOS. *The Journal of Clinical Endocrinology and Metabolism, 101*(8), 2966-2974.

Dumesic, D. *et al.*, (2015). Scientific statement on the diagnostic criteria, epidemiology, pathophysiology, and molecular genetics of polycystic ovary syndrome. *Endocrine, 36*(5), 487-525.

Eftekhar, T., Sohrabvand, F., Zabandan, N., Shariat, M., Haghollahi, F., Ghahghaei-Nezamabadi, A. (2014). Sexual dysfunction in patients with polycystic ovary syndrome and its affected domains. *Iran J Reprod Med, 12*(8), 539–46.

Elsenbruch, S., Hahn, S., Kowalsky, D., Offner, A.H., Schedlowski, M., Mann, K., *et al.* (2003). Quality of life, psychosocial well-being, and sexual satisfaction in women with polycystic ovary syndrome. *Journal of Clinical Endocrinology Metabolism, 88*(12), 5801–7.

Evans, T. and Riley, G. (1958). Polycystic Ovarian Disease (Stein-Leventhal Syndrome): Etiology and rationale for surgical treatment. *Obstetrics and Gynecology, 12*(2), 168-178.

Farrell, K., and Antoni, M.H. (2010). Insulin resistance, obesity, inflammation, and depression in polycystic ovary syndrome: biobehavioural mechanisms and interventions. *Fertility and Sterility*, *94*(5), 1565-1574.

Fauser, B.C.J.M., Tarlatzis, B.C., and Rebar, R.W., *et al.* (2012). Consensus on women's health aspects of polycystic ovary syndrome (PCOS): The Amsterdam ESHRE/ASRM-Sponsored 3rd PCOS Consensus Workshop Group. *Fertility and Sterility,* 97, 28–38.

Fauser, B. *et al.*, (2012). Consensus on women's health aspects of polycystic ovary syndrome (PCOS): The Amsterdam ESHRE/ASRM-Sponsored 3rd PCOS Consensus Workshop Group. *Fertility and Sterility, 97*(1), 28-38.

Fearnley, J. (2010). Exponential lower bounds for policy iteration. In *International Colloquium on Automata, Languages, and Programming*: Springer, Berlin, Heidelberg, 551-562.

Forshaw, M., Quick, C.R.G., Hubbard, C.S., and Day, N.E. (2002). Accuracy of serial screening for abdominal aortic aneurysms by ultrasound. *Journal of Medical Screening*, *9*(3), 125-127.

Franks, S. (2006). Diagnosis of polycystic ovarian syndrome: in defense of the Rotterdam criteria. *The Journal of Clinical Endocrinology and Metabolism, 91*(3), 786-789.

Franks, S., McCarthy, M. and Hardy, K., (2006). Development of polycystic ovary syndrome: involvement of genetic and environmental factors. *International Journal of Andrology, 29*(1), 278-285.

Franks, S., Stark, J. and Hardy, K. (2008). Follicle dynamics and anovulation in polycystic ovary syndrome. *Human Reproduction Update, 14*(4), 367-378.

Frankenburg, F.R. and Zanarini, M. (2011) Relationship between cumulative BMI and symptomatic, psychosocial, and medical outcomes in patients with borderline personality disorder. *Journal of Personality Disorders,* 25, 421–431.

Fr, D. and Tarlatzis, R. (2004). Revised 2003 consensus on diagnostic criteria and long-term health risks related to polycystic ovary syndrome (PCOS). *Fertility and Sterility, 81*(1).

Gambineri, A., Pelusi, C., Vicennati, V., Pagotto, U., and Pasquali, R. (2002). Obesity and the polycystic ovary syndrome. *International Journal of Obesity*, *26*(7), 883.

Geist, S. and Gaines, J. (1942). Diffuse luteinization of the ovaries associated with the masculinization syndrome. *American Journal of Obstetrics and Gynaecology, 43*(6), 975-983.

Gorry, A., White, D.M., and Franks, S. (2006). Infertility in polycystic ovary syndrome. *Endocrine*, *30*(1), 27-33.

Gottschau, M., Kjaer, S.K., Jensen, A., Munk, C., and Mellemkjaer, L. (2015). Risk of cancer among women with polycystic ovary syndrome: a Danish cohort study. *Gynecologic oncology*, *136*(1), 99-103.

Guidi, F., Raimondo, S. Di Segni, C., Silvestrini, A., Fato, R., Bergamini, C. and Mancini, A. (2017). Plasmatic and intracellular markers of oxidative stress in normal weight and obese patients with polycystic ovary syndrome. *Experimental and Clinical Endocrinology and Diabetes*, *125*(08), 506-513.

Halbreich, U., and Karkun, S. (2006). Cross-cultural and social diversity of prevalence of postpartum depression and depressive symptoms. *Journal of Affective Disorders*, *91*(2-3), 97-111.

Haoula, Z., Salman, M., and Atiomo, W. (2012). Evaluating the association between endometrial cancer and polycystic ovary syndrome. *Human Reproduction*, *27*(5), 1327-1331.

Harmanci, H., HergÜNer, S., Toy, H. (2013). Polikistik Over Sendromu olan Kadınlarda Psikiyatrik Belirtiler/Psychiatric Symptoms in Women with Polycystic Ovary Syndrome. *Dusunen Adam: The Journal of Psychiatry and Neurological Sciences.*

Hart, R., Hickey, M. and Franks, S. (2004). Definitions, prevalence and symptoms of polycystic ovaries and polycystic ovary syndrome. *Best Practice and Research Clinical Obstetrics and Gynaecology, 18*(5), 671-683.

Hahn, S., Benson, S., Elsenbruch, S., Pleger, K., Tan, S., Mann, K. and Janssen, O.E. (2006). Metformin treatment of polycystic ovary syndrome improves health-related quality-of-life, emotional distress and sexuality. *Human Reproduction*, *21*(7), 1925-1934.

Hillman, S.A. D.J. (2018). Polycystic ovarian syndrome: An under-recognised problem? *British Journal of General Practice, 68*(670), 244.

Himelein, M.J., and Thatcher, S.S. (2006). Polycystic ovary syndrome and mental health: A review. *Obstetrics Gynecology Survey, 61*(11), 723–32.

Hollinrake, E., Abreu, A., Maifeld, M., Van Voorhis, B.J., Dokras, A. (2007). Increased risk of depressive disorders in women with polycystic ovary syndrome. *Fertility and Sterility, 87*(6), 1369–76.

Hussain, A., Chandel, R.K., Ganie, M.A., Dar, M.A., Rather, Y.H., Wani, Z.A., and Shah, M.S. (2015). Prevalence of psychiatric disorders in patients with a diagnosis of polycystic ovary syndrome in Kashmir. *Indian Journal of Psychological Medicine*, *37*(1), 66.

Janssen, O.E., Hahn, S., and Elsenbruch, S. (2006). Psychosocial and quality-of-life consequences of androgen excess and the polycystic ovary syndrome. In *Androgen Excess Disorders in Women,* pp. 343-352, Humana Press.

Janssen, O.E., Mehlmauer, N., Hahn, S., Offner, A.H., and Gartner, R. (2004). High prevalence of autoimmune thyroiditis in patients with polycystic ovary syndrome. *European Journal of Endocrinology*, *150*(3), 363-369.

Jedel, E., Waern, M., Gustafson, D., Landen, M., Eriksson, E., Holm, G., *et al.* (2010). Anxiety and depression symptoms in women with polycystic ovary syndrome compared with controls matched for body mass index. *Human Reproduction, 25*(2), 450–6.

Joshi, B., Mukherjee, S., Patil, A., Purandare, A., Chauhan, S., and Vaidya, R. (2014). A cross-sectional study of polycystic ovarian syndrome among adolescent and young girls in Mumbai, India. *Indian Journal of Endocrinology and Metabolism*, *18*(3), 317.

Kachuei, M., Jafari, F., Kachuei, A., and Keshteli, A.H. (2012). Prevalence of autoimmune thyroiditis in patients with polycystic ovary syndrome. *Archives of Gynecology and Obstetrics*, *285*(3), 853-856.

Kahl, K.G., Greggersen, W., Schweiger, U., *et al.* (2013) Prevalence of the metabolic syndrome in patients with borderline personality disorder: Results from a cross-sectional study. *European Archives of Psychiatry and Clinical Neuroscience,* 263, 205–213.

Keegan, A., Liao, L.M., and Boyle, M. (2003). 'Hirsutism': A psychological analysis. *Journal of Health Psychology*, *8*(3), 327-345.

Keettel, W., Bradbury, J. and Stoddard, F. (1957). Observations on the polycystic ovary syndrome. *Obstetrical and Gynaecological Survey, 12*(5), 721-723.

Khadilkar, S. (2016). Polycystic Ovarian Syndrome: Is It Time to Rename PCOS to HA-PODS? *Journal of Obstetrics and Gynaecology of India, 66*(2), 81-87.

Knochenhauer, E. *et al.*, (1998). Prevalence of the polycystic ovary syndrome in unselected black and white women of the south eastern United States: A prospective study. *The Journal of Clinical Endocrinology and Metabolism, 83*(9), 3078-3082.

Kosari Moghadam, L., Hajloo, N. (2015). Comparison of anxiety, depression and stress in women with and without polycystic ovary syndrome (PCOS). *Int J Rev Life Sci, 5*(5), 249–52.

Krepula, K., Bidzinska-Speichert, B., Lenarcik, A., Tworowska-Bardzinska, U. (2012). Psychiatric disorders related to polycystic ovary syndrome. *Endokrynol Pol, 63*(6), 488–91.

Lam, P. and Raine Fenning, N. (2009). Polycystic ovarian syndrome: a misnomer for an enigmatic disease. *Ultrasound in Obstetrics and Gynecology: The Official Journal of the International Society of Ultrasound in Obstetrics and Gynecology, 33*(6), 621-627.

Lawton, M. (1991). A multidimensional view of quality of life in frail elders. *The Concept and Measurement of Quality of Life in the Frail Elderly.* California, USA: Academic Press, Inc. 4-27.

Learmonth, Y.C., Alwick, E.A., McAuley, E., and Motl, R.W. (2015). Quality of Life and Health-Related Quality of Life over 1 Year in Older Women: Monitoring Stability and Reliability of Measurement. *Social Indicators Research, 123*(1), 267-279.

Lee, J.S. (2015). It's not just physical: The adverse psychosocial effects of polycystic ovary syndrome in adolescents. *Women Health, 3*(1), 20–7.

Legro, R., Kunselman, A., Dodson, W. and Dunaif, A. (1999). Prevalence and predictors of risk for type 2 diabetes mellitus and impaired glucose tolerance in polycystic ovary syndrome: a prospective, controlled study in 254 affected women. *The Journal of Clinical Endocrinology and Metabolism,* 165-169.

Legro, R.S., Driscoll, D., Strauss, J.F., Fox, J., and Dunaif, A. (1998). Evidence for a genetic basis for hyperandrogenemia in polycystic ovary syndrome. *Proceedings of the National Academy of Sciences, 95*(25), 14956-14960.

Leichsenring, F., Leibing, E., Kruse, J., New, A.S., and Leweke, F. (2011). Borderline personality disorder. *The Lancet, 377*(9759), 74-84.

Leventhal, M. and Cohen, M., (1951). Bilateral polycystic ovaries the Stein syndrome. *American Journal of Obstetrics and Gynecology, 61*(5), 1034-1046.

Lewis, P.R., Travers, C.A., Esler, D.M., Guttikonda, K., and Dixon, A. (2007). The psychosocial experience of women with PCOS: A case control study. *Australian Family Physician, 36*(11), 965.

Lipton, G.M., Sherr, L., Elford, J., Rustin, H.A. and Clayton, W.J. (2006). Women living with facial hair: Psychological and behavioural burden. *Journal of Psychosomatic Research*, *61*(2), 161-168.

Lobo, R.A., Granger, L.R., Paul, W.L., Goebelsmann, U., Mishell, D.J. (1983). Psychological stress and increases in urinary norepinephrine metabolites, platelet serotonin, and adrenal androgens in women with polycystic ovary syndrome. *Am J Obstet Gynecol. 145*(4), 496–503.

Lujan, M.E., Jarrett, B.Y., Brooks, E.D., Reines, J.K., Peppin, A.K., Muhn, N., and Chizen, D.R. (2013). Updated ultrasound criteria for polycystic ovary syndrome: reliable thresholds for elevated follicle population and ovarian volume. *Human Reproduction*, *28*(5), 1361-1368.

Månsson, M., Holte, J., Landin-Wilhelmsen, K., Dahlgren, E., Johansson, A., and Landén, M. (2008). Women with polycystic ovary syndrome are often depressed or anxious—A case control study. *Psychoneuroendocrinology*, *33*(8), 1132-1138.

March, W. *et al.*, (2009). The prevalence of polycystic ovary syndrome in a community sample assessed under contrasting diagnostic criteria. *Human Reproduction, 25*(2), 544-551.

McCook, J.G., Bailey, B.A., Williams, S.L., Anand, S., and Reame, N.E. (2015). Differential Contributions of Polycystic Ovary Syndrome (PCOS) Manifestations to Psychological Symptoms. *Journal of Behaviour Health Service Research, 42*(3), 383–94.

McIntyre, R.S., Mancini, D.A., McCann, S., Srinivasan, J., and Kennedy, S.H. (2003). Valproate, bipolar disorder and polycystic ovarian syndrome. *Bipolar Disorders, 5*(1), 28–35.

Michelmore, KF, Balen AH, Dunger DB. (2001). Polycystic ovaries and eating disorders: Are they related? *Human Reproduction, 16*(4), 765–9.

Moran, LJ, Misso ML, Wild RA, *et al.* (2010). Impaired glucose tolerance, type 2 diabetes and metabolic syndrome in polycystic ovary syndrome: A systematic review and meta-analysis. *Human Reproduction Update,* 16, 347–363.

Morgan, C.L., Jenkins-Jones, S., Currie, C.J., and Rees, D.A. (2012). Evaluation of adverse outcome in young women with polycystic ovary syndrome versus matched, reference controls: a retrospective, observational study. *The Journal of Clinical Endocrinology and Metabolism*, *97*(9), 3251-3260.

National Institutes of Health. (2012). *Evidence-based Methodology Workshop on Polycystic Ovary Syndrome,* Maryland: National Institutes of Health.

Navaratnarajah, R., Pillay, O.C., and Hardiman, P. (2008). Polycystic ovary syndrome and endometrial cancer. In *Seminars in Reproductive Medicine, 26*(1), 062-071.

Norman, R., Dewailly, D., Legro, R. and Hickey, T. (2007). Polycystic ovary syndrome. *The Lancet, 370*(9588), 685-697.

Nisar, S., Shah, P.A., Kuchay, M.S., Bhat, M.A., Rashid, A., Ahmed, S., and Ganie, M.A. (2012). Association of polycystic ovary syndrome and Graves' disease: Is autoimmunity the link between the two diseases. *Indian Journal of Endocrinology and Metabolism*, *16*(6), 982.

Ong, K.J., Theodoru, E., and Ledger, W. (2006). Long term consequences of polycystic ovary syndrome. *Current Obstetrics and Gynaecology*, 16, 333-336.

Oláh, K.S. (2004). The modern management of hirsutism. *Reviews in Gynaecological Practice*, *4*(4), 211-220.

Plymate, S., Fariss, B., Bassett, M. and Matej, L. (1981). Obesity and Its Role in Polycystic Ovary Syndrome. *The Journal of Clinical Endocrinology and Metabolism, 52*(6), 1246-1248.

Podfigurna-Stopa, A., Luisi, S., Regini, C., Katulski, K., Centini, G., Meczekalski, B., *et al.* (2015). Mood disorders and quality of life in polycystic ovary syndrome. *Gynaecology Endocrinology*, *31*(6), 431–4.

PoLivy, J., and Herman, C.P. (2002). Causes of eating disorders. *Annual Review of Psychology*, *53*(1), 187-213.

Polson, D., Wadsworth, J., Adams, J. and Franks, S. (1988). Polycystic ovaries: A common finding in normal women. *The Lancet, 331*(8590), 870-872.

Power, M., Bullinger, M., and Harper, A. (1999). The World Health Organization WHOQOL-100: Tests of the universality of quality of life in 15 different cultural groups worldwide. *Health Psychology*, *18*(5), 495.

Rahiminejad, M.E., Moaddab, A., Rabiee, S., Esna-Ashari, F., Borzouei, S., Hosseini, S.M. (2014). The relationship between clinicobiochemical markers and depression in women with polycystic ovary syndrome. *Iran Journal of Reproductive Medicine, 12*(12), 811–6.

Rasgon, N.L., Altshuler, L.L., Fairbanks, L., *et al.* (2005). Reproductive function and risk for PCOS in women treated for bipolar disorder. *Bipolar Disorders*, 7, 246–259.

Rassi, A., Veras, A.B., dos Reis M., Pastore, D.L., Bruno, L.M., and Bruno, R.V., *et al.* (2010). Prevalence of psychiatric disorders in patients with polycystic ovary syndrome. *Comprehensive Psychiatry, 51*(6), 599–602.

Rees A.D., Jones S.J., and Morgan C.L. (2016). Contemporary Reproductive outcomes for Patients with Polycystic Ovary Syndrome: A Retrospective Observational Study. *Journal of Clinical Endocrinology and Metabolism, 101*(4), 1664-1672.

Richardson, M.R. (2003). Current perspective in polycystic ovary syndrome. *American Family Physician*, *68*(4), 697-705.

Sayyah-Melli, M., Alizadeh, M., Pourafkary, N., Ouladsahebmadarek, E., Jafari-Shobeiri M., Abbassi, J., *et al.* (2015). Psychosocial Factors Associated with Polycystic Ovary Syndrome: a Case Control Study. *Journal of Caring Science, 4*(3), 225–31.

Scaruffi, E., Gambineri, A., Cattaneo, S., *et al.* (2014). Personality and psychiatric disorders in women affected by polycystic ovary syndrome. *Frontiers in Endocrinology,* 5, 185.

Shafiee, M.N., Khan, G., Ariffin, R., Abu, J., Chapman, C., Deen, S., and Atiomo, W. (2014). Preventing endometrial cancer risk in polycystic ovarian syndrome (PCOS) women: could metformin help? *Gynecologic Oncology*, *132*(1), 248-253.

Sharma, T.R. (2015). Polycystic ovarian syndrome and borderline personality disorder: 3 case reports and scientific review of literature. *Journal of Psychiatry, 18*(6), 1–4.

Shakerardekani, Z., Nasehi, A., Eftekhar, T., Ghaseminezhad, A., Ardekani, M.A., and Raisi, F. (2011). Evaluation of depression and mental health status in women with poly cystic ovary syndrome. *Journal of Family Reproductive Health, 5*(3), 67–71.

Shoupe, D., Kumar, D. and Lobo, R., (1983). Insulin resistance in polycystic ovary syndrome. *American Journal of Obstetrics and Gynecology, 147*(5), 588-592.

Silva, J.S., Fonseca, A.M., Bagnoli, V.R., Cavalcanti, A.L., Soares, J.J., and Baracat, E.C. (2010). Sexuality in women with polycystic ovary syndrome: a pilot study. *Einstein (Sao Paulo), 8*(4), 397–403.

Sinha, U., Sinharay, K., Saha, S., Longkumer, T.A., Baul, S.N., and Pal, S.K. (2013). Thyroid disorders in polycystic ovarian syndrome subjects: A tertiary hospital based cross-sectional study from Eastern India. *Indian Journal of Endocrinology and Metabolism, 17*(2), 304.

Stein, I. and Cohen, M., (1939). Surgical treatment of bilateral polycystic ovaries—amenorrhea and sterility. *American Journal of Obstetrics and Gynecology, 38*(3), 465-480.

Stein, I. (1958). The Stein-Leventhal syndrome: A curable form of sterility. *New England Journal of Medicine, 259*(9), 420-423.

Stener Victorin, E., Yildiz, B.O., Duleba, A.J., Hoeger, K., Mason, H., and Balen, A. (2011). PCOS Forum: research in polycystic ovary syndrome today and tomorrow. *Clinical Endocrinology, 74*(4), 424-433.

Talbott, E., Guzick, D., Clerici, A., Berga, S., Detre, K., Weimer, K., and Kuller, L. (1995). Coronary heart disease risk factors in women with polycystic ovary syndrome. *Arteriosclerosis, Thrombosis, and Vascular Biology, 15*(7), 821-826.

Tan, S., Hahn, S., Benson, S., Janssen, O.E., Dietz, T., and Kimmig, R., *et al.* (2008). Psychological implications of infertility in women with polycystic ovary syndrome. *Human Reproduction, 23*(9), 2064–71.

Teede, H., Gibson-Helm, M., Norman, R. and Boyle, J., (2014). Polycystic ovary syndrome: Perceptions and attitudes of women and primary health care physicians on features of PCOS and renaming the syndrome. *The Journal of Clinical Endocrinology and Metabolism, 99*(1), E107-E111.

Testa, M., and Simonson, D. (1996). Assessment of quality-of-life outcomes. *The New England Journal of Medicine, 334*, 835-840.

Tomko, R.L., Trull, T.J., Wood, P.K., *et al.* (2014) Characteristics of borderline personality disorder in a community sample: Comorbidity, treatment utilization, and general functioning. *Journal of Personality Disorders*, 28, 734–750.

The Amsterdam ESHRE/ASRM-Sponsored 3rd PCOS Consensus Workshop Group. *Fertility and Sterility,* 97, 28–38e25.

Trent, M.E., Rich, M., Austin, S.B., Gordon, C.M. (2002). Quality of life in adolescent girls with polycystic ovary syndrome. *Arch Pediatr Adolesc,* 156, 556–560.

Vrbikova, J., and Hainer, V. (2009). Obesity and polycystic ovary syndrome. *Obesity Facts*, *2*(1), 26-35.

Weiner, C.L., Primeau, M., and Ehrmann, D.A. (2004). Androgens and mood dysfunction in women: Comparison of women with polycystic ovarian syndrome to healthy controls. *Psychosomatic Medicine*, 66, 356-362.

Wild, R., (2002). Long-term health consequences of PCOS. *Human Reproduction Update,* pp. 231-241.

Xita, N., Georgiou, I., and Tsatsoulis, A. (2002). The genetic basis of polycystic ovary syndrome. *European Journal of Endocrinology*, *147*(6), 717-725.

Yildiz, B. *et al.*, (2012). Prevalence, phenotype and cardiometabolic risk of polycystic ovary syndrome under different diagnostic criteria. *Human Reproduction, 27*(10), 3067-3073.

Zafari-Zangeneh, F., Naghizadeh, M., Abedinia, N., Haghollahi, F., Hezarehei, D. (2012). Psychological signs in patients with polycystic ovary syndrome. *Journal of Family Reproductive Health, 6*(4), 145–51.

13

Psychological and Lifestyle Correlates of Polycystic Ovarian Syndrome

An Overview

Ankita Ojha and *Dhananjay Kumar*

Introduction

Adolescent girls go through a difficult phase during menstrual disturbances. Mostly, they hesitate to discuss about it with their family members, doctor or gynecologist. Thc menstrual cycle involves a series of events by the hypothalamic–pituitary–ovarian axis. It is also affected by many psychological and physiological changes. Menstrual bleeding generally lasts 2 to 7 days in adolescent girls. Most cycles range from 21 to 45 days.

Polycystic ovarian syndrome (PCOS) is an endocrine disorder and believed to be the leading cause of female infertility worldwide (Goldenberg & Glueck, 2008). It affects 5 to 10 per cent of females at the reproductive age (Elsenbruch *et al.,* 2006) however, the rate of PCOS reported in various studies ranges from 2.2 per cent to as high as 26 per cent (Bruce, 2014). It is a heterogeneous syndrome characterized by features of anovulation (amenorrhea, oligomenorrhoea, and irregular cycles) combined with symptoms of androgen excess, e.g., hirsutism, acne, alopecia (Zawadzki & Dunaif, 1992). Amenorrhea is the absence of menstruation or one or more missed menstrual periods. The syndrome gets its name from multiple ovarian follicles, which look like cysts. In a normal menstrual cycle, dominant follicle releases matured egg. In PCOS, several follicles develop, but none of them becomes dominant (Soulez *et al.*, 1996). A polycystic ovary is defined as having 12 or more follicles (or cysts) within the 2-9 mm range under ultrasound (Balen *et al.*, 2009). There will be a lack of ovulation, or the menstrual cycle may be delayed or absent, resulting in subfertility. Stein and Leventhal (1935) were the first to distinguish the reproductive phenomenon that is known as PCOS.

Since 1935, several other symptoms have also been identified such as acne, male pattern balding, hirsutism, infertility, obesity, skin tags, and high androgen hormone levels (Fauser *et al.*, 2004). Most of the symptoms associated with PCOS found to be linked with high either androgen or insulin levels (Abbott *et al.*, 1998, 2002; Xita & Tsatsoulis, 2006). These symptoms were known as "Stein-Leventhal Syndrome" earlier, but the development of new scanning and measuring tools now made it easy to diagnose polycystic ovaries. The syndrome then began to be referred to as 'polycystic ovary syndrome' or 'PCOS' and polycystic ovaries were viewed as the cardinal trait for this syndrome (Balen, 2009; Rosenfield, 1997). These symptoms collectively are example of the broad spectrum of symptoms that are known as 'polycystic ovary syndrome'. This spectrum also entails symptoms that vary from mild to more severe, and some women may only have a few symptoms, while others have more.

After the joint meeting between experts from the European Society for Human Reproduction and Embryology and the American Society for Reproductive Medicine a revised diagnostic criteria for PCOS was opted. These are the so-called 'Rotterdam' criteria. The diagnosis depends on the presence of two of the three following features:

(1) hyperandrogenism (elevated levels of total or unbound hormone blood levels of testosterone), or clinical signs of hirsutism (excessive male patterned hair growth),
(2) intermittent or absent menstruation, and
(3) Polycystic ovaries visualized by ultrasound (Fauser *et al.*, 2004; Rotterdam, 2004).

Developmental Origin of PCOS

Studies suggest that there is an underlying predisposition to the typical ovarian abnormalities that would have been origins well before the onset of puberty. The probability is that the ovary is genetically predisposed to hypersecrete androgen, resulted condition of the activation of hypothalamic-pituitary axis, either in early post-natal life or at puberty (or indeed both). The consequences of this increased exposure to androgen include abnormalities of LH secretion, and insulin secretion and action, which will be manifested during adolescence (Abbott, Dumesic & Franks, 2002; Franks, McCarthy & Hardy, 2006). Normal puberty and adolescence are characterized by a physiological increase in insulin resistance along with an increase in serum concentrations of fasting insulin (Hannon,

Janosky & Arslanian, 2006). There will be a resultant fall in sex hormone-binding globulin, driven by higher brain centres and it is further amplify the effects of sex steroids. Insulin also has a direct gonadotropic action on ovarian steroidogenesis. These events are part of the normal cadence of puberty and provide a mechanism by which nutritional status can influence reproductive development. Higher than normal insulin levels, whether due to a genetic predisposition or excessive weight gain (or both), would be expected to exaggerate these potentially adverse effects (Franks, 2002).

Interaction of Genes and Environment in Etiology of PCOS

Genetic factors: There is now compelling evidence that genetic factor is important in the etiology of PCOS. There is familial clustering of cases and, significantly, a greater concordance of symptoms of PCOS in identical twins compared to non-identical twins (Franks & McCarthy, 2004; Vink, Sadrzadeh, Lambalk & Boomsma, 2006). There is also evidence for heritability of endocrine and metabolic features of PCOS (Legro, Bentley-Lewis, Driscoll, Wang & Dunaif, 2002). The more likely proposition is that PCOS is a complex endocrine disorder involving more than one, and probably several genes (Stewart, Dombroski, Urbanek, Ankener, Ewens & Wood *et al.*, 2006).

Obesity: Serves as both a symptom and a contributory factor and is associated with the worsening of other symptoms. The average proportion of overweight/obese subjects in the study was 35–40 per cent (Franks, 1995, 1989). Accumulating evidences suggest that overweight/obesity amplifies the clinical severity of PCOS and increases the risk of metabolic dysfunction. Increasing obesity gives rise to a disproportionate prevalence of metabolic abnormalities. Researchers argued that PCOS is a lifestyle disease in which genetic predispositions may in fact be activated by lifestyle factors (Balen *et al.*, 2009; Ehrmann, 2005; Franks, 1995).

PCOS in India

Media accounts have suggested that PCOS is on the rise in India and most common among the urban middle and upper classes because of their lifestyles (e.g., Garari, 2014; Pal, 2013; *Times of India*, 2012). The prevalence of obesity, overweight, and insulin resistance, which are all associated with PCOS pathogenesis, appears to be higher among members of higher socioeconomic strata living in urban areas. Medical researchers have attributed this to more sedentary lifestyles and access to more calorie-dense foods (Chopra *et al.*, 2013; Kalra & Unnikrishnan, 2012; Khandelwal & Reddy, 2013,). Although there have been no rigorous community-based epidemiological studies of PCOS published in India to date, a preliminary study among women aged 15-24 from the lower socioeconomic strata in Mumbai placed prevalence at near 22.5 per cent (around one in four women) (Joshi *et al.*, 2014). The study further observed that in other metabolic disorders and nutritional and physical activity patterns, this prevalence might be even higher among the higher socioeconomic strata. This contrast markedly seen with a prevalence of around 11 per cent in Australia, 8 per cent in the UK, and 4 per cent in the US (Wijeyaratne *et al.*, 2013). Irregular menstrual cycles and subfertility have long been of considerable concern in India (e.g., Leslie, 1996). Observations of several practitioners indicated that PCOS was rapidly increasing among urban middle-and upper-class women but now, increase also seen among women from the urban lower classes, and those who are living in urbanizing semi-rural areas.

Environmental, Occupational and Lifestyle Factors in PCOS

Kshetrimayum, Sharma, Mishra and Kumar (2019) conducted a review on environmental, occupational, lifestyle factors affect PCOS. It could have been linked with host factors (endogenous) and exogenous factors like lifestyle, and dietary, environmental or occupational factors. Genetic/host and environmental/lifestyle factors might be related to the pathophysiology of PCOS after prenatal exposure to androgen. March *et al.* (2010) drew attention to the important issue of PCOS non-diagnosis in the community and mentioned that about 68 per cent of women with PCOS had not been tested for PCOS in the past. The hazard factors of PCOS comprised menstrual cycle impairment, bad mood, and family history of diabetes, infertility in the family, mother menstrual irregularity and physical exercise deficiency. Srivastava, Bala and Verma (2018) conducted a study to know the association between socio-demographic factors and psychological distress levels among PCOS sufferers. One hundred fifty patients with PCOS recruited from various hospitals of Allahabad city and 150 controls of same age group were selected from university campus, girl's hostels and localities of Allahabad. The findings of the study revealed that PCOS subjects coming from high-income group to middle-income group manifested moderate to severe neurotic symptoms. Most of the severe neurotic patients were from highly educated group however, they were not employed anywhere. A significantly higher number of women in the PCOS group reported a family history of diabetes and some had a self-history of diabetes. In comparison to this, no women were diabetics in the control group (Moini *et al.*, 2009). The presence of type 2 diabetes in women with PCOS, suggests that body mass index, glucose, and sex hormone-binding globulin levels are connected to the risk factors of PCOS (Gambineri *et al.*, 2012).

Trace and Heavy Metals in Women with PCOS: Other studies well advocates that environmental factors might play an important role in deteriorating reproductive health including environmental toxins, diet and nutrition, socioeconomic status, and geography. Industrial chemicals may also contribute to unveil PCOS characteristics in genetically susceptible individuals (Palioura *et al.*, 2013). Human body needs some metals in trace quantities for various physiologically essential functions. These metals are called essential trace metals. Some studies aimed to investigate the role of these essential trace and heavy metals in human subjects with PCOS. Serum copper, and zinc concentrations were found to be significantly higher, whereas manganese and lead values were lower in subjects with PCOS. It appears that metals such as copper and nickel might be linked in the causation of PCOS and with impairment of reproductive hormone levels (Zheng *et al.*, 2015). The relationship between hormonal impairments and the fluctuation of trace element (manganese), macro elements (magnesium and calcium), and heavy metals such as cadmium, and lead in both obese and non-obese subjects with PCOS was studied. They were significantly found to be related with the subjects with PCOS (Mhaibes *et al.*, 2017). Taher and Mhaibes (2017) reported that serum copper and nickel levels were considerably elevated in subjects with PCOS, whereas the concentration of serum zinc was declined in subjects with PCOS (obese and non-obese) in comparison with controls (obese and non-obese). The data on lifestyle, diet, and some metals suggest that these factors may also have some role in the occurrence of PCOS phenotypic symptoms and weight management. Healthy lifestyle and regular exercise might be beneficial in the reduction of PCOS linked features in young adult girls.

Modern Lifestyles and PCOS

"Modern" market-driven urban middle-class lifestyles association with PCOS is relatively recent to India. There is a shift in nutrition intake with a tendency to consumption of more fats, oils, and sugars (Griffiths & Bentley, 2001; Nagesh, 2012). Increased access to helping devices and vehicles reduced physical activity. Resulting increased risk factors escalated the prevalence of diabetes and cardiovascular disease among India's middle classes, especially in urban areas (Celermajer *et al.*, 2012; Khandelwal & Reddy, 2013). Increased opportunities for urban middle-class women in terms of employment, jobs requiring educational achievement, occupation of important social, economic, and symbolic position (Radhakrishnan, 2009), the public visibility and their freedom to pursue careers is considered markers of new middle-class identity (Gangulye Scrase, 2003). However, domestic tasks, child-rearing, and household tasks seen as the responsibility of women, they must take on the responsibility of being modern without foregoing the traditional. Therefore, increased opportunities for middle-class women place additional burdens upon them. Students face high degrees of parent supervision for several activities such as socializing, television viewing, or play. Eating is the only sanctioned source of pleasure preferably junk food and sugary things. New work structures result in very little time for exercise, skipped or late lunches (at 4 or 5 pm), long hours, and late dinners (up to 11 pm). At the same time, new communications technologies, such as email and mobile phones, allow individuals to be constantly accessible for work.

Dietary Factors: Exposure to dietary factors has been linked with the appearance of PCOS in girls who are susceptible to PCOS. Weight gain and obesity worsen the characteristic features of PCOS, whereas weight loss, reduces the characteristic features of PCOS (Moran *et al.*, 2010). The appropriate weight loss through lifestyle change, regulate menstrual cycle in women with PCOS. A moderate diet with carbohydrates, poly- and mono-unsaturated fats, and a high content of fiber with lean protein sources, reported to be beneficial to overall health parameters in women with PCOS. Further, the exercise in daily life showed a positive effect on the clinical representations of PCOS (Krystock *et al.*, 2014).

The clinical and biochemical abnormality is increased by overweight and obesity (Franks, 1995; Ehrmann, 2005). Approximately 300 women with PCOS observed on different measures and it was found that the prevalence of hirsutism and ovulatory dysfunction was significantly greater in overweight and obese women than in lean subjects (Kiddy *et al.* & Bray *et al.*, 1990), leading to higher concentrations of free testosterone. Nevertheless, total testosterone is also positively correlated with BMI, (Conway, Honour & Jacobs, 1989; Conway & Jacobs, 1993) probably reflecting the effect of insulin on theca cell androgen production. Smyka, Grzechocińska, and Wielgoś (2017), found that a change in lifestyle, well-balanced diet and physical activity are the most effective medical way contributing to weight reduction, which reactivates regular ovulation and facilitates getting pregnant. Vitamin D supplementation as well as inosital is of great importance as well. Adding them to a daily diet contributes to improving carbohydrate metabolism and reducing insulin resistance. Additionally, they accelerate weight loss, regulate menstrual cycles and enhance reinstating regular ovulation.

The increasing prevalence of overweight and obesity in children has given rise to numerous concerns about short and longer-term effects. Overweight and obese girls with PCOS have at least a threefold increase in risk of developing type-2 diabetes in later life and, alarmingly impaired glucose tolerance (IGT), and even overt diabetes, have been reported in teenagers with PCOS (Palmert, Gordon, Kartashov, Legro, Emans, & Dunaif, 2002). Another alarming, but not all together unexpected, finding from the northern Finland cohort study, was that girls who were obese at the age of 14 were very likely to be obese at age 31; those who were obese at age 14 had a greater chance of developing symptoms of PCOS in at age 31. The highest free androgen index was found in adults who were obese at the age of 14 (Laitinen, Taponen, Martikainen, Pouta, Millwood & Hartikainen *et al.*, 2003).

Psychological Factors Related with PCOS

Many psychological symptoms have been correlated with PCOS, however it is still unclear that, whether these factors have only correlation or they have at least some causal role in PCOS. Most studies have shown only correlation of psychological factors with PCOS, but some studies have investigated the causal role also, although the number is little, but they are able to demonstrate that there are some evidences that suggested the causal role of psychogenic factors in the PCOS. Some studies are able to demonstrate that these psychological factors will have a mediating effect or a role to aggravate the symptoms of PCOS.

Lorencatto and associates (2006) study to compare the prevalence of depression in women surgically diagnosed with endometriosis into the conditions of presence or absence of pelvic pain. Hundred women were sampled receiving care at the outpatient's clinic for endometriosis, from Sao Paulo, Brazil. The Beck Depression Inventory used in order to measure depression. Depression detected in 86 per cent and 38 per cent of the women with and without chronic pelvic pain respectively. Complaints of depression, such as somatic concerns, work inhibition, dissatisfaction, and sadness, observed at a significantly higher rate in the group with pain.

To investigate the psychological difference between women with symptomatic as compared to asymptomatic mild endometriosis, Waller *et al.* (1995) conducted a study on 44 women with minimal or mild endometriosis. A group of normal controls and another group with complaints of pelvic pain having no organic pathology studied also. Women with pelvic pain symptoms, whether they had mild endometriosis or a normal pelvis, scored similar on the Beck Depression Inventory. These scores were significantly higher in comparison to those of women with asymptomatic disease and normal women. According to the findings of several studies in this area, 28 per cent to 64 per cent of patients with PCOS had depression (Scaruffi *et al.*, 2014). Compared to the healthy population; bipolar patients experience mental and physical issues (Davari-Tanha *et al.*, 2014).

Depression has been associated with increased cortisol levels, increased sympathetic activity and decreased serotonin levels in the central nervous system. These features also associated with insulin resistance (Hollinrake *et al.*, 2007). Depression is about twice as common in people with diabetes compared with healthy individuals and treating depression can improve glucose control, although this is not a consistent finding (Brown, 2004). Roos *et al.,* (2007) reported the relationship between insulin resistance and psychiatric distress in PCOS group.

Açmaz *et al.* (2013) studied depression, anxiety, low self-esteem, and social worry by classifying PCOS according to symptoms. The first group consisted of 86 patients diagnosed with PCOS and the second group consisted of 47 healthy volunteers. Depression scores of infertile group found to be higher while anxiety scores of the obese group were found to be higher than other groups. It was the obesity group, which received the lowest score in self-esteem and trust in people and the highest score in sensitiveness to criticism. The most affected group was oligomenorrhoea-hirsutism group in terms of physical functioning, physical role function, pain, social functioning, emotional role function, and emotional well-being.

Personality and PCOS

Tan, Grigg and Kulkarni (2018) conducted a review to identify the common etiological mechanism of borderline personality disorder (BPD) and PCOS. The literature suggested that women with (BPD) had higher than expected serum androgen levels and incidence of polycystic ovaries, which can be key features of polycystic ovary syndrome.

Scaruffi *et al.*, (2019) assess personality characteristics, body image, and alexithymia in women with PCOS. Fifty-nine women with PCOS and 38 healthy controls were administered the tests. The PCOS group showed higher values of alexithymia and a higher body uneasiness. They also showed higher values on many clinical, content, and supplementary scales of the Minnesota Multiphasic Personality Inventory-2. It seems that physical appearance and bodily functions have a central place in the minds of women with PCOS, as well as in their relationships. However, it is their body, they find it hard to feel and, with which they mostly feel uncomfortable. Their approach to the outside world seems to be characterized by a certain degree of immaturity, anger, hostility, and distrust. Low self-esteem also seems to be connected to a certain tendency toward introversion and, withdrawal. This leads to problems in social, professional, and intimate relationships.

Dag, Oguzturk, Isik, Turkel & Bulcun (2015), investigated the personality traits of patients with polycystic ovary syndrome. Forty-nine patients with PCOS and 34 healthy controls enrolled in the study. Psychometric evaluation made with the Minnesota Multiphasic Personality Inventory. Additionally, Short Form-36 (SF-36), Hospital Anxiety and Depression Scale (HADS) were also performed. Polycystic ovary syndrome patients had significantly higher, absolute and clinical elevation scores on depression, hysteria, psychasthenia and hypomania compared with the controls. Patients with PCOS had lower SF-36, physical and mental health summary scores, and higher HADS anxiety and depression subscale scores. Polycystic ovary syndrome patients seem to have depressive, hysterical, psychasthenic and hypomanic personality traits.

Scaruffi, Gambineri, Cattaneo, Turra, Vettor & Mioni (2014) investigated relationship of hyper-androgenic syndrome with psychopathological personality. Sixty PCOS subjects were evaluated on anthropometric, metabolic, hormonal, clinical, and psychological parameters. The Rorschach test (Exner's comprehensive system) and the Millon Clinical Multiaxial Inventory-III (MCMI-III) were also administered to each patient. Results evidenced the prevalence of personality disorders and other psychopathology in patient group [schizoid, depressive, sadistic, negativistic (passive–aggressive), and masochistic, avoiding, dependent, histrionic, narcissistic, obsessive–compulsive], in various degrees and further, anxiety, somatoform disorder and bipolar disorder, and major depressive disorder. Finally, they found delusional disorder and thought disorder. Rorschach test's results show 53.1 per cent reduced coping abilities and social skills, 55.1 per cent depression, 30.6 per cent perceptual distortion and cognitive slippage, 24.5 per cent constantly alert and worry, 8.1 per cent at risk for suicide, and finally about 50 per cent of patients had chronic stress.

Psychosomatic Aspects of Polycystic Ovarian Syndrome

To know the psychosomatic linkage with polycystic ovarian syndrome, Azizi and Elyasi (2017) did a review. It was concluded that a number of disorders are associated with PCOS, including impaired body image and body dissatisfaction, eating disorder, sexual dysfunction, and reduced quality of life. Based on a tendency to use helplessness, self-blame, and accepting responsibility, which are unwillingly applied in their daily life that are mostly characterize as emotion focused coping. Compared to problem-focused coping emotion focused coping strategies are considered as passive methods. These passive patterns of patients with PCOS in response to stressful situations may play a primary role in developing psychosomatic disorders (Lobo RA *et al.*, 1983; Özenl Y *et al.*, 2009). Bensona *et al.* (2009) conducted a study to know neuroendocrine and immune cell responses to psychosocial stress in PCOS subjects. Results suggested that in response to public speaking stress, both groups showed significant, but comparable increases in state anxiety, and blood pressure. The ACTH and cortisol stress responses were significantly enhanced in PCOS. In addition, heart rate was significantly higher in PCOS subjects. PCOS patients were characterized by increased psychological distress. Further, these patients showed enhanced HPA-axis and heart rate reactivity as well as a reduced up regulation of IL-6 in response to stress. The altered stress reactivity in PCOS patients may constitute a link between depressions, overweight, and the cardiovascular and diabetes risks associated with the diagnosis. Jansen *et al.*, (2008), also concluded that PCOS is associated with psychosocial problems, including chronic stress, depression, social fears, and reduced quality-of-life. Psychological factors likely to contribute to the development, progression, and maintenance of fat accumulation, (Pasquali *et al.*, 2006). Zangeneh *et al.* (2012) conducted a study in which 81 patients with PCOS were recruited. The descriptive results showed that 9.9 per cent participants did not have any signs of stress, 39.5 per cent had neurotic stress, 35.8 per cent had high and 14.8 per cent showed extremely high levels of stress. The high levels of anxiety with hirsutism, obsession in overweight patients, high levels of worries in patients with touchy personality were found to be related with PCOS group.

Bajpai, Mishra and Ghai (2015) found in their study that PCOS group reported irregular menstruation, obesity, infertility, acne and hair growth on the face, chest, and back (hirsutism) and ovarian cysts. Some have Type 2 diabetes and most of them have effects of androgenic (masculinizing) hormones. Serum insulin levels were significantly higher in subjects having PCOs. Androgens, specifically testosterone, and often less estrogen and progesterone than normal were also found. Many other associated health problems such as dyslipidemia, autoimmune thyroiditis, high blood pressure were present among the patient group.

Elsenbruch et al. (2003), investigated the impact PCOS of health-related quality of life and sexuality. Patients showed greater disturbances on the dimensions of obsessive-compulsive, interpersonal sensitivity, depression, anxiety, aggression, and psychoticism, along with a lower degree of life satisfaction scales of health, self, and sex. Health related quality of life revealed significantly decreased scores for physical role function, bodily pain, vitality, social function, emotional role function, and mental health in patients with PCOS. Although patients had the same partner status and frequency of sexual intercourse, they were significantly less satisfied with their sex life and found themselves less attractive. Most of the differences were not affected by correction for body weight. In conclusion, PCOS causes a major reduction in the quality of life and severely limits sexual satisfaction.

Gul, Gul, Ergur, & Ozen, (2018) examined the relationship between anger and anxiety in adolescents with PCOS compared to the healthy controls. Twenty-eight adolescents with PCOS and 16 healthy adolescents were recruited to the study. Results indicated that anxiety and anger types, except for internalized anger, were higher and anger control was lower in adolescents with PCOS than controls. In addition, state and trait anxiety were negatively associated with anger control in adolescents with PCOS, while there were no such associations in healthy controls. They demonstrated that, there was a unique relationship between anxiety and anger in adolescents with PCOS than controls.

Conclusion

The review brought many factors in focus related with PCOS that need to further verification. Based on this body of knowledge new researches can also be planned to investigate the correlating as well as the causal link of lifestyle and psychological factors with PCOS. Like other chronic diseases, PCOS have also a mediating link of HPA axis and involvement of autonomic nervous system as well as lifestyle and dietary habits. Thus, the present authors are of opinion that studies should be planned towards investigating the psychogenic origin of PCOS. In addition, this literature will also help to the counselors who are actively engaged in counseling of distress and other psychological condition.

References

Abbott D.H., Dumesic D.A., and Franks S. (2002). Developmental origin of polycystic ovary syndrome—A hypothesis. *Journal of Endocrinology,* 174, 1–5.

Abbott, D.H., D.A. Dumesic, J.R. Eisner, R.J. Colman, and J.W. Kemnitz, (1998). Insights into the Development of Polycystic Ovary Syndrome (PCOS) from Studies of Prenatally Androgenized Female Rhesus Monkeys. *Trends in Endocrinology and Metabolism, 9*(2), 62-67.

Açmaz, G., Albayrak, E., Acmaz, B., Başer, M., Soyak, M., Zararsız, G., and İpekMüderris, İ. (2013). Level of anxiety, depression, self-esteem, social anxiety, and quality of life among the women with polycystic ovary syndrome. *The Scientific World Journal*, Hindawi Publishing Corporation, Article ID 851815, 7 pages http://dx.doi.org/10.1155/2013/851815.

Azizi, M., and Elyasi, F. (2017). Psychosomatic aspects of polycystic ovarian syndrome: A review. *Iranian Journal of Psychiatry and Behavioural Science, 11*(2), e6595.

Bajpai, P., Mishra, S., and Ghai, S. (2015). Effect of Stress and Anxiety on Polycystic Ovarian Syndrome and related health problems in Chhattisgarh women. *International Journal of Researches in Social Science and Information Studies* (*IJRSSIS*), Volume-I, Issue-III *Online Journal* ISSN No. 2347-8268.

Balen, A., R. Homburg, and S. Franks (2009). Defining Polycystic Ovary Syndrome. *BMJ* (*Clinical Research Ed.*) 338.

Balen, Adam, Homburg, Roy, Franks, Stephen (2009). Defining polycystic ovary syndrome. *British Medicine Journal,* 338 (7692), 426.

Benson, S., Arck, P.C., Tan, S., Hahn, S., Mann, K., Rifaie, N. and Elsenbruch, S. (2009). Disturbed stress responses in women with polycystic ovary syndrome. *Psychoneuroendocrinology*, *34*(5), 727-735.

Brown, A.J. (2004). Depression and insulin resistance: applications to polycystic ovary syndrome. *Clinical Obstetrics and Gynecology*, *47*(3), 592-596.

Bruce LA., (2014). Body mass and depression among Mississippi women with polycystic ovarian syndrome. The University of Southern Mississippi.

Celermajer, D.S., Chow, C.K., Marijon, E., Anstey, N.M., and Woo, K.S. (2012). Cardiovascular disease in the developing world: Prevalences, patterns, and the potential of early disease detection. *Journal of the American College of Cardiology*, *60*(14), 1207-1216.

Chopra, S., Misra A., Gulati, S., Gupta R. (2013). Overweight, obesity and related noncommunicable diseases in Asian Indian girls and women. *European Journal of Clinical Nutrition,* 67 (7), 1-9.

Conway, G.S., and Jacobs, H.S. (1993). Clinical implications of hyperinsulinaemia in women. *Clinical Endocrinology*, *39*(6), 623-632.

Conway, G.S., Honour, J.W., and Jacobs, H.S. (1989). Heterogeneity of the polycystic ovary syndrome: Clinical, endocrine and ultrasound features in 556 patients. *Clinical Endocrinology*, *30*(4), 459-470.

Davari-Tanha, F., Hosseini, R.B., Ghajarzadeh, M., and Noorbala, A.A. (2014). Bipolar disorder in women with polycystic ovarian syndrome (PCO). *Acta Med Iran*, *52*(1), 46–8.

Ehrmann, D.A. (2005). Polycystic ovary syndrome. *New England Journal of Medicine,* 352, 1223–1236.

Elsenbruch S., Benson S., Hahn S., Tan S., Mann K., Pleger K. *et al.* (2006). Determinants of emotional distress in women with polycystic ovary syndrome *Hum Reprod; 21*(4): 1092-9.

Elsenbruch, S., Hahn, S., Kowalsky, D., Öffner, A.H., Schedlowski, M., Mann, K., and Janssen, O.E. (2003). Quality of life, psychosocial well-being, and sexual satisfaction in women with polycystic ovary syndrome. *The Journal of Clinical Endocrinology and Metabolism*, *88*(12), 5801-5807.

Fauser, B.C.J.M., Tarlatzis, Fauser, Chang, Aziz, Legro, Dewailly, Franks, Balen, Bouchard, Dahlgren, Devoto, Diamantı, Dunaif, Filicori, Homburg, Ibanez, Laven, Magoffin, Nestler, Norman, Pasquali, Pugeat, Strauss, Tan, Taylor, Wild, Wild, Guzik, Ehrmann, and Lobo (2004). Revised 2013 Consensus on Diagnostic Criteria and Long-Term Health Risks Related to Polycystic Ovary Syndrome. *Human Reproduction, 19*(1), 41-47.

Franks S. (2002). Adult polycystic ovary syndrome begins in childhood. *Best Practice Research Clinical Endocrinology Metabolism,* 16, 263–272.

Franks S., McCarthy MI., Hardy K. (2006). Development of polycystic ovary syndrome: involvement of genetic and environmental factors. *International Journal of Andrology,* 29, 278–285.

Franks, S. (1989). Polycystic ovary syndrome: A changing perspective. *Clinical Endocrinology,* 31, 87–120.

Franks, S. (1995). Polycystic ovary syndrome. *New England Journal of Medicine,* 333, 853–861.

Gambineri A., Patton L., Altieri P., Pagotto U., Pizzi C., Manzoli L., *et al.* (2012). Polycystic ovary syndrome Is a risk factor for Type 2 diabetes. Results from a long-term prospective study. *Diabetes*, 61, 2369-74.

Ganguly-Scrase, R. (2003). Paradoxes of globalization, liberalization, and gender equality: The worldviews of the lower middle class in West Bengal, India. *Gender and Society*, *17*(4), 544-566.

Garari, Kaniza. (2014). PCOSd All You Need to Know. *Asian Age,* Jun 30.

Goldenberg, N., Gleuck, C., (2008). Medical therapy in women with polycystic ovarian syndrome before and during pregnancy and lactation. *Minerva Ginecol.* 60 (1), 63-75.

Griffiths, P.L., and Bentley, M.E. (2001). The nutrition transition is underway in India. *The Journal of Nutrition, 131*(10), 2692-2700.

Gul, A., Gul, H., Ergur, A.T., and Ozen, N.E. (2018). Anxiety-anger relationship in hyperandrogenemia: A comparative study with polycystic ovary syndrome (PCOS) and healthy control adolescents. *Psychiatry and Behavioural Sciences, 8*(1), 27.

Hannon, T.S., Janosky, J., and Arslanian, S.A. (2006). Longitudinal study of physiologic insulin resistance and metabolic changes of puberty. *Pediatric Research, 60*(6), 759-763.

Hollinrake, E., Abreu, A., Maifeld, M., Van Voorhis, B.J., and Dokras, A. (2007). Increased risk of depressive disorders in women with polycystic ovary syndrome. *Fertility and Sterility, 87*(6), 1369-76.

Janssen, O.E., Hahn, S., Tan, S., Benson, S., and Elsenbruch, S. (2008, January). Mood and sexual function in polycystic ovary syndrome. In *Seminars in Reproductive Medicine*, 26, (1), 045-052.

Joshi, B., Mukherjee, S., Patil, A., Purandare, A., Chauhan, S., and Vaidya, R. (2014). A cross-sectional study of polycystic ovarian syndrome among adolescent and young girls in Mumbai, India. *Indian Journal of Endocrinology and Metabolism, 18*(3), 317.

Kalra, S., and Unnikrishnan, A.G. (2012). Obesity in India: The weight of the nation. *Journal of Medical Nutrition and Nutraceuticals, 1*(1), 37.

Khandelwal, S., and Reddy, K. (2013). Eliciting a policy response for the rising epidemic of Overweight Obesity in India. *Obes. Rev. 14 (Suppl. 2),* 114-125.

Khandelwal, S., and Reddy, K.S. (2013). Eliciting a policy response for the rising epidemic of overweight–obesity in India. *Obesity Reviews, 14*, 114-125.

Kiddy, D.S., Sharp, P.S., White, D.M., Scanlon, M.F., Mason, H.D., Bray, C.S., and Franks, S. (1990). Differences in clinical and endocrine features between obese and non-obese subjects with polycystic ovary syndrome: An analysis of 263 consecutive cases. *Clinical Endocrinology, 32*(2), 213-220.

Krystock, A. (2014). Role of lifestyle and diet in the management of polycystic ovarian syndrome. In *Polycystic Ovary Syndrome,* pp. 147-164, Springer, New York, NY.

Kshetrimayum, C., Sharma, A., Mishra, V.V., and Kumar, S. (2019). Polycystic ovarian syndrome: Environmental/occupational, lifestyle factors; an overview. *Journal of the Turkish German Gynecological Association, 20*(4), 255.

Laitinen, J., Taponen, S., Martikainen, H., Pouta, A., Millwood, I., Hartikainen, A.L., and Järvelin, M.R. (2003). Body size from birth to adulthood as a predictor of self-reported polycystic ovary syndrome symptoms. *International Journal of Obesity, 27*(6), 710-715.

Legro, R.S., Bentley-Lewis, R., Driscoll, D., Wang, S.C., and Dunaif, A. (2002). Insulin resistance in the sisters of women with polycystic ovary syndrome: Association with hyperandrogenemia rather than menstrual irregularity. *Journal of Clinical Endocrinology Metabolism,* 87, 2128–2133.

Leslie, J. (2014). *Myth and Mythmaking: Continuous Evolution in Indian Tradition.* Routledge.

Lobo, R.A., Granger, L.R., Paul, W.L., Goebelsmann, U., and Mishell, D.J. (1983). Psychological stress and increases in urinary norepinephrine metabolites, platelet serotonin, and adrenal androgens in women with polycystic ovary syndrome. *American Journal of Obstetrics Gynecology, 145*(4), 496-503.

Lorencatto, C., Alberto Petta, C., José Navarro, M., Bahamondes, L., and Matos, A. (2006). Depression in women with endometriosis with and without chronic pelvic pain. *Acta Obstetricia et gynecologica Scandinavica, 85*(1), 88-92.

March, W.A., Moore, V.M., Willson, K.J., Phillips, D.I., Norman, R.J., and Davies, M.J. (2010). The prevalence of polycystic ovary syndrome in a community sample assessed under contrasting diagnostic criteria. *Human Reproduction, 25*(2), 544-551.

Mhaibes, S.H., Taher, M.A., and Badr, A.H. (2017). A Comparative study of blood levels of manganese, some macroelements and heavy metals in obese and non-obese polycystic ovary syndrome patients. *Iraqi Journal of Pharmaceutical Sciences, 26*(2), 85-94.

Moini, A., and Eslami, B. (2009). Familial associations between polycystic ovarian syndrome and common diseases. *Journal of Assisted Reproduction and Genetics, 26*(2-3), 123-127.

Moran, L.J., Lombard, C.B., Lim, S., Noakes, M., and Teede, H.J. (2010). Polycystic ovary syndrome and weight management. *Women's Health, 6*(2), 271-283.

Nagesh, B. (2012). The food and grocery market. *Business World Marketing White book* 2012e2013. ABP, New Delhi, 187-205.

Ozcan Dag̀, Z., Oguzturk, O., Isik, Y., Turkel, Y., and Bulcun, E. (2015). Personality profile in patients with polycystic ovary syndrome. *Gynecological Endocrinology, 31*(7), 540-542.

Özenl, Y., Haydardedeoğlu, B., Mıcozkadioğlu, İ., Şımşek, E., Kiliçdağ, E.B., and Bağiş, T. (2009). Anxiety, Depression and Ways of Coping Skills by Women with Polycystic Ovary Syndrome: A Controlled Study. *Journal of the Turkish-German Gynecological Association, 10*(4).

Pal, Somita. (2013). PCOS Hitting the Young. Daily News and Analysis, Mar 8.

Palioura, E., and Diamanti-Kandarakis, E. (2013). Industrial endocrine disruptors and polycystic ovary syndrome. *Journal of Endocrinological Investigation, 36*(11), 1105-1111.

Palmert, M.R., Gordon, C.M., Kartashov, A.I., Legro, R.S., Emans, S.J., and Dunaif, A. (2002). Screening for abnormal glucose tolerance in adolescents with polycystic ovary syndrome. *The Journal of Clinical Endocrinology and Metabolism, 87*(3), 1017-1023.

Pasquali, R., and Gambineri, A. (2006). Insulin-sensitizing agents in polycystic ovary syndrome. *European Journal of Endocrinology, 154*(6), 763-775.

Pasquali, R., Vicennati, V., Cacciari, M., and Pagotto, U. (2006). The hypothalamic-pituitary-adrenal axis activity in obesity and the metabolic syndrome. *Annals of the New York Academy of Sciences, 1083*(1), 111-128.

Radhakrishnan, S. (2009). Professional women, good families: Respectable femininity and the cultural politics of a "new" India. *Qualitative Sociology*, *32*(2), 195-212.

Roos C., Lidfeldt J., Agardh CD., Nyberg P., Nerbrand C., Samsioe G., *et al.* (2007). Insulin resistance and self-rated symptoms of depression in Swedish women with risk factors for diabetes: The Women's Health in the Lund Area study. *Metabolism, 56*(6), 825-9.

Rosenfield, R.L., (1997). Current Concepts of Polycystic Ovary Syndrome. *Baillière's Clinical Obstetrics and Gynaecology, 11*(2), 307-333.

Rotterdam, I. (2004). Revised 2003 consensus on diagnostic criteria and long-term health risks related to polycystic ovary syndrome (PCOS). *Hum Reproduction, 19*, 41-47.

Scaruffi, E., Franzoi, I.G., Civilotti, C., Guglielmucci, F., La Marca, L., Tomelini, M. and Granieri, A. (2019). Body image, personality profiles and alexithymia in patients with polycystic ovary syndrome (PCOS). *Journal of Psychosomatic Obstetrics and Gynecology*, *40*(4), 294-303.

Scaruffi, E., Gambineri, A., Cattaneo, S., Turra, J., Vettor, R., and Mioni, R. (2014). Personality and psychiatric disorders in women affected by polycystic ovary syndrome. *Frontiers in Endocrinology*, *5*, 185.

Smyka, M., Grzechocińska, B., and Wielgoś, M. (2017). The role of lifestyle changes in the treatment of polycystic ovary syndrome. *Neuroendocrinology Letters*, *38*(8).

Soulez, B., Dewailly, D., and Rosenfield, R.L. (1996). Polycystic Ovary Syndrome: A Multidisciplinary Challenge. *The Endocrinologist*, *6*(1), 19-29.

Srivastava, R., and and Anisha Verma, N.B. (2018). Psychological distress levels and its relationship with Socio-demographic factors of polycystic ovarian syndrome population in Allahabad city. *Journal of Pharmacognosy and Phytochemistry*, *7*(6), 92-96.

Stewart, D.R., Dombroski B.A., Urbanek, M., Ankener W., Ewens K.G., Wood, J.R. *et al.* (2006). Fine mapping of genetic susceptibility to polycystic ovary syndrome on chromosome 19p13.2 and tests for regulatory activity. *Journal of Clinical Endocrinology Metabolism,* 91, 4112–4117.

Taher, M.A., and Mhaibes, S.H. (2017). Assessment of some trace elements in obese and non-obese polycystic ovary syndrome (PCOS). *International Journal of Science and Research*, *6*(9), 1333-1341.

Tan, R.Y., Grigg, J., and Kulkarni, J. (2018). Borderline personality disorder and polycystic ovary syndrome: A review of the literature. *Australian and New Zealand Journal of Psychiatry*, *52*(2), 117-128.

Times of India, (2012). Modern Lifestyle Increases PCOS Cases. *Times of India*, Jan 20.

Vink, J.M., Sadrzadeh, S., Lambalk, C.B., and Boomsma, D.I. (2006). Heritability of polycystic ovary syndrome in a Dutch twin-family study. *The Journal of Clinical Endocrinology and Metabolism*, *91*(6), 2100-2104.

Waller, K.G. and Shaw, R.W. (1995). Endometriosis, pelvic pain, and psychological functioning. *Fertility and Sterility*, *63*(4), 796-800.

Wijeyaratne, C.N., Dilini Udayangani, S.A., and Balen, A.H. (2013). Ethnic-specific polycystic ovary syndrome: Epidemiology, significance and implications. *Expert Review of Endocrinology and Metabolism*, *8*(1), 71-79.

Xita, N., and A. Tsatsoulis. (2006). Review: Fetal Programming of Polycystic Ovary Syndrome by Androgen Excess: Evidence from Experimental, Clinical, and Genetic Association Studies. *Journal of Clinical Endocrinology and Metabolism, 91*(5), 1660-1666.

Zangeneh, F.Z., Jafarabadi, M., Naghizadeh, M.M., Abedinia, N., and Haghollahi, F. (2012). Psychological distress in women with polycystic ovary syndrome from Imam Khomeini Hospital, Tehran. *Journal of Reproduction and Infertility*, *13*(2), 111.

Zawadzki, J., and Dunaif, A. (1992). Diagnostic criteria for polycystic ovary syndrome: towards a more rational approach. *Polycystic Ovary Syndrome*, 377-384.

Zheng, G., Wang, L., Guo, Z., Sun, L., Wang, L., Wang, C. and Qiu, H. (2015). Association of serum heavy metals and trace element concentrations with reproductive hormone levels and polycystic ovary syndrome in a Chinese population. *Biological Trace Element Research*, *167*(1), 1-10.

14

Down to the Roots

Understanding the Mental Health of Women with Post-Menstrual Syndrome (PMS)

Akansha Pandey and *Anubhuti Dubey*

Introduction

The women of 21st century are outperforming men in many sectors of work and life. They are consistently trying to be free from the bondage of male dominance and establishing themselves with their own identity. Meanwhile, all these women are seen with an eye in almost every endeavour of theirs and hence this proves the apt time to discuss what changes a woman goes through every month with their menstrual cycle which takes the hold of their physical as well as psychological build.

Menstrual cycle is a normal process that females go through as their bodies prepare themselves for potential pregnancy. It is a part of this monthly menstrual cycle that occurs in the female reproductive system and makes pregnancy possible. The reproductive age for women lasts for about 30 years which begins with their puberty and the menopause marks its end. This age of fertility comes with a roller coaster ride of various health issues for the women. The WHO assessed in 2008 that reproductive and sexual ill-health accounts for 20 per cent of the global burden of ill-health for women and 14 per cent for men. There exist various reproductive health issues which a woman may face in her life such as Endometriosis, Uterine Fibroids, Sexually Transmitted Diseases, Polycystic Ovary Syndrome (PCOS), Premenstrual Syndrome (PMS), etc.

Before the onset of the menstrual cycle, women experience a lot of changes in them commonly referred as premenstrual changes. These changes can be positive as well as negative. The positive changes are often overlooked and it includes increase in energy efficiency and better performances at times. Premenstrual symptoms have been a part of normal ovulatory cycle and for majority of women these symptoms are so mild that they act as mere markers of their onset of menstrual cycles. But for a considerable proportion of women, these symptoms get so grave to interfere with, their psychic and physical wellbeing. The term 'Premenstrual syndrome' are reserved for such group of women for whom these premenstrual changes are adverse and also sustains for a sufficient duration to impair their activities in almost all the sectors of life.

Premenstrual Syndrome (PMS) is a common health problem associated with women in their reproductive age. It is a cluster of physical as well as emotional symptoms that appear on a regular basis before the onset of menstrual bleeding. There are several psychological features that characterize the occurrence of PMS in an individual and it includes anger, irritability, anxiety, stress (Deuster, Adera, & South-Paul; 1999), depressed mood, oversensitivity, difficulty in concentration as well as social withdrawal. Besides these, it is marked by the several physical symptoms like acne, headache, bloating, fatigue, weight gain, food cravings, and appetite change and breast tenderness. It often marks various severe symptoms like mood swings, irritability and anxiety with the greatest impairment in the home/family domain (Vichnin, Freeman, Lin, Hillman & Bui, 2006). These physical and emotional symptoms can be severe enough to impair various aspects of women's life.

Premenstrual dysphoric disorder (PMDD) is a severe, sometimes disabling extension of premenstrual syndrome (PMS). Although regular PMS and PMDD both have physical and emotional symptoms, Premenstrual dysphoric disorder causes extreme mood shifts that can disrupt the work and damage the relationships. The preponderance of this extreme condition is not as much as PMS; rather 8 to 10 per cent of women all across put up with such maximal conditions.

In both PMDD and PMS, symptoms usually begin seven to ten days before the period starts and continue for the first few days that women have their period. Both of these disorders lead to some common physical and psychological issues such as bloating, breast tenderness, fatigue, and changes in sleep and eating habits. However, premenstrual dysphoric disorder establishes itself with at least one of the emotional and behavioural symptoms standing majestically out to ruin the condition even more. These symptoms can be Sadness or Hopelessness, Anxiety or Tension, Extreme Mood swings, Excessive irritability or Anger.

Majority of the female population experience these premenstrual changes during their reproductive age. The pervasiveness of PMS is much higher than that of PMDD. Various researchers affirm this postulate in various parts of the world be it India (Banerjee, Roy & Takkar, 2000), Europe (Wittchen, Becker, Lieb & Krause, 2002), Canada, USA, Nigeria (Ogebe, Abdulmalik, Mojeed, Holder, Jones, Ogun & Omigbodun, 2011) and Japan (Takeda, Tasaka, Sakata & Murata, 2006). The prevalence of PMS or PMDD was meta-analyzed and the results show that prevalence of PMS is highest in Asia and lowest in Europe (Moghadam, Sayehmiri, Delpisheh & Kaikhavandi, 2014). Nevertheless, PMS or PMDD is still under-recognized in large published epidemiological studies, as well as assessments of burden of the disorder.

This monthly recurrence of hormonal variations gulfs the life of women into two different non-identical beings, especially for those who are in the catch of PMS or PMDD. It not only compels them to feel physical pain from mild to severe rather it also holds the entire behavioural aspect of them. Number of researches have already affirmated the disaster such cohorts go through. Halbreich, Borenstein, Pearlstein, & Kahn (2003) explored the extent of impact of PMS as well as PMDD and found that the impairment and lowered quality of life for PMDD is similar to that of dysthymic disorder and is not much lower than major depressive disorder. This disorder not only interrupts social activities of the person but also decreases educational productivity and even impairs family relations. A strong and consistent relationship exist between the symptoms of PMS and interference in quality of life of women in almost all the spheres of her life (Nisar, Zehra, Haider, Munir & Sohoo, 2007). Therefore, the recognition and identification of the symptoms becomes a necessity and demands a treatment which may otherwise interfere with the daily living of the individual.

The etiology of PMS or PMDD remains unexplored and the emphasis is entirely upon the after effects of these disorders wherein what issues such women go through while experiencing these life traumatizing symptoms. It has been generally told that these disorders may lead to various physical as well as psychosocial consequences but this isn't a one way mirror unlike other disorders. It has been found that past as well as present history of some psychiatric disorders also leads to severe exacerbation of premenstrual symptoms as the severity ascends then (Severino, Hurt & Shindledecker; 1989). Kornstein et al. (2005) also validated this notion by observing an induced exacerbation of premenstrual tension in the women suffering from major depressive disorders. The researchers have amplified the situation to the extent whereby it was also found that the prevalence of such symptoms can be frequently seen in women who are less educated and has past depression history (Cohen, Soares, Otto, Sweeney, Liberman & Harlow, 2002).

This paper reviews all the psychological assaults be it emotional, social, familial, marital as well as negative self-evaluation that a woman confronts while she is dealing with a enormous menstrual pain and trying hard to put everything in place with her life.

Extent of Emotional Ramification

Various streams of studies were focused upon the emotional states of women pre- or peri-menstrual. As already mentioned, PMS as well as PMDD induce varied emotional assaults marking from mood shifts to anxiety or depression. Eggert, Witthöft, Hiller and Kleinstäuber (2016) found that women with PMS employ emotional dysfunctional strategies and negative affective reaction when compared to non-PMS group. Harsher emotional state of the woman may indicate the grave symptoms. The severity of Premenstrual syndrome depends upon the appraisal of the situation (Wu, Lian, Wang, Zhao & Zhou, 2016). Wu and associates in their study on Chinese women found that the greater and habitual use of cognitive reappraisal in everyday life was related to a less experience of premenstrual symptoms, especially emotion-related symptoms. Whereas, the suppression of emotions as a habitual practice led to various premenstrual symptoms such as tension and insomnia. Some researchers even suggest that not only the premenstrual phase but throughout the menstrual cycle, women develop stress sensitivity and this induces the severe perception of symptoms (Ossewaarde, Hermans, Van, Kooijman, Johansson, Bäckström, & Fernández, 2010). Gonda *et al.* (2010) mentioned in their study that women with more premenstrual symptomatology have a trait-like negative bias in perception of life events which may play a significant role in the experience and emergence of PMS or PMDD and this negative biased perception may even worsen the symptoms further. That is to say if one is agonized with the harsh symptomatology of this disorder, she develops an inclination towards negative evaluation of the world around.

Another stream of studies has proved the role of altered timing of Cortisol (our body's main stress hormone) secretion which segregates women with PMS/PMDD from others (Parry, Laughli, Hauge & Clopton, 2000). Cortisol works with parts of our brain to control our mood, motivation and fear. And hence an altered timing of this hormone tends to affect the responsiveness of the individual regarding any observed situation. A very recent study by Izadi & Amiri (2019) reveals that the existence of Premenstrual syndrome or Premenstrual dysphoric disorder is synchronous to the trait of neuroticism in such women. These grounds the presence of negative like attitude and difficulty in coping with the stress perceived during those days. This perceived stress in turn enhances the severity of the symptomatology and when combined together, they tend to impair the cognitive appraisal of such cohorts.

Cognitive Repercussions

Women with PMS are found to be affected and impaired not only physiologically but cognitively as well (Rapkin, Chang & Reading, 1989). The symptomatic conditions in PMS influences the retrieval capabilities of the individual to the extent in which she may encode the information well but could not access them easily (Keenan, Lindamer & Jong, 1995) and this dissociation of memory performance prevails throughout the cycle in every hormonal state.

Resnick, Perry, Parry, Mostofi and Udell (1998) investigated the impact of severity of PMDD on various neuro-cognitive tasks and found that there does not exist any discernable difference between the performances of women with or without PMDD on any such tasks rather they observed mere slowing down of neuro-cognitive performance. They reasoned this poor performance as the outcome of negative self-evaluation during those days because of depressive states. Thus, they neglected the poor capabilities of women with PMS/PMDD in areas of attention, memory or verbal learning aspects. This work received affirmation from another work of Man, MacMillan, Scott and Young (1999). In contrast to this, a recent study of Reed, Levin and Evans (2008) supports the conviction of cognitive impairment as they established it with their research work and adduced that women with PMDD performed significantly poorer than the control women on various psychomotor tasks during their luteal phase. Besides, Yen, Chang, Long, Tang, Chen and Yen (2012) not only explored the poorer cognitive performance due to Working memory deficit in women with PMDD but also established that this cognitive deficit further leads to irritability as well as difficulty in concentrating during their luteal phase. This shows that the women with Premenstrual dysphoric disorder lives a difficult phase of life when dealing with such severe symptomatic influences. Altered cognitive abilities not only decrease their intellectual and memory performances rather they also impact the self-regulation of emotions (Schmeichel, Volokhov & Demaree, 2008), hence making it difficult for the such women sustain a sound life having experiencing those manifestations.

The gravity of this concern lies here where it was found that recipient of PMS/PMDD gradually fall victim to their lack of educational productivity. Soares, Cohen, Otto and Harlow (2001) provided a conceivable explanation that women with PMDD and a life history of depression may have suffered greater functional impairment which resulted in lower educational level, thus impacting the intellectual living thereafter.

Social Aftermath

A major proportion of our life is indulged in society and social interactions whether it is a work place or the institution we are the part of. Premenstrual syndrome pulls the strings of productivity of the cohorts in addition to its other impacts. Women with PMS have to deal with social, interactional and economical ramifications apart from their emotional intrusions. PMS can be seen muddling the life in different phases, be it the absenteeism from schools, colleges or the work places. The productivity of these corps were found impaired in their school as well as office works upto 50 per cent and was also seen to be significantly attached with the increase in intensity of the symptoms (Dean & Borenstein, 2004). Even this impacts the social interaction and relationships of the individual. Robinson and Swindle (2000) have distinctly shown the level of interference and influence of symptom burden has on different domains like household activities, school or work productivity, social life and relationship with husband and kids. It is easily comprehensible that women with PMS or PMDD tend to suffer in all these domains the most in comparison to their non-affected counterparts. Various retrospective and prospective studies have verified that the relationship issues of such individual increases with the increase in the severity of the symptoms. Thus, the emerging picture clarifies that apart from emotional disturbance this PMS or PMDD condition adds to the productivity loss and occupational absenteeism. Izadi and Amiri (2019) when tried to establish relation between this etiology and the personality traits found that these women with premenstrual syndrome or premenstrual dysphoric disorder tend to score low on the trait of agreeableness. This trait reflects personality characteristics such as kind, sympathetic, cooperative and social harmony which shows that such women manifest lesser of these desirable traits in turn providing ample support to the fact of social withdrawal and seclusion. Eissa (2010) discerned the presence of elevated perfectionist thinking concurrent with the severity of these symptoms. This perfectionism is inclined towards self-sacrifice and excessively unfavourable comparison with others whereby women tend to perceive negatively the errors in the task or unresolved relationship issues and feeling alone. The same study also concluded that the presence of these symptoms was negatively correlated with the social support perceived by them. That is to say, if provided with ample support maybe from society or their family or even the partner, such women would be able to evaluate themselves positively during these days of sheer need of affection and support.

Dismantling Relationships

The gravity of consequences which PMS or PMDD furnishes the individual with can be seen in the form of marital dissatisfaction which is reported not only by the women suffering from these but also their partners. A number of women with PMS reported higher on amount of conflicts and lesser emotional expressiveness in family than the non-PMS counterparts (Kuczmierczyk, Labrum & Johnson, 1992). In a prospective study (Robinson & Swindle, 2000) women were found to be reporting that the interference of premenstrual syndrome was much high with their personal bond or relationship which they share with their husband and also the kids. They seemed to accept that apart from all other world known impacts of PMS, their interpersonal relationship which defines their personal world suffers the most. These findings gain validation from another study by Brown and Zimmer (1986) who found that not only females but also their male partners can feel this premenstruum symptomatology and in order to deal with them they seek different coping strategies from supporting their partner, expressing anger, seeking outside help or avoiding the partner to seeking counselling. The study emerged with several themes underlying it which are increased conflicts, decreased family participation in enjoyable or social tasks, damaged cohesion among family members and friction in relationships. Many instances of men reacting with physical abuse or anger or hitting the women can also be seen, whereas some of the partners were also found seeking more information regarding these problems. The potential of destruction that can be caused by these syndromes can be vividly visualized by higher number of divorce seeking partners which disrupts the entire family system (Cortese & Brown, 1989).

Contemporary Perspective

Everything till now is just one side of the coin. When we are headed to understand the mental health of these women we need to flip it and discover the underlying concerns. An entirely distinct point of view for all these situations has also been provided. It is already established that premenstrual changes are negotiated to be distressing by some females i.e., it is not PMS that causes distress rather it is the distress itself that is appraised as an exacerbation of such symptoms and this appraisal depends upon the relationship the lady shares (Jones *et al.,* 2000).

Ussher (1999, 2000) described the occurrence of PMS as not fixed rather through the interaction of materials, discursive and intra-psychic factors which includes hormonal changes, cultural construction of the reality and evaluation of the self respectively. Women reported that the changes which they were experiencing became problematic only when expressed outside and hence attributed as PMS. Number of studies addressed the relationship issues such as marital dissatisfaction influencing PMS. Kuczmierczyk, Labrum and Johnson (1992) found that women with PMS scored lesser on expressiveness of their emotions in the family. This is because expressing that anger and panics lead to relationship deterioration, and hence the female suppresses all those to herself. The expected groomed personality with all the responsibilities tend to ruin her situation more as this is once in the month she could not idealize the feminine expectations thus causing self-pathology (Ussher, 2003). While accounting for premenstrual distress in lesbian couple Ussher and Perz (2008) found that none of those women expressed or considered themselves as 'monstrous feminine' or 'loony tune' or 'mad' which was very common feeling among the women in a heterosexual relationship as the society has already framed the criteria of women being caring, responsible and loving whereas angry, anxious and irritated ones are bad. This exhibits that the positioning of PMS is entirely different for a lesbian relationship. The openness to communicate, getting support from the partner, awareness of the partner regarding the situation the other one is going through and using a positive tone to deal with the premenstrual changes helped women to accept themselves with no attempts to lead an unrealistic idealized life. Thus, such women showed lesser symptom of premenstrual distress as they had more openness to talk with and could focus on self-care and can avoid self-guilt as well as self-blame. Women who possess a negative attitude towards PMS or PMDD were found to seek lesser medical attention (Robinson & Swindle, 2000). This negative attitude was no where related to the severity of the symptoms rather it felt as if other factors are inhibiting them from coming front and discussing their health issues. It may be they feel embarrassed or consider it as their personal weakness that they do not want to reveal or discuss such grave issues and over the time they fall in accepting these traumatizing symptoms as the part of their daily life.

SUPPORT: The Need of the Hour

The aforementioned studies distinctly clarifies that PMS or PMDD is not only biological or psychological pathogenesis rather the cultural context plays the equally important role in its expression. For years, the women alone have been attributed for the manifestation of this symptomatology but the contribution of the society they live in, the family they live in or the partner they live with has been no less. It is the time that women must be given a voice among their significant others to express about the changes they are going through rather than just overburdening them with their gender roles and responsibilities.

The aspect of emotional regulation during PMS or PMDD shows that if women are provided with ample support to assess the situations of their life as well as during those menstrual cycles positively, then they can manage their symptoms efficiently and even the extent of severity of PMS would be less. In other words, if women could be taught or enabled to assess and appraise their circumstances cognitively then they can supervise their own intense or mild symptoms.

It was found that female with PMS or PMDD exhibit less of agreeableness trait in comparison to mild or non sufferers. This can be fixed by providing extra social and moral support to them. If greater support is added to high agreeableness, this may result to lower exacerbation of PMDD symptom severity.

Psychosocially, life events such as problems in family and work life can make a woman more susceptible to hormonal changes and thus play a part in causing variations in premenstrual symptoms. The familial expectations and relationships prove to be essential in determining PMS. Therefore, not only the women must be the core concern of intervention rather the entire family must be considered for it. Moreover, if those women accept their fallibility of this once in a month and free themselves from all the superwomen expectations then definitely they may grab some time for themselves enabling better dealing with this condition. Besides, the family members must also accept her during all her ups and downs of her life and must provide an environment to her free enough to talk about her hard times.

Conclusion

The existence of premenstrual changes in women makes them prone to a number of unruly situations which not only affect their mental peace but also their significant others. It interferes with their occupational functioning and dealing with others to an extent that their daily life cohesion gets disturbed. This review presented the emotional, social, interpersonal torments these women experience during their premenstrual or perimenstrual phase of life. It could be clearly seen that the severity of the symptoms which these women experience, possess a direct relation with the support and reverence the people in their life give to them. Because, when not able to deal with all the expectations simultaneously that this world loads on them, they develop the feeling of self-pathologization which turns them down or irritate them. Hence, the family members, especially the partners own the liability of being there for them and understand them in such difficult times.

References

Banerjee, N., Roy, K.K., and Takkar, D. (2000). Premenstrual dysphoric disorder—A study from India. *International Journal of Fertility and Women's Medicine*, *45*(5), 342-344.

Brown, M.A., and Zimmer, P.A. (1986). Personal and family impact of premenstrual symptoms. *Journal of Obstetric, Gynecologic, and Neonatal Nursing*, *15*(1), 31-38.

Cohen, L.S., Soares, C.N., Otto, M.W., Sweeney, B.H., Liberman, R.F., and Harlow, B.L. (2002). Prevalence and predictors of premenstrual dysphoric disorder (PMDD) in older premenopausal women: the Harvard Study of Moods and Cycles. *Journal of Affective Disorders*, *70*(2), 125-132.

Cortese, J., and Brown, M.A. (1989). Coping responses of men whose partners experience premenstrual symptomatology. *Journal of Obstetric, Gynaecologic, and Neonatal Nursing*, *18*(5), 405-412.

Dean, B.B., and Borenstein, J.E. (2004). A prospective assessment investigating the relationship between work productivity and impairment with premenstrual syndrome. *Journal of Occupational and Environmental Medicine*, *46*(7), 649-656.

Deuster, P.A., Adera, T., and South-Paul, J. (1999). Biological, social, and behavioural factors associated with premenstrual syndrome. *Archives of Family Medicine*, *8*(2), 122.

Direkvand-Moghadam, A., Sayehmiri, K., Delpisheh, A., and Kaikhavandi, S. (2014). Epidemiology of premenstrual syndrome (PMS)—A systematic review and meta-analysis study. *Journal of Clinical and Diagnostic Research: JCDR*, *8*(2), 106.

Eggert, L., Witthöft, M., Hiller, W., and Kleinstäuber, M. (2016). Emotion regulation in women with premenstrual syndrome (PMS): Explicit and implicit assessments. *Cognitive Therapy and Research*, *40*(6), 747-763.

Eissa, M. (2010). Personality and psychosocial factors affecting premenstrual syndrome. *Current Psychiatry*, *17*(1), 55-62.

Gonda, X., Fountoulakis, K.N., Csukly, G., Telek, T., Pap, D., Rihmer, Z., and Bagdy, G. (2010). Association of a trait-like bias towards the perception of negative subjective life events with risk of developing premenstrual symptoms. *Progress in Neuro-Psychopharmacology and Biological Psychiatry*, *34*(3), 500-505.

Halbreich, U., Borenstein, J., Pearlstein, T., and Kahn, L.S. (2003). The prevalence, impairment, impact, and burden of premenstrual dysphoric disorder (PMS/PMDD). *Psychoneuroendocrinology*, *28*, 1-23.

Izadi, M., and Amiri, S. (2019). Personality characteristics in female students with premenstrual dysphoric disorder and premenstrual syndrome. *Advances in Nursing and Midwifery*, *28*(3), 40-45.

Keenan, P.A., Lindamer, L.A., and Jong, S.K. (1995). Menstrual phase-independent retrieval deficit in women with PMS. *Biological Psychiatry*, *38*(6), 369-377.

Kornstein, S.G., Harvey, A.T., Rush, A.J., Wisniewski, S.R., Trivedi, M.H., Svikis, D.S. and Harley, R. (2005). Self-reported premenstrual exacerbation of depressive symptoms in patients seeking treatment for major depression. *Psychological Medicine*, *35*(5), 683-692.

Kuczmierczyk, A.R., Labrum, A.H., and Johnson, C.C. (1992). Perception of family and work environments in women with premenstrual syndrome. *Journal of Psychosomatic Research*, *36*(8), 787-795.

Man, M.S., MacMillan, I., Scott, J., and Young, A.H. (1999). Mood, neuropsychological function and cognitions in premenstrual dysphoric disorder. *Psychological Medicine*, *29*(3), 727-733.

Nisar, N., Zehra, N., Haider, G., Munir, A.A., and Sohoo, N.A. (2008). Frequency, intensity and impact of premenstrual syndrome in medical students. *J Coll Physicians Surg Pak*, *18*(8), 481-4.

Ogebe, O., Abdulmalik, J., Bello-Mojeed, M.A., Holder, N., Jones, H.A., Ogun, O.O., and Omigbodun, O. (2011). A comparison of the prevalence of premenstrual dysphoric disorder and comorbidities among adolescents in the United States of America and Nigeria. *Journal of Paediatric and Adolescent Gynaecology*, *24*(6), 397-403.

Ossewaarde, L., Hermans, E.J., van Wingen, G.A., Kooijman, S.C., Johansson, I.M., Bäckström, T., and Fernández, G. (2010). Neural mechanisms underlying changes in stress-sensitivity across the menstrual cycle. *Psychoneuroendocrinology*, *35*(1), 47-55.

Parry, B.L., Javeed, S., Laughlin, G.A., Hauger, R., and Clopton, P. (2000). Cortisol circadian rhythms during the menstrual cycle and with sleep deprivation in premenstrual dysphoric disorder and normal control subjects. *Biological Psychiatry*, *48*(9), 920-931.

Rapkin, A.J., Chang, L.C., and Reading, A.E. (1989). Mood and cognitive style in premenstrual syndrome. *Obstetrics and Gynaecology*, *74*(4), 644-649.

Reed, S.C., Levin, F.R., and Evans, S.M. (2008). Changes in mood, cognitive performance and appetite in the late luteal and follicular phases of the menstrual cycle in women with and without PMDD (premenstrual dysphoric disorder). *Hormones and Behaviour*, *54*(1), 185-193.

Resnick, A., Perry, W., Parry, B., Mostofi, N., and Udell, C. (1998). Neuropsychological performance across the menstrual cycle in women with and without premenstrual dysphoric disorder. *Psychiatry Research*, *77*(3), 147-158.

Robinson, R.L. and Swindle, R.W. (2000). Premenstrual symptom severity: Impact on social functioning and treatment-seeking behaviours. *Journal of Women's Health and Gender-based Medicine*, *9*(7), 757-768.

Schmeichel, B.J., Volokhov, R.N., and Demaree, H.A. (2008). Working memory capacity and the self-regulation of emotional expression and experience. *Journal of Personality and Social Psychology*, *95*(6), 1526.

Severino, S.K., Hurt, S.W., and Shindledecker, R.D. (1989). Spectral analysis of cyclic symptoms in late luteal phase dysphoric disorder. *American Journal Psychiatry*, *146*(9), 1155-1160.

Soares, C.N., Cohen, L.S., Otto, M.W., and Harlow, B.L. (2001). Characteristics of women with premenstrual dysphoric disorder (PMDD) who did or did not report history of depression: A preliminary report from the Harvard Study of Moods and Cycles. *Journal of Women's Health and Gender-based Medicine*, *10*(9), 873-878.

Takeda, T., Tasaka, K., Sakata, M., and Murata, Y. (2006). Prevalence of premenstrual syndrome and premenstrual dysphoric disorder in Japanese women. *Archives of Women's Mental Health*, *9*(4), 209-212.

Ussher, J.M. (2003). The ongoing silencing of women in families: An analysis and rethinking of premenstrual syndrome and therapy. *Journal of Family Therapy*, *25*(4), 388-405.

Ussher, J.M., and Perz, J. (2008). Empathy, egalitarianism and emotion work in the relational negotiation of PMS: The experience of women in lesbian relationships. *Feminism and Psychology*, *18*(1), 87-111.

Vichnin, M., Freeman, E.W., Lin, H., Hillman, J., and Bui, S. (2006). Premenstrual syndrome (PMS) in adolescents: severity and impairment. *Journal of Paediatric and Adolescent Gynaecology*, *19*(6), 397-402.

Wittchen, H.U., Becker, E., Lieb, R., and Krause, P. (2002). Prevalence, incidence and stability of premenstrual dysphoric disorder in the community. *Psychological Medicine*, *32*(1), 119-132.

Wu, M., Liang, Y., Wang, Q., Zhao, Y., and Zhou, R. (2016). Emotion dysregulation of women with premenstrual syndrome. *Scientific Reports*, *6*, 38501.

Yen, J.Y., Chang, S.J., Long, C.Y., Tang, T.C., Chen, C.C., and Yen, C.F. (2012). Working memory deficit in premenstrual dysphoric disorder and its associations with difficulty in concentrating and irritability. *Comprehensive Psychiatry*, *53*(5), 540-545.

Yonkers, K.A., O'Brien, P.S., and Eriksson, E. (2008). Premenstrual syndrome. *The Lancet*, *371*(9619), 1200-1210.

15

From Private to Public

Marital Conflicts, Litigation and Psychological Distress in Women

Aparna Joshi, Amrita Joshi, Ipsita Chatterjee, Chinmayee Kantak and *Anushree Puntambekar*

Introduction

The institution of marriage is regarded as "a social, religious, spiritual, and/or legal union of individuals…in which interpersonal relationships (usually intimate and sexual) are acknowledged by the state, by religious authority, or both" (Dhar, 2013, p. 1). Indian marriage systems create organisational hierarchies built on age, gender and extended family precedence (Sonpar, 2005), where power often rests with the husband and his family. Further, the perceived permanence of marriage does not permit separation due to marital instability (Mullatti, 1995).

In the Indian context, a majority of marriages are arranged marriages (Banerji, Martin & Desai, 2013). Arranged marriages are preferred over love marriages in the Indian society since they preserve the norms of partner selection as well as family ideals. A study conducted by Allendorf and Pandian (2016) notes that arranged marriages are strongly linked majorly to endogamy of caste, and sometimes to consanguinity of marriage. However, mis marriages, which are love marriages permitted and arranged by elders, are being increasingly permitted lately (Mahapatro, Gupta & Gupta, 2012).

Marriage and Marital Conflicts

Research on marriage and individual well-being in the western countries has consistently reported that married individuals experience better psychological health than unmarried individuals (Kim & McKenry, 2002).

Proulx, Helms and Buehler (2007) found that in addition to marital status, marital quality and psychological well-being, too, were positively related, indicating that better marital quality is associated with greater individual well-being.

One of the primary indicators of marital quality is marital conflict (Stanley, 2007). Marital conflicts are widely accepted as a natural part of marital interactions and in fact considered healthy (Ashford, LeCroy, & Lortie, 2006). However, while some conflicts are avoidable and healthy, there arises a problem in the Indian context, as Indian marriage systems are based on the norms of patriarchy and collectivism. This results in the creation of organisational hierarchies built on age, gender and extended family precedence (Sonpar, 2005). In these patriarchal systems, power rests with the husband and his family, while the wife remains subservient (Fernandez, 1997).

Subsequently, marital conflicts too are found to have gendered patterns. Common causes for conflicts in marriage found in the West are, the wife not complying to traditional expectations about division of labour, alcohol consumption by the husband, and due to the wife being educationally more qualified than her husband (Hotaling & Sugarman, 1990). In addition to all this, marital conflicts can also stem from personal characteristics and behaviours of the spouse, unequal burden of household chores, differences of opinion relating to financial expenditures and extra-dyadic relationships by either spouse. Women, especially, report their husband's jealousy and unnecessary financial expenditures as stressors that lead to conflict between the couple (Fincham, 2003). Studies have found that women who hold more egalitarian gender role beliefs report higher marital instability than those who held more traditional gender role beliefs (Guilbert, Vacc & Pasley, 2000; Heise, 1998). Walker (2009) suggests that in traditional gendered marriages, gender roles are neatly aligned with patriarchal belief patterns. Therefore, when women comply with their traditional gender roles, they meet the husband's expectations of an ideal wife.

Western literature has indicated that marital discord has also been found to be an indicator for possible violence meted against women (Coleman & Strauss, 1986). However, in India violence is systemic and structural at the hands of family. Owing to large-scale presence of patriarchy, violence is typically directed towards the woman at the hands of all family members including the partner (Fernandez, 197; Sonpar, 2005).

Domestic Violence against Women

In the Western societies, intimate partner violence in heterosexual marriages largely occurs majorly at the hands of the husband (Johnson, 2006). Johnson (1995) uses the term "intimate terrorism" for what is known as intimate partner violence and explains it as a general pattern of control and domination exerted by the husband over the wife in various ways including violence.

Unlike the west, in the Indian context, intimate partner violence is conceptualized as "domestic violence". The Indian society socialises women to ally with men and their interests, resulting in women too, turning into oppressors and perpetrators of violence (Fernandez, 1997). This leads to violence against the woman happening at the hands of the mother-in-law, along with other members of the extended family. At the same time, the daughter-in-law is also important for the family's status in the society and hence, most likely to be controlled and dominated upon, even through the use of physical violence. In the event of the family status or honour being compromised, she is held accountable and it is considered acceptable for her to be "punished" for the same (Fernandez, 1997). Furthermore, the strong enmeshed relationships within the matrimonial house give the couple little privacy to develop their own relationship. The daughter-in-law is targeted as the source of these strained relationships and is subjected to violence (Sonpar, 2005; cited in Gangoli & Rew, 2011).

Therefore, the Protection of Women from Domestic Violence Act (2005) in India classifies violence against women into physical, verbal, emotional, sexual and financial violence. Physical violence includes acts of violence perpetrated physically against the woman that may comprise of "assault, battery, serious injuries or burns, etc." (Sharma, 2005, p. 376). An unequal power balance within the family (Coleman & Strauss, 1986), sexual jealousy and allegations of adultery (Wilson & Daly, 1993), as well as dowry, play a key role in the perpetration of violence against women (Ahmed-Ghosh, 2004).

Several studies suggest that emotional violence too can bc a significant part of physically abusive relationships (Follingstad, Rutledge, Berg, Hause & Polek, 1990). Verbal and emotional abuse are understood as, verbal humiliation, isolation, possessiveness and accusations of infidelity, in addition to threats of abuse, divorce, abandonment, extra-dyadic relationship, and damage or destruction of the personal property of the victim, which are some other ways used by the perpetrator to ensure the victim's compliance and subordination (Walker, 1984).

Sexual violence ranges from lewd verbal comments and derogatory remarks to forced sexual intimacy and rape. The husband expects his wife's sexual availability based on his desire, and thus, rationalizes her rape in event of her denial to give consent (Frieze, 1983). In India, despite widespread presence, marital rape remains unrecognized as a criminal offence (Singh, 2013).

Financial or economic abuse, another form of domestic violence, is inflicted by withholding money, monitoring expenditure, taking away the wife's salary, or stopping her access to work and gain financial independence. Holding a job outside the house, while simultaneously caring for young children creates difficulties for women, leading to women's dependence on their husbands being augmented. As a result, women who are financially dependent on their husbands are unable to leave abusive marriages, especially when they have children (Kalmuss & Strauss, 1982).

Understanding Domestic Violence and Why Women Stay

Given its complexity, several theories have been developed to explain the phenomenon of domestic violence. Psychological theories related to understanding developmental and personality factors contributing to men perpetuating domestic violence.

However, these theories were largely unidimensional, thereby creating a need for a more holistic, nuanced understanding of domestic violence. Heise (1998) thus proposed the ecological model influenced by a gendered lens. This model focused on the interplay between personal history and larger social and structural factors, at several levels. Individual factors related to experiencing or witnessing abuse. The interpersonal context focused on male dominance, male control of wealth, alcohol use, and marital and verbal conflict, in which the abuse often takes place. The exosystem included social networks and socioeconomic background of the family, including low socioeconomic development, isolation of women and delinquent peer relationships. Each of these factors was influenced by overall societal norms and structures, such as rigid gender roles, acceptance of violence, male entitlement. The model postulates interaction between various levels resulting in violence against women. The understanding has thus moved from single factorial theories to more complex and ecological models.

The question that then follows is-why do women continue to stay in abusive relationships? Walker (1977) proposed that the concept of learned helplessness (Seligman, 1975) was applicable here, such that battered women who were repeatedly exposed to violent experiences felt powerless to stop them. Often, they eventually ceased to make any attempts to escape or change the abusive situation. Walker (1979) also highlighted the cyclic nature of violence which contributed towards keeping the women in abusive relationships. The model suggested three phases, starting with an initial escalation of tension, moving towards a full-blown violent episode, and eventually an apology and promise of improvement from the perpetrator. This last phase provides women the positive reinforcement to remain in the relationship. Dutton and Painter (1981) coined the term "traumatic bonding" to describe the emotional attachment style between survivor and perpetrator of domestic violence, wherein the perpetrator alternated between episodes of violence and rage, and episodes of warmth and care.

In the Indian context in particular, stigma related to divorced women also played an important factor in contributing to women's decision to stay. Societal norms dictate that married women must live with their husband—a societal belief also mirrored in their own natal family's mindsets. Some women's families urge them to return to their matrimonial homes despite conflicts and violence, to preserve the family's honour socially (Fernandez, 1997). This stems from the social belief that the onus of making the marriage successful lies upon the woman (Strube, 1988). As a result, in several cases, women choose not to take decisions that might threaten their family's honour in the society, or their own identity as a married woman, given how significant marriage is, as an aspect of women's identity (Thapan, 2003).

Separation and Litigation

Despite the norms of secrecy, maintenance of family honour, and the normalization of abuse as a part of marriage, some women do raise their voices against the domestic violence they are subjected to. Women experiencing marital conflicts as well as those who are subjected to domestic violence often also seek the help of community stakeholders, non-governmental organizations and family counselling centres, in order to seek redressal. They finally approach legal settings looking for assistance to resolve their grievances or to end the marriage. Approaching the legal space is often a last resort for women given the stigma against marital conflicts, separation from spouse and legal spaces carry.

Seeking separation or litigation is one of the many outcomes of matrimonial disputes. Marital separation is one of the most stressful life events in an individual's life (Holmes-Rahe Life Stress Inventory). It often results when the couple is unable to reconcile following marital conflicts and can cause severe emotional impact (Weiss, 1976).

In India, the physical separation of a married couple does not necessarily cease the legal marital relationship, and the lack of legal separation does not ensure continuation of the couple's cohabitation either (Parry, 2001). The presence of multiple respective laws for people of different religious groups and the availability of multiple avenues to resolve matrimonial discords (Vatuk, 2013a; cited in Dommaraju, 2016) has led to the co-presence of religion-oriented family laws (personal laws) and constitutional central government laws in India (Dommaraju, 2016).

Owing to the growing need to resolve familial disputes outside the conventional legal system the Family Courts Act was passed in 1984. It provided for every state to formulate its own set of procedures, allowing litigants to be self-represented, forsaking the need for lawyers and advocates. Family courts were established in the country, to ensure that there is a safe and sensitive legal space for matrimonial disputes. The Family Courts Act aimed to resolve family-related conflicts by hiring gender-sensitized personnel, thereby, setting up couples' counselling as a significant part of the Family Court process (Maitra & K.R., 2015). Hence, it introduced the position of marriage counsellors. According to the rules of the Code of Civil Procedure, a case in any Family Court can precede "only after the preliminary meeting with the marriage counsellor" (Maitra *et al.,* 2015, p. 1).

Furthermore, Family Courts brought together civil and criminal disputes relating to families under one roof, and dealt with issues of divorce, maintenance, restitution of conjugal rights, and child custody. Women, as compared to men, report greater incidences of violence, of physical, verbal, emotional and sexual nature, and hence, the Act gave special attention to ensure gender sensitivity (Basu, 2012).

Difficulties Faced and Impact on Life During Litigation

The Indian society actively discourages bringing one's intimate discord into the purview of the legal system. Given Indian society's collectivist, conservative nature, the impact of litigation is social, as well as emotional. The population of individuals who have undergone marital separation in India is almost three times that of the divorced population, according to Census 2011 (Jacob & Chattopadhyay, 2016). This trend could be a result of the stigma associated with reporting divorce (Belliappa, 2013) and the time-consuming nature of litigation in India (Kumar, 2012), which aggravate the emotionally burdensome processes of separation and divorce. The lengthy litigation process results in distress which often manifests through a variety of psychological and physical symptoms such as sleeplessness, anger, frustration, humiliation, headaches, difficulty concentrating, loss of self-confidence, indecision, anxiety, despondency: commonly associated with mental health concerns like post-traumatic stress disorder and impact on mood (Strasburger, 1999). Since these emotional consequences of litigation are often disregarded by the law, the term "critogenic harms" was coined by Gutheil, Bursztajn, Brodsky and Strasburger (2000) to define the emotional harms that are caused by the legal process itself. The term thus addressed the trauma resulting from the legal process, describing it as "distressing and disruptive" (p. 10).

Furthermore, the legal process also requires litigants to recount incidents of marital conflicts at various stages of filing complaint, interrogations and trials, putting them at a risk of re-traumatization (Gutheil *et al.*, 2000) which involves an increase in post-traumatic stress reactions in response to the original trauma (Orth & Maercker, 2004). Women who have experienced intimate partner violence are particularly at risk during the litigation process because it requires re-living traumatic events repeatedly (Katirai, 2019).

To sum it up, experiencing emotional distress, humiliation, and stigma becomes a part of the process of seeking divorce. Individuals who get a divorce, themselves feel excluded and devalued (Gerstel, 1987). This is even worse for women since the society respects married women who abide by the societal notions that support patriarchal power dynamics. Unmarried, separated or divorced women become victims of gossip in the society as they suggest autonomy from these power dynamics (Fernandez, 1997). Initiating a divorce process is an important indicator of mental health of the litigants. There are some marked differences in the way women react to divorce. When divorce is initiated by the spouse, it aggravates the stress felt by the other spouse who was not a part of this decision-making process (Pledge, 2008). Contrarily, at the same time, women who commence the divorce process may feel respite at the thought of the end of the unhappy marital relationship (Leopold, 2018).

Impact of Separation on Women

The Marriage law in India aims to work on gender inequality in the Indian institutions of law and marriage. While there is an assumption of equality among both partners in the marriage, in reality, this is often not true as women continue to depend on their husbands due to a lack of financial independence. As a result, although men and women are considered equal in divorce laws, women tend to be more adversely impacted in the economic aspect of divorces (Basu, 2012). The financial impact of separation is worse for women than for men (Kincaid & Cladwell, 1995). In the Indian context, this is because women are traditionally expected to be financially dependent on their husbands. Following separation, this primary source of financial support is removed and women are either forced to depend on their parents or explore working opportunities themselves. Therefore, women face a more significant decline in household income and are at a greater poverty risk post their separation, compared to their husbands (Smock & Manning, 1999) due to a rise in financial needs but limited possibilities and opportunities to be employed given their custody of children, inadequate child or spousal maintenance, and an economic shortfall resulting from gender roles in the marriage (Bröckel & Andress, 2015; Holden & Smock, 1991).

Furthermore, the loss of a marital relationship causes individuals "anger, bitterness and resistance in accepting the painful reality" (Shair & Shear, 2005, p. 253). These distress-causing thoughts and difficulty in coming to terms with the end of the marriage might also lead to the individuals avoiding situations and/or activities which might remind them of their loss, leading to them having a reduced interest and engagement in their life's daily activities (Shair & Shear, 2005).

Given the importance of marriage in India, the role of a wife is an important part of women's identity. Cross and Madson (1997) explored the possibility of women defining their identity and self-concept in terms of their relationships as compared to men, who were less likely to do so. During marital separation, this identity is in crisis. Thoits (1991) has proposed that the threat from stressors related to an important identity is higher as compared to threat to a less important identity, and leads to identity disruption (DeGarmo & Kitson, 1996).

Consequently, given the large scale impacts that divorce has on every aspect of women's lives, starting life anew after the divorce is not easy for women. Adjustment to the reality of divorce or separation for a woman is explained by Goode as the process of "once more, finding her own identity as a person" (Goode, 1956, p. 241). According to the study, women face more difficulties while adjusting to life post-divorce, as compared to men, which could stem from their subordinate status in the marriage, their dependency on their husband, a general passiveness, and difficulty perceiving themselves as productive or useful outside of the marital role (Pledge, 2008).

Although remarriages are not uncommon in the Indian society anymore, they are considerably more acceptable for men than for women, since women who have been married previously are considered impure (Holden, 2008; cited in Dommaraju, 2016). As a result, women in India do not often remarry especially when they have children (Amato, 1994. Therefore, divorce is a process of major transitions in an individual's life and leads to tremendous amounts of stress.

Rationale

Women experience marital conflicts as well as conflicts which also include domestic violence. This violence, depending on its nature, has severe short-term and long-term impacts on women, ranging from physical and sexual health related issues to mental health related difficulties. Furthermore, there is an economic impact on the woman given her dependence on her husband for financial requirements. Along with all these impacts, women also experience social repercussions such as losing identity as a married woman and stigma.

When all channels of help fail, individuals turn to Family Courts to seek redressal. Entering the legal space for a private conflict intensifies the stigma and difficulties experienced by women attempting to seek justice and fulfilment of their rights. Lack of legal awareness, combined with the intimidating and confusing legal structures and processes, further elevate women's mental stress.

The impact of this process is thus social, emotional, and physical in nature. The aim of the study, which is a part of a larger state-wide research study, is to understand this impact in detail by utilising the General Health Questionnaire. Through this paper, the authors aim to bridge the gap in literature, providing insights into women's lived experiences of distress and hope in the aftermath of marital conflicts, separation and the litigation process.

Methods

The paper is based on a state-wide (Maharashtra) research conducted with the aim of exploring litigants' and counsellors' views on the nature of marital concerns and stressors experienced by litigants, and of articulating effective elements of the counselling interventions offered to address the same. The present paper employs part of the data collected during the process of this larger study, and aims to describe the nature of marital conflicts and distress experienced by women litigants, along with its impact on their lives. The study used a quantitative approach and a cross-sectional design. Quantitative approach is a descriptive research that employs formal measures of behaviours; and offers the advantage of studying ongoing behaviours of the participants in its original form (Stagnor, 2011). Given the aim of studying the nature of marital conflicts and distress experienced by women litigants, quantitative methodology was deemed to be appropriate.

Methods of Data Collection

The data was collected using a set of standardised and self-constructed questionnaires. Details of these questionnaires were as follows:

(1) *Self-constructed Questionnaire for litigant*—A questionnaire was designed to assess five primary domains: socio-demographic details, the nature of marital conflicts faced by the litigants, the litigants' general help seeking patterns, the perceived impact of the marital conflicts and the process of litigation, and finally, their subjective experience with marriage counselling. Out of these five domains, the present paper focused on three domains—socio-demographic profiles, nature of marital conflicts which was measured by pre-designed checklist and the impact of marital conflicts and the process of litigation, which was assessed by an open ended question. The check-list carried 14 categories of marital conflicts, and the participants could choose all that they found relevant to their history. These categories were created based on the researchers' prior intervention work with the family courts.

(2) *The General Health Questionnaire* (*GHQ, Goldberg & Williams, 1988*)—The twelve-item General Health Questionnaire was introduced by Goldberg and Williams (1988) as a screening tool for assessing psychological distress. The scale consists of six positively phrased and six negatively phrased items. The items are answered using the revised CGHQ (Goodchild & Duncan-Jones, 1985) four-point scale, which is particularly suited for assessing chronic conditions, making it more appropriate for legal settings. On this scale, the categories for scoring positive items were, "0 = better than usual", "0 = same as usual", "1 = less

than usual" and "1 = much less than usual", and those for negative items were "0 = not at all" "1 = no more than usual", "1 = rather more than usual" "1 = much more than usual", thus resulting in 0-0-1-1 scale for positive items and 0-1-1-1 scale for negative items. Herein, 0 indicated the absence and 1 indicated the presence of symptomatic behaviours and emotional responses. For the purpose of scoring, the response of 0 or 1 for each item was added to obtain a cumulative score for the participant, with the lowest score possible being 0 and the highest score possible being 12, with higher scores indicating greater distress. After calculating the cumulative score for each participant, the sample mean was found. This mean GHQ score for the sample population was used as the cut-off score, as suggested by Goldberg, Oldehinkel and Ormel (1998). For the present study, both the tools were translated in local language for participants's understanding, since majority of the litigants who approach family courts, do not speak English.

Sample and Sampling Strategy

The technique of convenience sampling was employed to approach the litigants. Convenience sampling, also known as Haphazard Sampling or Accidental Sampling is a type of non-probability or non-random sampling, where members of the target population that meet certain practical criteria, such as easy accessibility, geographical proximity, availability at a given time, or the willingness to participate, are included for the purpose of the study (Dörnyei, 2007). In case of the current research, practicality was of utmost importance for participant selection, given the busy schedules of the court and the litigants. Hence convenience sampling method was used to select the research participants.

The questionnaire was administered to 150 women litigants, across two Family Courts in two metropolitan cities in Maharashtra. Women litigants who had at least one on-going or closed case in family court, including divorce petitions (petition A or F), restitution of conjugal rights, child custody, nullity and maintenance cases and had completed at least one session with the marriage counsellor, were included in the research study.

Data Collection Process

Permission to collect the data from various family courts across the state of

Maharashtra was first sought from the Bombay High Court, and then from respective family courts where the data were collected. The participants were women litigants with on-going cases at two major Family Courts in Maharashtra. Both courts are located in urban, metropolitan cities. Court A, deals with an approximate yearly caseload of 1000 cases per year and Court B, with 3383 cases filed in 2018. The process of data collection, involved the research assistants contacting individual litigants within family court premises, seeking informed consent and administering the questionnaires.

Ethical Considerations

Approval for the study was obtained from the University Institutional Review Board (Tata Institute of Social Sciences, Mumbai). Care was taken to maintain anonymity and confidentiality of the participants by masking any details that reveal their identity. Further, data collection was conducted with sensitivity so as not to aggravate participants' distress. Inclusion of only those participants who had accessed at least one counselling session with the marriage counsellor based in the family court, helped researchers to ensure that the women litigants were connected with helping professionals. Participants were also provided with a list of help-lines and mental health professionals in the neighbouring regions, in case they wanted to access additional help.

Data Analysis

Data collected through the questionnaires were analysed using descriptive statistics in the form of frequency and percentages. The data collected in response to the open-ended question assessing the impact of the marital conflicts and the process of litigations was entered verbatim and analysed using thematic analysis. Thematic analysis can be defined as a method for identifying, analysing, and reporting patterns (themes) within data. It minimally organizes and describes data set in rich detail. However, it also goes further than this, and interprets various aspects of the research topic (Boyatzis, 1998).

Overall, a feminist perspective was adopted during the study to understand the impact of marital conflict and litigation on women's overall well-being. A feminist perspective is a gender-sensitive socio-political view that acknowledges the gender-power dynamics in patriarchal societies, and is pivotal to understanding women's subjective personal experiences and live realities. The feminist view helped the researchers to understand the nuances in the women's stories.

Results

The following section first elaborates upon the profile of research participants. It then moves on to present findings related to the nature of marital conflicts reported by women litigants and the distress experienced by them.

Participants' Profile

An overwhelming majority of women litigants (95.3%) lived in urban areas. Most participants (47.3%) belonged to the 30-39 **age** group, and almost majority (47.3%) had studied up to graduation. While 43.2 per cent women litigants worked in the service sector, 25.7 per cent were homemakers. Reflective of the state's (Maharashtra state) demographics, 86.7 per cent women litigants were followers of Hinduism, followed 6 per cent Christian followers and 3.3 per cent followers of Buddhism and Islam.

Table 15.1: Age of Participants Group

Age of Litigant	*Total*	
	Frequency	*Percentage*
20–29	56	37.3
30–39	71	47.3
40–49	20	13.3
50–59	3	2.0
Total	**150**	**100.0**

Table 15.2: Educational Qualification of thc Litigants

Educational Qualification	*Total*	
	Frequency	*Percentage*
Below 10th	4	2.7
10th Pass	17	11.3
12th Pass	25	16.7
Graduation	71	47.3
Other	33	22
Total	**150**	**100**

Table 15.3: Occupation of the Litigant

Occupation	*Total (N=150)*	
	Frequency	*Percentage*
Service	64	43.2
Business	10	6.8
Home-maker	38	25.7
Others	36	24.3
Total	**150**	**100**

Table 15.4: Religion of the Litigant

Religion of the Litigant	*Total*	
	Frequency	*Percentage*
Hinduism	130	86.7
Islam	5	3.3
Christianity	9	6
Buddhism	5	3.3
Sikh	1	0.7
Total	**100**	**100**

Table 15.5: Living Arrangement Post-separation

Current Place of Residence	*Total*	
	Frequency	*Percentage*
With spouse	4	2.7
With natal family	116	77.3
With matrimonial family	1	0.7
Living independently	28	18.6
Other	1	0.7
Total	**150**	**100**

The present study found that during marital conflicts and consequent separation, majority of the women (77.3%) live with their natal families while they approach the family courts, while 18.6 per cent women lived independently.

Details of Marriage

Majority of the women litigants (74.7%) reported that they were in an arranged marriage, while 13.3 per cent reported being in a love marriage. Another concept unique to the Indian context was love-arranged marriage (love marriage which was later arranged by respective families), which was reported by 10.7 per cent of the litigants. 82 per cent women litigants reported that they married a partner who belonged to the same caste and 88 per cent reported that their partner belonged to the same community. This is also linked to the widespread prevalence of arranged marriages which tend to be caste and community endogamous. A total of 96 per cent of marriages were within religion, reflective of traditional marital norms where inter-religious marriages are largely forbidden as they are viewed to be a threat to one's community and religious upbringing (Gupta, 1976).

Table 15.6: Duration of Marriage

Total Number of Years Married to Each Other	*Total*	
	Frequency	*Percentage*
> 1 year	8	5.3
1–5	55	36.7
6–10	45	30.0
11–15	20	13.3
16–20	19	12.7
21–25	1	0.7
26–30	2	1.3
Total	**150**	**100.0**

Table 15.6 demonstrates that most couples seeking help/divorce/separation within 1 to 5 years of the marriage.

Nature of Litigation

The start of the litigation process at Family Court marked the formal transition of women's marital lives entering the public realm of legal system. The nature and duration of litigation varied, along with the number of on-going cases. These cases varied from divorce of contested and mutual nature, to maintenance and child custody.

Nature of Petition

It was not uncommon for individuals to have more than one on-going cases at Family Court. A closer look at the nature of litigation filed by women showed that the highest number of cases were filed for maintenance (54.7%), closely followed by divorce of a contested nature (49.3%).

Table 15.7: Nature of Petitions Filed

Nature of Petition	*Total*	
	Frequency	*Percentage*
Divorce–Contested	74	49.3
Mutual Consent Divorce	47	31.3
Judicial Separation	4	2.7
Child Custody	12	8.0
Annulment	4	2.7
Restitution of Conjugal Right	5	3.3
Maintenance	82	54.7
Total	**150**	**100.0**

Table 15.8: Duration of Petition

Duration of Petition	*Total*	
	Frequency	*Percentage*
Less than 1 year	74	49.7
1-5 years	62	41.6
6–10 years	9	6.0
More than 10 years	3	2.0
Over	1	0.7
Total	**150**	**100.0**

Table 15.9: Case filed by Self or Spouse

Case Filed by	*Total*	
	Frequency	*Percentage*
Self	65	43.3
Spouse	70	46.7
Both	15	10.0
Total	**150**	**100.0**

While 43.3 per cent women had filed court petitions themselves, a similar proportion of women (46.7%) were at the receiving end of the court order, with their spouses having approached the court first. In a smaller proportion (10%), usually in instances of mutual consent divorces, both the husband and the wife had approached the court together.

Having looked at the participants' profile, details of their marriages and details of the petitions filed by them, the next section explores the nature of marital conflicts reported by women litigants.

Nature of Marital Conflicts

As mentioned in the earlier section, women litigants were presented with a checklist of 14 areas of marital conflicts and were requested to respond to the same. Each response was coded as 'Yes or No', which indicated the presence or absence of that particular conflict within the litigant's marital life. Needless to say that the litigants were requested to report as many areas of conflicts as they found applicable to their marital history. The following table shows the findings.

Table 15.10: Nature of Marital Conflicts

Marital Conflict	*Presence of Conflict*	
	Frequency	*Percentage*
Communication	49	32.7
Physical violence	93	62.0
Verbal violence	110	73.3
Time spent Together	19	12.7
Financial abuse	65	43.3
Household responsibilities	45	30.0
Child Care	25	16.7
Husband's out of marriage relationship	49	32.7
Alcohol/Drug	38	25.3
Interference by in-laws	78	52.0
Sexual issues	34	22.7
Husband being suspicious	30	20.0
Intellectual differences	19	12.7
Cultural differences	26	17.3

As can be seen in the table, the majority of women reported experiencing verbal (73.3%) and physical violence (62%) in their marriages. Interference by in-laws (52%) and conflicts due to lack of access and control over economic resources (43.3%) were also reported to be common areas of marital conflicts by women litigants.

Having looked at the nature of marital conflicts reported by women litigants, the next section throws light on the distress experienced by them,

Nature of Distress Experienced by Women

The nature of distress was assessed through the administration of the General Health Questionnaire (Goldberg *et al.*, 1988) as well as an open-ended question. It is important to note that the source of distress at the moment of data collection did not stem from the conflict itself as most were separated. The current focus was thus on post-separation living, along with litigation and societal changes.

As mentioned in the methods section, women litigants were asked to respond to the twelve-item General Health Questionnaire (Goldberg *et al.,* 1988) to understand the distress experienced by them. Participants were asked to respond to each of these items by choosing a category from a four point scale mentioned in the methods section. They were asked to choose a category based on the distress experienced by them in the recent past (one month), as a response to the marital conflicts and the process of litigation. The scoring procedure followed for each item and per participant, too, has been mentioned in the methods section. The following table demonstrates item-wise break-up of participants' responses to the GHQ. The column zero denotes absence of distress related to the respective item, while column one denotes presence of distress related to that particular item.

Table 15.11: Statement-wise Break-up of the GHQ

GHQ statement	*0 (positive)*		*1 (negative)*	
	Frequency	*Percentage*	*Frequency*	*Percentage*
Concentration	40	26.7	110	73.3
Loss of sleep	72	48.0	78	52.0
Playing a useful role	96	64.0	54	36.0
Feeling capable of making decisions	104	69.3	46	30.7
Constant stress	76	50.7	74	49.3
Cannot overcome difficulties	72	48.0	78	52.0
Enjoy normal activities	53	35.3	97	64.7
Ready to face problems	116	77.3	34	22.7
Unhappy and depressed	74	49.3	76	50.7
Losing confidence	72	48.0	78	52.0
Consider self-worthy	68	45.3	82	54.7
Happy	53	35.3	97	64.7

As seen in the table, distress was most observed in women's difficulty in concentrating at work or at home (73.3%). Further, majority women (64.7%) also reported reduced enjoyment of normal activities. In spite of this distress, 69.3 per cent women now felt capable of making decisions for themselves, and a higher proportion of women (77.3%) now felt ready to face their problems.

As mentioned in the methods section, in order to calculate an overall score per participant, the response scores for each item were added. Thus, a total score was obtained for each participant. A sample mean was calculated and used as a cut-off point to indicate the proportion of the litigants who are psychologically healthy and those who are vulnerable to experience psychological distress.

The mean GHQ score for the sample was 6.03 (SD=2.38). Based on the mean, the cut-off point 6/7 was used. The study revealed that 62 (41.3%) of the participants scores 7 and above on the GHQ-12, while 88 (58.7%) others obtained scores 6 and lower. These findings seem to indicate that the proportion of the litigants who are psychologically healthy was just slightly higher than those vulnerable to experience psychological distress. However, the results do indicate that a high proportion of women litigants are still vulnerable to experience psychological distress.

To further elaborate on the findings from the GHQ, responses to the open-ended questions were explored to understand the impact of marital conflicts and process of litigation on various aspects of women's lives. The following section focuses on these findings, corroborating with the item-wise analysis of the GHQ.

Impact on Physical Health

Impact on physical health was evident with 52 per cent women reporting sleeping difficulties with symptoms often aggravating around court dates. Women also recounted how prolonged stress and lifestyle related health issues such as weight gain, high blood pressure and thyroid had occurred.

> "*The stress has given me thyroid.*" (Suvarna)

The pressure of the ongoing court case and abusive behaviour from the women's matrimonial family towards the natal family also impacted their physical health and emotional health, with women reporting cardiac issues and suicides in the family post-litigation.

Contrarily, litigation sometimes validates women's difficulties and facilitates change in a process that was stuck and is, therefore, viewed by women more optimistically. For some women, litigation alleviated their stress symptoms and women were now in better physical health. But this was a slightly lesser percentage of the sample (48%).

> "*I am sleeping and eating better now on the contrary...*" (Shivani)

Emotional Impact

The emotional impact of separating from partner and consequently coming to court was varied, with some women benefiting from the process while most being left emotionally reeling. Litigation itself caused distress for women because of procedural issues. The delays caused by court resulted in women feeling confused about their decision. Court process required women meeting their spouses in court, resulting in irritation, frustration and anger. This also negatively affected their perception of justice in courts, leading them to believe that the process was pointless.

> *"I feel very depressed. I feel angry. I see him, and I think he destroyed my life. I feel very angry at him."* (Sameera)

Further, as a part of litigation, women were forced to repeatedly retell stories about their conflicts at court, leading them to relive those memories and associated emotions. Retraumatization was particularly intense when marital details included violence.

> *"The biggest trauma is to repeat the story again and again. It reminded me of everything."* (Karishma)

Cognitive impact was observed through reduced concentration as reported by 73.3 per cent women. This was particularly heightened around court dates. The inability to concentrate affected their productivity at the workplace and their success therein.

> *"I lose concentration before court dates. I cannot take decisions at work too."* (Sindhu)

Overall, women reported feeling lost, stuck, anxious, and angry in response to court proceedings surrounding their marriage. In certain instances of abusive marriages, women were concerned about spouses refusing to give them a divorce. Losing a partner also brought along a sense of loneliness.

> *"Sometimes, I feel very lost, I don't know what to do in life."* (Bhagyashree)

An accumulation of intense stress, sadness and despair often resulted in diagnosed or undiagnosed mental health concerns for women. Depression was common, along with suicide ideations.

> "*I can't kill myself, that is why I have to live*" (Sangita)

Women also experienced panic attacks at the court. Distressing experiences like being able to hear the spouse or constantly dreaming of him were also reported. Most women (64.7%) reported difficulty enjoying normal activities. An overall sense of hopelessness and helplessness was predominant. Consequently, 64.7 per cent of women reported experiencing a lack of an overarching sense of happiness.

> "*I have lost interest in everything. There is no excitement anymore.*" (Sindhu)

Conversely, for some women, the emotional impact was predominantly positive. With regard to making decisions in general, 69.3 per cent litigants actually believed that they are now capable of the same. For 35.3 per cent women, separation and consequent litigation was a source of relief and escape from an abusive matrimonial home to a safer natal or independent home. Further, some also perceived courts as a source of hope, and believed in its fairness and sense of justice.

Impact on Sense of Self

Women's perception of themselves was also changed in the process of litigation. In the recent past, negative repercussions on one's confidence were reported by 52 per cent of women. Some women became doubtful of their decision-making ability. They also began isolating themselves from their social circles, unable to hold conversations, and constantly worried about the societal repercussions. This resulted in 52 per cent women perceiving themselves incapable of dealing with future obstacles. The sense of helplessness often emerged from financial dependence on others. Consequently, poor perception of one's worth was reported by a little over majority women (54.7%),

> "*I don't consider myself worthy–absolutely zero.*" (Sara)

On the other hand, positive changes in their sense of self were also observed. In the recent past, 64 per cent women experienced a sense of usefulness in their lives. For some, it was related to the presence of a neutral party at court to handle one's marital problems. For most others, this sense of usefulness was driven by trying to accomplish something for themselves—be it maintenance, child custody and/or divorce.

Almost half the litigants (48%) were determined to overcome difficulties they may be faced with, exhibiting a belief in the court system, along with an intense resolve to seek justice for themselves and their children.

> *"...I will fight till I live. I will not let him escape."* (Netra)

A similar percentage of women (48%) reported that their self-confidence had remained steady or improved in the recent past. Further, 45.3 per cent women reported steady or improving self-worth as well.

Thus, in spite of being bogged down by marital distress and litigation, 77.3 per cent felt ready to face their problems, coming from a space of determination and purpose. The litigants elaborated by sharing that approaching the courts was the most courageous step which provided them with confidence to proceed with their litigation. This narrative was echoed especially by women who wanted to right a wrong, and sought justice following an abusive relationship.

> *"But I will fight till I live. I will not let him escape. He has ruined my life. I will not allow him to escape."* (Netra)

Women also acquired strength from their will to show their husbands that they were capable of looking after themselves and their children without any help from the husband.

> *"I learnt a lot in life. I have freedom. I can stand on my own feet and take care of my children"* (Prema)

This increase in confidence and personal strength also reflected in women's decision-making abilities which they noted, had improved since the litigation process had begun. Another factor that contributed to increasing their self-worth was financial independence.

> *"My self-worth has increased. I used to be dependent...Ever since I started working, I have become happier."* (Aastha)

Social Impact

The impact on social life as a result of the public nature of the litigation was also evident. Women were harassed by neighbours and extended family members with repeated questions about the absent spouse. The women's natal families were perceived in a negative light by society at large, with parents often being at the receiving end of societal flak.

Women were often held responsible for the breakdown of the marriage, irrespective of the husband's actions. Women also consistently noticed the gendered nature of this stigma with differential treatment meted out to them in the aftermath of marital conflicts and separation as against the treatment received by their husbands.

> "*Society tortures me. I can see my parents' troubles. The society's view of me is wrong. Men can do whatever they want, but if girls do anything, it is wrong.*" (Sameera)

These women were treated differently from women who continued to live with their spouses and were excluded from certain religious and social ceremonies. The resultant mental distress from such social ostracization became a part of everyday life for several women.

Impact on Work and Finances

The financial impact of the court process was heavily felt by women, who face significant decline in household income as compared to their husbands post separation. Consequently savings were exhausted in an effort to pay for court along with paying rent and looking after children, as women are usually the custodial parent. Women were often also dependent on their natal family for financial aid, some in spite of being educated. The issue was further aggravated by women's employment opportunities being significantly hindered because of an on-going court case. As a consequence of needing regular leaves, women reported losing out on promotions, and losing jobs altogether.

> "*My work life has been affected a lot. I lost 3 jobs because of court dates/process*" (Nabila) "*Even I go for interviews for jobs...I am not accepted because I have court process going on.*" (Ishita) "*Have to lie at work—cannot tell people that a divorce case is going on.*" (Ujjwala)

> *"My work has been affected. I am required to come to court and holidays are hard to get."* (Sangeet)

Impact on Children

Women reported that parenting was adversely affected as constant court dates and other litigation related stressors reduced the time women could spend with their children. Financial issues were at the fore.

> *"I have tension about what to eat, how to pay rent, how to take care of kids."* (Anokhi)

Women were also worried about the impact of parental separation on the child's future. Concerns relating to whether the child would have his father's name or handling situations when the child starts questioning parental separation were common. Women were also worried about separation affecting the manner in which their children perceived them.

In one instance of an abusive marriage, the child often served as a reminder of the perpetrator, causing the woman distress.

> *"I was so depressed. When I looked at my daughter, I would get angry thinking that this was his daughter."* (Namrata)

Gendered Nature of Impact

Gender roles and expectations were also clearly visible, in terms of societal treatment and internalised gender norms. Few women reported distress about delayed or denied motherhood if the divorce came through, displaying societal beliefs about a woman's true worth being measured only by her ability to bear children. Some women did not want a divorce, irrespective of the treatment meted out to them by the matrimonial house, because it was imperative to *"think as a woman"* (Pratima) displaying an understanding that society treated divorced women differently. Sometimes women's narratives around their emotional distress, marital distress, as well as separation/divorce were dismissed by the society. For instance, they faced gender insensitive comments which suggested that the onus of the separation was often placed on the women, irrespective of the man's actions. Additionally, they also faced ablest and patriarchal statements which indicated that were also held responsible for their own well-being.

> *"In the society, my image has reduced. People keep telling me it is my mistake."* (Sameera)

Further, women who were undergoing divorce proceedings were labelled as burdens on the natal family by society. The financial dependence on the natal family often resulted in women internalising the narrative of being burdens for their parents and siblings, leaving them feeling helpless. Consequently, women often limited social interactions.

> *"They keep saying how I am a divorcee who is a burden on how parents and I have started feeling the same."* (Pratima)

While internalised gender norms were recurring in women's narratives, experiences in their marriages and litigation process played an important role in bringing about change. Women noted the gender disparity in treatment, acknowledged the unfairness of the same, and started veering away from the normative. Opinions about divorce had evolved, and it was perceived as more acceptable in the face of violence.

> *"These days everyone gets divorced. It is better to get divorced than getting beaten every day."* (Payal)

The necessity of marriage for living a fulfilling life was questioned, with "marriage should not be compulsory" emerging as an important learning for some women. The entire process of marital conflicts leading up to litigation had changed women's beliefs about marriage, often advocating for a more liberal stance and focusing on shifting the blame away from women.

Discussion

The present findings are a part of a larger study conducted across Maharashtra. The larger study seeks to understand gendered patterns in divorce/separation, effects of matrimonial distress on litigants, nature of litigation, help-seeking behaviours, and effective elements of counselling to address divorce/separation. This paper emphasizes the effect of litigation on the overall health of female litigants using the GHQ. In order to understand the prevalence of distress among litigants, it is important to place them within their socio-economic context. Most women in the current study were in their thirties, had completed their graduation and were currently employed in the service sector. The trend indicates increased educational status and a shift in the overall participation of women in the workforce. Both factors contribute to the empowerment of women, posing a challenge to the traditional subservient role ascribed to women in Indian marriages. Studies have found that working women are in fact more likely to divorce their partners as compared to non-working women (Schoen, Astone, Kim, Rothert & Standish, 2002). While the empowerment hypothesis has not been extensively studied in India, similar results were also found by Maitra *et al.* (2015), and was thus considered while understanding the data from the present study.

The present study found that marriages are largely arranged, and thus, are caste and community endogamous. However, all kinds of marriages, arranged, love, or love-arranged seemed to have prevalence of violence. The use of force and violence was more widely prevalent within the marriage itself in the form of emotional, verbal, physical and financial violence with an overwhelming majority reporting such experiences in their marriage. This reflected the constant effort by men to preserve their dominance and control over women through aggression and violence (Bonisteel & Green, 2005; cited in Naidu, 2011). Women often explained how the violence was not only meted out by spouses but matrimonial families as well, which suggests that violence in the Indian context is familial rather than interpersonal.

The familial nature of violence was closely linked to another recurrent reason for conflict-interference from in-laws, most often the mother-in-law. Such interference ranged from decision making regarding everyday life to sexual life, conceptualised by Naidu (2011) as a "three person triadic unit". It is explained as married couples being forced to conceptualize their unit as a "three person triadic unit" which included the mother-in-law, in addition to the couple, instead of the couple being a two-person dyadic unit. This often acted as a trigger in marital conflicts and discord.

When these conflicts were unresolvable and recurrent, separation occurred. As a result, one of the most preliminary findings to emerge from the present study was the process within the marital journey leading up to litigation. Marital conflicts marked the initiation into the process, which when unresolvable and recurrent, resulted in separation. Following separation, the decision to reconcile, separate or acquire child custody was made by the husband and/or wife. When this decision was legally acted upon, litigation ensued, thereby marking the entry of one's personal life into the public realm. Often, the process was not linear, with multiple instances of separation and reconciliation occurring before the legal system was approached. This is in line with modern literature which has also begun to view divorce and marital separation as a process, rather than as a single event (Pledge, 2008).

Thus, given the lengthy nature of the process, marital distress and litigation had a significant impact on women's lives, even when women in the present study were not in active marital conflicts. Overall, the adverse impact on the emotional well-being of women was heavily felt, as was reflected in the GHQ scores. Physical issues like high blood pressure and sleeplessness were also common. This is in line with Strasburger (1999) who found that the lengthy litigation process severely affected physical and emotional health.

One of the major stressors negatively affecting women's emotional and physical health was financial difficulties. Women repeatedly vocalised distress arising out of financial concerns relating to everyday survival, paying rent and looking after children. Saving depletion and dependence on natal family was also common. This was aggravated by women's employment opportunities being significantly hindered because of an on-going court case. This is not surprising, with studies showing that the financial impact of the court process is heavily felt by women (Amato, 1994), who face significant decline in household income as compared to their husbands post separation (Smock & Manning, 1999). Conventionally, women after marriage are expected to depend on their husbands as "breadwinners" (Agnes, 2009). Following separation, women are often left bereft of any financial backing. Emotional consequences in terms of lack of concentration, reduced confidence, and a sense of helplessness were thus evident in the GHQ. Women then turned to maintenance for basic financial aid, as is reflected in the high number of maintenance cases filed by women in the present study.

Moreover, majority women post separation resided with their natal families. This raised the issue of financial dependence in a patrilocal society that detaches women from their natal homes after marriage. Societal criticism of separated women as burdens on the natal family was often so heavily emphasised that it resulted in women internalising the label and heightening their sense of despair, as was reflected in women's reduced sense of self-worth in the GHQ. Ahmed-Ghosh (2004) explains the public shame attached to married women returning to their natal homes, which often threatens the chances of the younger siblings' marriage. The woman is perceived as not only an economic burden but also a social liability. In this setting, women were also worried for the well-being of the children, which was in jeopardy because of financial constraints as well as because of the social and legal implications of being raised by a single mother.

Further, marital separation and litigation resulted in women's private lives now entering the public space. Their social lives were impacted, as women reported harassment from neighbours and extended family members incessantly enquiring about the absent spouse and the litigation. Women were left with no space to escape from their prying eyes, making them feel frustrated, and with their personal lives being reduced to a news item meant for the public gaze. Gutheil *et al.* (2000) has similarly elaborated upon blurring of public and personal boundaries resulting in stress because of the disclosure of conflicted or shameful aspects of an intimate relationship. Further, Fernandez (1997) situates the same in the Indian context, where unmarried or separated women become the primary subject of societal gossip as they suggest autonomy from the normative gendered power dynamics of the society.

However, certain aspects of the normative societal beliefs were often internalised by women, particularly with regard to the institute of marriage itself. The permanence of marriage was viewed as central to the institute, and termination of the same was unimaginable (Holden, 2008). Consequently, separation was not a linear process, instead involving several attempts to repair the marriage before separating. In these instances, when a divorce process was initiated by the spouse, women's unhappiness stemmed from being unable to give their marriage another chance, irrespective of the violence and other marital conflicts. Because some women perceived their marriage as a failure, they also experienced a sense of shame, and reduced self-worth, as reported in the GHQ. Given the social conditioning and women's self-identity being significantly more relational, (Ahmed-Ghosh, 2004), a threat to their identity as a wife thus was extremely unsettling for several women.

Beyond these aspects, the court process itself often augmented women's distress. Repeated dates, procedural delays, missing days at work because of the court process, the possibility of retraumatization, and the uncertainty of the verdict, all acted as stressors for women. Most women stated that their distress was significantly higher around court dates because of these reasons. Singh (2013) commented about the lengthy court process to award maintenance, the cost involved in fighting litigation and losing a day's wage because of court dates being primary sources of court-related stressors for women. Thus, for slightly more than half the women, the GHQ indicated that this period was marked with unhappiness.

Overall, the results of the current study indicated that almost half the women were vulnerable to experience psychological distress, as assessed by the GHQ. The pressure of a court case, the social dimensions of bringing the personal into the public, the financial burden of the process, impact on work, and the emotional turmoil of marital distress and litigation, all contributed towards it.

On the other hand, there were also several women whose lives in fact improved post-separation and litigation. This stemmed from a sense of empowerment and relief that women experienced following the separation and legal process. For some women, financial independence was the most important shift. Guru (2009) noted that women post-separation were financially self-sufficient, enhancing their overall sense of independence and scope for decision-making. This improved scope for decision-making ability was observed in the present study. Given the power dynamics of an Indian marriage system, decision-making was largely considered the domain of the man. Post-separation, women now had better scope to make decisions for themselves, giving them agency in shaping their own journey.

Further, and most importantly, women who had experienced violence at matrimonials homes felt safer in their natal homes, living without the constant fear of a physical or verbal attack, which improved emotional and physical health. The relief was also significant when women themselves initiated the decision to end an unhappy, abusive marriage (Leopold, 2018). This was reflected in the present study with some women reporting an improved sense of happiness following separation.

Consequently, several women reported less stress in the recent past. In addition to the aforementioned factors, previously developed stress management techniques in response to marital discord and an overall familiarity with the court process also reduced stress. Even in instances were violence was not involved in the marriage, living away from the spouse and his family ensured that the major sources of stress were avoided. Social support was also found to be one of the critical determinants of distress management post separation. Support from natal family was the primary positive factor, with additional protective factors also including support from friends, counseling at court and current employment. Thus, distress management, sense of happiness, and an improved sense of self were interlinked, in which finding supportive networks played a large role.

An insightful change in the course of women's journey through conflict and litigation was the development of critical consciousness. Freire (1972) defined critical consciousness as "the development of a critical awareness of oppressive social structures and cultural norms and a resistance against these" (Guru, 2009, p. 296). In the present study, women reported an understanding of the differential treatment meted out to men and women in the face of marital litigation, with Guru (2009) noting that such cultural hostility post separation often served as an impetus to question the gendered structural oppression.

Conclusion

As the study suggests, marriages in India continued to follow the traditional values of abiding to caste and religion, albeit less strictly. Gender norms that perpetuate the institute were also dominant, with women being consistently expected to adhere to the role of the submissive obedient wife. Intimate terrorism, motivated by exerting controlling over the wife, was experienced by an overwhelming majority. While the frequency and intensity varied, the impact involved short-term and long-lasting negative consequences on women's emotional, physical and social well-being.

In most cases, separation occurred following a series of unresolved conflicts and intense violence. Litigation was equally initiated by men and women, with the nature of cases varying from divorce to restitution and maintenance. While the conflicts themselves were described as painful, for most women, the public nature of litigation further compounded their agony. Marital distress and litigation together affected various aspects of women's lives, both positively and negatively.

The society placed the onus of maintaining a marriage entirely on the woman and actively ostracised women who did not adhere to the role of the ideal Indian wife. Further, the society also portrayed women who had returned to the natal home as a burden on the parents, thus failing to perform the duties of a wife and a daughter. In certain instances, this sense of burden was internalised and women were doubly inflicted with pain and agony. The gendered experience of stigma was particularly heightened for women who realised that their husbands were not subject to similar societal humiliation.

Further, the court process itself was riddled with triggers, requiring women to meet their spouse and retell stories of marital conflict and violence. Re-traumatisation was thus a recurrent theme in women's narratives, emphasising how efforts to forget their troubled past would falter within the court set-up. An overwhelming sense of stress manifested through sleeplessness, loss of concentration, reduced excitement for normal activities and a general sense of sadness. Many women also reported an increase in physical ailments along with undiagnosed mental health concerns.

Conversely, for some women, litigation offered a sense of hope and reassurance because of perceived fairness of the legal setting, resulting in improved physical and emotional well-being. Although stigmatised, women showed also signs of resilience and determination to seek justice. A sense of usefulness was experienced by pursuing litigation for self and children.

Through the hardships of conflicts, separation and litigation, there were certain factors that worked towards mitigating the negative consequences of marital distress on women. The primary factor was the support of the natal family, particularly during separation and litigation. Natal families provided women with emotional and financial support and sustenance, allowing women the space to cope and heal in the aftermath of marital distress. Further, women who were financially independent and were currently employed were less dependent on the natal family and felt more empowered to deal with litigation and the consequent distress. In certain instances, counselling provided at court and support from the litigation strengthens women in the face of constant stress.

Overall, it would be important to acknowledge that women's experiences of marital conflicts, separation and litigation were diverse, influenced by nature of conflicts and litigation, social support, and individual resilience.

It was evident in the course of this paper that ingrained gender norms contributed greatly to the elevated distress experienced by women. There is a need to work towards creating equalitarian social norms so as to ensure fair treatment of women. Such a societal shift would work at the preventive level, and ensure gendered equality within social institutions such as marriage. To achieve this, studies have shown that working with men, who the current beneficiaries of the system, with regard to gender sensitivity and equality are particularly helpful.

Further, studies have found that sources of help-seeking, both informal and formal, play an important role in processing marital trauma (Sen, 1999). Most importantly, it has been noted that many women do not seek immediate help when maritals conflicts emerge. It has also been found that support from the natal family is in fact the most significant protective factor in dealing with post separation living and litigation distress. Thus, it would be important to bridge this gap by sensitising natal families to violence, and accepting daughters back home without heeding to societal pressure of leaving daughter in abusive matrimonial homes. At a broader community level, institutes like Society for Nutrition, Education and Health Action (SNEHA) and Special Cell for Women and Children works towards removing women from violent situations and ensuring safety in times of reconciliation. In fact, studies have shown that women's shelter and counseling centres were the most effective source of help during marital violence (Panchanadeswaran & Koverola, 2005). There is thus a need to strengthen this secondary level chain as well.

Most relevant to the current paper is the role of formal settings like family courts in women's experiences of distress. While certain aspects of family court were perceived as potential stressors, the legal settings were also a source of hope to many. Building on this, family courts can provide certain services which can ease the process and the consequent distress. Given limited access of finances and education, most women do not have a comprehensive understanding of the law. Offering resources which would simplify the law and enhance its accessibility to women would be beneficial in aiding their understanding of their case. Further, the limited financial resources also prevent women from seeking financial aid. Thus, provision of good legal aid for such individuals would be uplifting.

Moreover, it is important to focus on their emotional journeys within the court system as well. Women, as documented in the present study, experience intense distress through post separation living and litigation. Providing stress management services at courts can thus be very helpful. One such endeavour is Sukoon, a field action project by School of Human Ecology, Tata Institute of Social Sciences, Mumbai (Bhosle, 2019). It provides psychosocial support to individuals, couples and families approaching legal settings for matrimonial conflicts. Additionally, Sukoon also works on issues of violence and marginalization through interventions informed by a strengths-based and gender sensitive framework. Sukoon attempts to create a safe space for the well-being of litigants experiencing personal and relational distress, and prescribes to a gendered and strengths-based framework. Projects like these are extremely important in absorbing women's distress and empowering women's journeys during a highly public, socially stigmatised and litigious process.

References

Agnes, F. (2009, October 31-November 6) Conjugality, Property, Morality and Maintenance. *Economic and Political Weekly*. *44*(44). 58-64.

Ahmed-Ghosh, H. (2004). Chattels of Society. *Violence Against Women*, *10*(1), 94–118. doi: 10.1177/1077801203256019.

Allendorf, K. (2013). Schemas of Marital Change: From Arranged Marriages to Eloping for Love. *Journal of Marriage and Family*, *75*(2), 453–469. doi: 10.1111/jomf.12003.

Allendorf, K., and Pandian, R.K. (2016). The Decline of Arranged Marriage? Marital Change and Continuity in India. *Population and Development Review*, *42*(3), 435–464. doi: 10.1111/j.1728-4457.2016.00149.x

Amato, P.R. (1994). The Impact of Divorce on Men and Women in India and the United States. *Journal of Comparative Family Studies*, *25*(2), 207–221. doi: 10.3138/jcfs.25.2.207.

Ashford, J.B., LeCroy, C.W., and Lortie, K.L. (2006). *Human Behaviour in the Social Environment: A Multidimensional Perspective* (3rd Edition). California: Thomson Brooks.

Banerji, M., Martin, S., and Desai, S. (2013). Are the young and educated more likely to have 'love' than arranged marriage? A study of autonomy of partner choice in India. *Working Paper Series,* pp. 1-43, New Delhi: NCAER.

Basu, S. (2012). Judges of Normality: Mediating Marriage in the Family Courts of Kolkata, India. *Signs: Journal of Women in Culture and Society*, *37*(2), 469–492. doi: 10.1086/661712.

Belliappa, J.L. (2013). *Gender, Class and Reflexive Modernity in India*. Basingstoke: Palgrave Macmillan.

Bhosle, P. (2019, June 2). Bombay HC prioritises mental health of litigants. Mid-Day. Retrieved from https://www.mid-day.com/articles/bombay-hc-prioritises-mental-health-of-litigants/21065156

Boyatzis, R.E. (1998). *Transforming Qualitative Information: Thematic Analysis and Code Development*. Thousand Oaks, California: SAGE Publications, Inc.

Bröckel, M., and Andreß, H. (2015). The Economic Consequences of Divorce in Germany: What Has Changed since the Turn of the Millennium?. *Comparative Population Studies, 40*(3). Retrieved from http://www.comparativepopulationstudies.de/index.php/CPoS/article/view/182/200

Coleman, D.H., and Straus, M.A. (1986). Marital Power, Conflict, and Violence in a Nationally Representative Sample of American Couples. *Violence and Victims*, *1*(2), 141–157. doi: 10.1891/0886-6708.1.2.141

Crocker, J., Major, B., and Steele, C. (1998). Social stigma. In: J. Crocker, B. Major, C. Steele, D. Gilbert, and S. Fiske (Eds.), *The Handbook of Social Psychology,* pp. 504–553, Boston, MA, USA: McGraw-Hill.

Cross, S. and Madson, L. (1997). Models of the self: Self-construals and gender. *Psychological Bulletin. 122*(1). 5-37. doi: 10.1037//0033-2909.122.1.5.

DeGarmo, D.S., and Kitson, G.C. (1996). Identity relevance and disruption as predictors of psychological distress for widowed and divorced women. *Journal of Marriage and the Family*, 58, 983–997.

Dhar, R.L. (2013). Intercaste Marriage: A Study from the Indian Context. *Marriage and Family Review*, *49*(1), 1–25. doi: 10.1080/01494929.2012.714720.

Dommaraju, P. (2016). Divorce and Separation in India. *Population and Development Review*, *42*(2), 195–223. doi: 10.1111/j.1728-4457.2016.00127.x

Dutton, D.G., and Painter, S.L. (1981). Traumatic bonding: The development of emotional attachments in battered women and other relationships of intermittent abuse. *Victimology: An International Journal,* 6, 139–155.

Fernandez, M. (1997). Domestic Violence by Extended Family Members in India. *Journal of Interpersonal Violence, 12*(3), 433–455. doi: 10.1177/088626097012003008.

Fincham, F. (2003). Marital Conflict. *Current Directions in Psychological Science. 12*(1). 23–27. doi:10.1111/1467-8721.01215.

Follingstad, D.R., Rutledge, L.L., Berg, B.J., Hause, E.S., and Polek, D.S. (1990). The role of emotional abuse in physically abusive relationships. *Journal of Family Violence, 5*(2), 107–120. doi: 10.1007/bf00978514.

Freire, P., (1972). *Pedagogy of the Oppressed.* London: Penguin Books.

Frieze, I.H. (1983). Investigating the Causes and Consequences of Marital Rape. *Signs: Journal of Women in Culture and Society, 8*(3), 532–553. doi: 10.1086/493988.

Gerstel, N. (1987). Divorce and Stigma. *Social Problems, 34*(2), 172–186. doi: 10.1525/sp.1987.34.2.03a00050.

Goodchild, M.E., and Duncan-Jones, P. (1985). *Chronicity and the General Health Questionnaire. The British Journal of Psychiatry, 146*(*1*), *55–61.* doi:10.1192/bjp.146.1.55.

Goldberg D.P. and Williams P. (1988). *A User's Guide to the General Health Questionnaire*. Basingstoke NFER-Nelson.

Goode, W. (1956). *Women in Divorce.* New York: The Crowell-Collier Publishing Company.

Guilbert, D.E., Vacc, N.A., and Pasley, K. (2000). The Relationship of Gender Role Beliefs, Negativity, Distancing, and Marital Instability. *The Family Journal, 8*(2), 124-132. doi:10.1177/1066480700082003.

Gutheil, T.G., Bursztajn, H., Brodsky, A., and Strasburger, L.H. (2000). Preventing "Critogenic" Harms: Minimizing Emotional Injury from Civil Litigation. *The Journal of Psychiatry and Law, 28*(1), 5–18. doi:10.1177/009318530002800102.

Gupta, G.R. (1976). Love, Arranged Marriage, and the Indian Social Structure. *Journal of Comparative Family Studies, 7*(1), 75–85. doi: 10.3138/jcfs.7.1.75.

Guru, S. (2009). Divorce: Obstacles and Opportunities–South Asian Women in Britain. *The Sociological Review, 57*(2), 285–305. doi:10.1111/j.1467-954x.2009.01830.x

Heise, L.L. (1998). Violence against Women: An Integrated, Ecological Framework. *Violence against Women, 4*(3), 262–290.

Holden, L. (2008). Hindu Divorce: A Legal Anthropology, Aldershot, England; Burlington, Vermont: Ashgate.

Holden, K.C., and Smock, P.J. (1991). The Economic Costs of Marital Dissolution: Why Do Women Bear a Disproportionate Cost? *Annual Review of Sociology, 17*(1), 51–78. doi: 10.1146/annurev.so.17.080191.000411.

Hotaling, G.T., and Sugarman, D.B. (1990). A risk marker analysis of assaulted wives. *Journal of Family Violence, 5*(1), 1–13. doi: 10.1007/bf00979135.

Jacob, S., and Chattopadhyay, S. (2016, August 13). Marriage Dissolution in India. *Economic and Political Weekly, 1*(33), 25-27.

Jeyaseelan, L., Kumar, S., Neelakantan, N., Peedicayil, A., Pillai, R., and Duvvury, N. (2007). Physical Spousal Violence against Women in India: Some Risk Factors. *Journal of Biosocial Science, 39*(5), 657-670. Doi:10.1017/S0021932007001836.

Johnson, M.P. (1995). Patriarchal Terrorism and Common Couple Violence: Two Forms of Violence against Women. *Journal of Marriage and the Family, 57*(2), 283. doi: 10.2307/353683.

Johnson, M.P. (2006). Conflict and Control. *Violence Against Women, 12*(11), 1003–1018. doi:10.1177/1077801206293328.

Kalmuss, D.S., and Straus, M.A. (1982). Wife's Marital Dependency and Wife Abuse. *Journal of Marriage and the Family, 44*(2), 277. doi: 10.2307/351538.

Katirai, N. (2019, May 7). Retraumatization in Family Courts. 62 *Arizona Law Review* (2020, Forthcoming); Arizona Legal Studies Discussion Paper No. 19-10.

Kim, H.K., and Mckenry, P.C. (2002). The Relationship Between Marriage and Psychological Well-being. *Journal of Family Issues, 23*(8), 885–911. doi: 10.1177/019251302237296

Kincaid, S.B., and Cladwell, R.A. (1995). Marital Separation, Journal of Divorce and Remarriage, 22: 3-4, 109-128, DOI: 10.1300/J087v22n03_07.

Kumar, V.A. (2012). Judicial Delays in India: Causes and Remedies. *Journal of Law, Policy and Globalization. 4*, 16–21.

Leopold, T. (2018). Gender Differences in the Consequences of Divorce: A Study of Multiple Outcomes. *Demography, 55*(3), 769–797. doi: 10.1007/s13524-018-0667-6.

Maitra, S., and K.R., Gayathri. (2015). Divorce Trends and its Implications for Children's Well-being: A Study of Family Court in Mumbai. Mumbai: School of Social Work, Tata Institute of Social Sciences.

Naidu, M. (2011). Indian women in marriage: When the sacred marriage thread becomes a noose. *Agenda, 25*(1), 84–92. doi: 10.1080/10130950.2011.575587.

Orth, U., and Maercker, A. (2004). Do Trials of Perpetrators Retraumatize Crime Victims? *Journal of Interpersonal Violence, 19*(2), 212–227. doi: 10.1177/0886260503260326.

Panchanadeswaran, S., and Koverola, C. (2005). *The Voices of Battered Women in India. Violence Against Women, 11(6), 736–758* doi: 10.1177/1077801205276088.

Parry, J.P. (2001). Ankalus Errant Wife: Sex, Marriage and Industry in Contemporary Chhattisgarh. *Modern Asian Studies, 35*(4), 783–820. doi: 10.1017/s0026749x01004024.

Pledge, D.S. (2008). Marital Separation/Divorce. *Journal of Divorce and Remarriage, 17*(3-4), 151–182. doi: 10.1300/j087v17n03_10.

Proulx, C.M., Helms, H.M., and Buehler, C. (2007). Marital Quality and Personal Well-being: A Meta-Analysis. *Journal of Marriage and Family, 69*(3), 576–593. doi: 10.1111/j.1741-3737.2007.00393.x

Rao, N., and Rao, P.V. (1990). Desired Qualities in a Future Mate in India, *International Journal of Sociology of the Family, 20*(2), 181-198.

Schoen, R., Astone, N.M., Kim, Y.J., Rothert, K., and Standish, N.J. (2002). Women's employment, marital happiness, and divorce. *Social Forces, 81*(2), 643-662.

Seligman, M.E.P. (1975). *Helplessness: On Depression, Development and Death.* San Francisco, CA: Freeman.

Sen, P. (1999). Enhancing women's choices in responding to domestic violence in Calcutta: A comparison of employment and education. *European Journal of Development Research*, 11, 65-86.

Sharma, B. (2005). Social etiology of violence against women in India. *The Social Science Journal, 42*(3), 375–389. doi: 10.1016/j.soscij.2005.06.009.

Shear, K., and Shair, H. (2005). Attachment, loss, and complicated grief. *Developmental Psychobiology, 47*(3), 253–267. doi: 10.1002/dev.20091.

Singh, A. (2013). Marital rape: A socially and legally justified crime in India. In: K. Jaishankar, and N. Ronel (Ed.), *Second International Conference On The South Asian Society On Criminology And Victimology,* pp. 19-31, Tirunelveli, Tamil Nadu, India: Department of Criminology and Criminal Justice.

Singh, K. (2013). *Separated and divorced women in India: Economic rights and entitlements.* Ottawa, Ont.: International Development Research Centre.

Smock, P.J., Manning, W.D., and Gupta, S. (1999). The Effect of Marriage and Divorce on Women's Economic Well-Being. *American Sociological Review, 64*(6), 794-812. doi: 10.2307/2657403.

Sonpar, S. (2005). Marriage in India: Clinical Issues. *Contemporary Family Therapy, 27*(3), 301–313. doi: 10.1007/s10591-005-6211-z.

Stanley, S. (2007). Assessing couple and marital relationships: Beyond form and toward a deeper knowledge of function. In: S. Hofferth, and L. Casper, *Handbook of Measurement Issues in Family Research,* pp. 85–99, Mahwah, NJ: L. Erlbaum.

Strube, M.J. (1988). The decision to leave an abusive relationship: Empirical evidence and theoretical issues. *Psychological Bulletin, 104*(2), 236–250. doi: 10.1037//0033-2909.104.2.236.

Stagnor, C. (2011). *Research Methods For The Behavioural Sciences.* Belmont, CA: Wadsworth, Cengage Learning.

Strasburger, L.H. (1999). The Litigant-Patient: Mental Health Consequences of Civil Litigation. *J Am Acad Psychiatry Law. 27*(2). 203-211.

Thapan, M. (2003). Marriage, well-being, and agency among women, *Gender and Development, 11(2),* 77-84, DOI: 10.1080/741954320.

Walker, L.E. (1977-1978). Battered women and learned helplessness. *Victimology, 2*(3-4), 525-534.

Walker, L.E. (1984). *The Battered Woman Syndrome.* New York: Springer.

Walker, L.E. (2009). *The Battered Woman.* New York: Harper and Row.

Weiss, R. (1976). The Emotional Impact of Marital Separation. *Journal of Social Issues, 32*(1), 135–145. doi:10.1111/j.1540-4560.1976.tb02484.x.

Wilson, M., and Daly, M. (1993). An Evolutionary Psychological Perspective on Male Sexual Proprietariness and Violence Against Wives. *Violence and Victims*, *8*(3), 271–294. doi: 10.1891/0886-6708.8.3.271.

Legislation Cited

The Protection of Women from Domestic Violence Act, 2005 (No. 43 of 2005), Government of India.

The Family Court Act, 1984 (No. 66 of 1984), Government of India.

16

Physical Wounds and Psychological Repercussions of Rape

Rupali Joshi and *Aradhana Shukla*

Introduction

In the aftermath of a sexual assault or rape, survivors can face extremely difficult and painful emotions and experiences. Every survivor responds to traumatic events in their own way. The effects of the trauma can be short-term or last long after the sexual assault or rape. Rape is one of the most severe of all traumas, causing multiple long-term negative outcomes such as posttraumatic stress disorder (PTSD), depression, substance abuse, suicidality, repeated social victimization and chronic physical health problems (Kilpatric & Acierno, 2003; Koss, Bailey, Yuan, Herrera & Licher, 2003).

Law defines rape as vaginal or anal penetration in the absence of lawful consent. However, the source of penetration (e.g. Penis, finger or objects), object of perpetrator and victim and definition of consent varies greatly across jurisdictions. Rape is considered to have occurred when her consent has been obtained by putting her (or any person in whom she is interested, e.g. children, close relatives) in fear of death or of hurt, the administration by him personally or through another of any stupefying or unwholesome substance (so-called "date-rape") or when the age of the victim is below 16 years. Moreover, Indian Law (section 375 of Indian Penal Code) specifically states that if a woman consents to sex, that consent is invalid and rape is still considered to have taken place if the woman is suffering from "unsoundness of mind or intoxication" so that she is unable to understand the nature and consequences of that to which she gives consent.

Types of Rape

1. **Penetrative Rape:** The vagina is penetrated by penis, finger or other objects.
2. **Statutory Rape:** The penis is touched on vagina but no penetration takes place. This type of rape does not exist in Indian statutes yet.
3. **Marital Rape:** When rape occurs within a marriage. This is not yet recognized in Indian law.
4. **Gang Rape:** When more than one person rapes the victim.
5. **Date Rape:** When rape occurs during an exploratory platonic romantic meaning between man and woman, where often an intoxicating agent is mixed in the food or drink of the victim.

Rape, sexual assault and verbal abuse of females of all ages and socio-economic strata have become common incidents in India. Such crime distresses countless women and challenges their well-being. A new U.N. report has highlighted around 20 million girls around the world, close to one in 10, have been raped or seriously assaulted by the time they turn 20 years (UNICEF, 2014). United Nations Statistical report has shown about 65 countries completed data from government sources (registered cases only) that annually more than 25000 cases of rape or attempted rape were recorded by police (UNO, 2000).

According to Indian express dated on 15th Dec., 2013, National Crime Records Bureau of India reveals that there has been an eight-fold increase in the number of rapes in the last four decades. The rise in the number of rape cases is the most rapid compared to other serious crimes such as murder, robbery and kidnapping (Sardar, 2013). For every one hour, 2.84 cases of rape were reported in country in which, on an average, 3.55 persons were arrested during the year 2012 (NCRB, 2012). JAGORI (Non-government organization working for women safety in Delhi) and UN Women report 2010 have found that, in New Delhi about 66 per cent of women's reported experiencing sexual harassment between two to five times during the past year (JAGORI and Women, 2010). Rape cases day by day increase in major cities of India. Generally people believe that the primary cause of rape is an aggressive desire to dominate the victim rather than an attempt to achieve sexual fulfillment (JAGORI and Women, 2010). It is significant to note that on 16 December 2012 a 23 years old girl was raped and brutally hurt in Delhi while the rapists including the bus driver gave lift to girl and her boy friend returning to their homes.

After gang raping the girl and brutally assaulting her they threw the girl and her boy friend out of bus at roadside. The girl died from her virginal injuries after thirteen days undergoing emergency treatment in Singapore. The incident created a widespread nationwide and worldwide coverage and criticized by common people, various non-profit organization, social workers and women's groups, both in India and abroad. Subsequently, public protests especially girls/women's against the Government of Delhi and India for not providing appropriate protection for girls and women's took place in New Delhi (*The Economic Times*, 2012). Priority treatment is essential to be given in the rest of the country too, although equally serious crimes against women in outlying areas typically get less media attention. Numerous rape cases in India received widespread media attention and activated protests since 2012 (*The Telegraph*, 2012; Perceived government inaction over rape and murder of two teenage girls sparks public anger" India'sNews.Net). After this big issue rape cases suddenly increased due to women awareness and mass media exposure in India. According to the official statistics of NCRB India, incidents of crime against women (both under IPC and Special and Local Laws) These crimes have continuously increased during 2007-2011 with 185, 312 cases in the year 2007, 195,856 cases in the year 2008, 203,804 cases in the year 2009 and 213,585 cases in the year 2010 and 228,650 cases in the year 2011. A large number of studies have suggested the effective measures to prevent violence against women by fully enforcing their legal and constitutional rights and there by rehabilitating them in the 17977 Ramu Rawat and Tadapatri Masthanaiah, Explosion of rape cases in India: A study of last one decade society as its respect figure members (http://ncrb.gov.in/index.htm) Although, women being a victims of any of the general crimes such as rape, kidnapping and abduction for different purposes, torture-both mental and physical, molestation and sexual harassment. As crime against women various new legislation have been enacted and amendments have been made in existing laws with a view to handle these crimes effectively. n almost 94 per cent of the cases, the offenders were known to the victims-family members, friends, live-in partners, employers or others, the data showed.

Data of National Crime Report Bureau (2018)—According to National Crime Report Bureau (2018) 33,356 incidents of rape were reported during 2018 involving 33,977 victims, an average 89 rapes daily. In 2017, 32,559 rape cases were registered, while in 2016 the number stood at 38,947, the data stated. Overall, 72.2 per cent of rape victims were above 18 years and 27.8 per cent below 18, the data stated (National Crime Report Bureau, 2018). In 2018, 51.9 per cent rape victims (17,636) were aged between 18 and 30 years, 18 per cent (6,108) above 30 and below 45 years, 2.1 per cent (727) above 45 and below 60 years and 0.2 per cent (73) above 60 years, it showed. According to the NCRB, 14.1 per cent rape victims (4,779) were aged above 16 years and below 18 years, followed by 10.6 per cent (3,616) who were between 12 and 16 years, 2.2 per cent (757) who were between 6 years and 12 years and 0.8 per cent (281) were below 6 years. Among states, Madhya Pradesh reported the highest (5,433) such cases in 2018, followed by Rajasthan (4,335), Uttar Pradesh (3,946), Maharashtra (2,142), Chhattisgarh (2,091), Kerala (1,945), Assam (1,648), Delhi (1,215), Haryana (1,296), Jharkhand (1,090) and West Bengal (1,069).The NCRB data also showed that in almost 94 out of 100 rape cases, the victim were known to the offenders. In 15,972 of the total 33,356 rape cases, the offenders were either family friends or neighbour or employer or other known person, while in 12,568 cases, the offenders were friends or online friends or live-in partner on pretext of marriage or separated husband, the data stated. In 2,780 cases, the victims were violated by their own family members, while only in 2,036 cases the offenders were unknown to them, according to the statistics. The NCRB, under the Union Ministry of Home Affairs, is responsible for collecting and analysing crime data as defined by the Indian Penal Code and special and local laws in the country.

Despite the fact that rape is regarded heinous and criminal in nature, the number and the level of inhumanity of this crime has been on a rise. Be it in affluent or frugal, educated or non-educated contexts; or open or closed societies, this crime is on a rise. Studies that have continued to assess rape victims over time (Resick, 18 months, Kilpatrick & Veronen, 1983 for 3 years) or have assessed women after an extended period (Burgers & Holmstrom, 1978 after 6 years, Elis, Atkinson & Calhoun, 1981 from 16 years have found continued problems with fear of depression. The psychological consequences of sexual trauma among survivors have been widely studied. The National Violence against Women Survey reported that 18 per cent of women experienced a completed or attempted rape during their lifetime (Tjaden & Thoennes, 2000). Majority (54%) of the rape survivors were less than 18 years old when they experienced their first attempted or completed rape. The responses of survivors to the trauma of rape are complex and unique (Brier & Jordon, 2000).

Indian Studies on Status and Consequences of Rape

Madan and Sinha (2013) addressed dynamics of rape with particular reference to India and examined recently introduced Indian law to reduce rape incidents. They applied correlations to rape data from all the 35 regions of India with eleven socio-economic demographic predictor variables to find the effect of the variables of incidents of rape. It was found that only literary status as a proxy for male and female in urban population indicated significant desirable effect on the number of rape incidents.

Rawat and Masthanaiah (2015) examined the rape trends and situations in India and its states during last one decade by age and religion. They used National Crime Records Bureau (NCRB) of India data for the year 2004-2013. During study period they found rape cases significantly increased in all states. They also found the rape cases committed by the blood relatives remarkable increased over time period and age group 18-30 years have been found more venerable group.

Davey (2020) studied rape against girls and women and found rape is the fourth most common crime in India and also found that 97 cases were committed by someone known to victim and said this leads various physical and mental problems among rape victims. The Indian studies also indicate that rape is very serious problem in India. It marked that girls are not safe even in their house and more vulnerable group was found 18-30 years. However, it is also essential to understand as to what are types of psychological repercussions females feel after being the victim of rape.

Psychological Repercussions of Rape

Rape and sexual violence frequently results in many negative consequences for women. Consequently psychological mechanisms to motivate rape-avoidance behaviours in women have evolved. Rape is traumatic for women due to fear of serious physical injury or death. Psychological repercussions of Rape include several serious consequences like negative self belief, anxiety, depression, low self-esteem etc.

Depression is a common and serious medical illness that negatively affects how you feel, the way you think and how you act. Depression causes feelings of sadness and or loss of interest in activities once enjoyed. It can lead to a variety of emotional and physical problems and can decrease a person's ability to function at work and home.

Two groups of researchers have focused primarily on the assessment of depression in rape victims.

Frank, Turner and Duffy (1979) administered the Beck Depression Inventory (BDI, Beck, Ward, Mendelsohn, Mock & Rebought, 1961) to 34 rape victims within one month of their assaults. They found that 44 per cent scored in the moderately or severely depressed range. A later study with a larger sample (n = 90) resulted in similar findings (Frank & Stewarch, 1984). On the BDI, 56 per cent of those subjects fell in to the moderately or severely depressed range and 43 per cent of the women were diagnosed as suffering from a major depression based on a semi structured interview.

Atkinson *et al.* (1982) examined depressive reactions in rape victims compared to non-victims over a one-year period using the BDI and the Hamilton Psychiatric Rating scale for Depression (HPRS, Hamilton, 1960). They found that both the BDI and HPRS scores for the rape victims were significantly different than non-victims at 2 weeks, 1 month and 2 months post-assault but not at the later assessment periods. On the BDI, at 2 weeks post crime 75 per cent of the victims reported from mild to severe symptoms of depression.

Other studies have found similar levels of depression initially (Kil Patrick & Veronen, 1984; Resick, 1988; Rothbaum *et al.*, 1992) using the BDI, the Depression-Dejection scale from the Profile of Mood States Scale (POMS, McNair, Lorrr & Droppleman, 1971) on the Depression subscale from SCl-90R or BSI. However, Kilpatrick and Veronen (1984) continued to find differences between victims and non victims for 1 year after the crime on both the depression subscales between robbery and rape victims at the 1, 3, 6 and 18 month sessions but not the 12-month session, on a cross sectional analysis, but found no differences at any session on a longitudinal analysis with a smaller sample.

Finally, the level of suicidal ideation and attempts among rape victims is notable. Although the rates of suicidal behaviour are not very high in the first month after victimization, Elis *et al.* (1981) found that 50 per cent of their long term sample had considered suicide. Kilpatrick, Best *et al.* (1985) found in their random survey that 44 per cent of rape victims had suicidal ideation and that 19 per cent had suicide attempt.

Rothbaum, Foa, Murdock, Riggs and Walsh (1992) have studied early patterns of reaction by assessing 95 victims of rape or attempted rape weekly for 12 weeks following the crime. They found a consistent pattern with most of the assessment measures they used. At 1-week post crime, 94 per cent of the subjects met the symptoms of criterion for posttraumatic stress disorder, stress disorder and were clinically depressed.

Abrahamas, Jewkes and Mathews (2012) interviewed 140 participants who were recruited from public hospital service medication. A structured questionnaire was used to collect data on socio-demographic and sexual assault characteristics including perpetrator. Depressive symptomatology was measured using the Centre for Epidemiological Studies Depression Scale. Results showed 84.3 per cent (95%) women were found to have high level of depressive symptoms but lower levels were found among women raped in circumstances in which there was a lesser likelihood of blame such as those raped by stranger rather than intimate partners. Receiving support and severe sexual assault were not associated with depression.

Patrica (1993) studied to review the literature on the psychological impact of rape on adult female victims. Typical patterns of recovery were all reviewed. The problems were fear and anxiety, post-traumatic stress disorder, depression, poor self-esteem, social adjustment issues and sexual dysfunctions.

Choudhary, Smith and Bossarte (2011) aimed to identify patterns in the associations between sexual violence victimization and depression and anxiety symptoms using data from the sexual violence and DA Behavioural Risk Factor Surveillance System (BRFSS) modules. Among all 61,187 participants more than 5 (n = 3, 240) were victims of sexual violence, out of which 18.82 per cent reported being diagnosed with depression and anxiety, 8.37 per cent reported an anxiety disorder and 29.28 per cent reported being diagnosed with Depression and Anxiety Disorder.

Self-esteem reflects an individual's overall subjective emotional evaluation of his or her own worth. It is the decision made by an individual as an attitude toward the self. Self-esteem encompasses beliefs about oneself, as well as emotional states. Self-esteem is attractive as a social psychological construct because researchers have conceptualized it as an influential predictor of certain outcomes. Psychologists usually regard self-esteem as an enduring personality characteristic.

Given the debilitating psychological impact of rape, it is a reasonable to hypothesize that victimization would have a negative impact on victim's self-esteem. Janoff-Bulman and Friezee (1983) have identified self-esteem as a relevant clinical issue for rape victims.

While several authors have suggested that rape victims experience a reduction in self-esteem (Wortman, 1983), there are few data available in this area. Data that are available are limited by an absence of comparison groups of non victims; nevertheless, they provide preliminary support for low self-esteem among rape victims. Resick (1987a) administered the Tennessee Self Concept Scale (TSCS; Fitts, 1965) to rape-robbery victims. She found that overall; rape-robbery victims had lower self-esteem than both the other groups at all assessment sessions up to and until one-year post-rape.

Murphy *et al.* (1998) conducted a study on 204 recent rape victims and a matched comparison group of 173 women to determine the short and long term effects of rape victim's self-esteem. Research participants were assessed at 6-21 days, 1 month, 3 months, 6 months, 1 year, 18 months and 2 years post-assault. Findings suggest that victims experience short and long term problems in self-esteem, relationships with others, work satisfaction, relationship with authority, hope for the future and happiness with life, reality and parents compared with non-victims. Victims reported impaired relationships with significant others at 1 year, post-assault significantly, lower self-esteem and 18 months post-assault and lower satisfaction in relation with their parents at the 2-year post-assault assessment.

Abdullah, Sallesh, Mahmud, Ahmad and Ghani (2011) investigated the relationship among cognitive distortion, depression and self-esteem. Self-Cognitive Distortion Scale (CDS), Beck Depression Scale (BDI) and Rosenberg Self-Esteem Scale (RSES). Correlation indicated a positive correlation between cognitive distortion and depression with self-esteem. Results also concluded that rape victims are likely to experience a certain degree of cognitive distortion.

Periloux, Duntley and Boss (2012) examined costs experienced by victims of completed rape (n = 49) and attempted sexual assault (n = 91) using quantitative analysis of domains: health, self-esteem, self-perceived attractiveness, self-perceived mate value, family relationship, work life, social life, social reputation, desire to have sex, frequency of sex, enjoyment of sex and long term committed relationship. Compared to victims of an attempted sexual assault, victims of rape reported significantly more negative outcomes in 11 of 13 domains. The most negatively affected domains were self-esteem, sexual reputation, frequency of sex, desire to have sex and self-perceived mate values.

Krahe (1988) presented a longitudinal analysis of the links between sexual assault, victimization, depression and sexual self-esteem by examining their cross-legged paths among both men and women. The sample comprised of 2,425 male and female college students. The study consisted of three data waves in their first, second and third year of university separated by 12 months' interval, with sexual assault at one-T1 since the age of 14 and at T2 and T3 for the last of 12 months. Depression and sexual self-esteem were measured at each level. Random intercept cross-legged panel analysis controlling for individual differences in depression and sexual self-esteem showed that sexual assault at T1 predicted depression whereas T2 predictor is associated with depression and lower self-esteem. The T3 predictor is related with sexual assault victimization as such as well as sexual assault victimization by undergoing depression at T2. Both depression and lower sexual esteem at T1 were indirectly linked to sexual victimization at T3. Sexual assault victimization was shown to be a risk factor for both depression as a general mental health indicator and lowered sexual self-esteem as a specific outcome in the domain of sexuality.

Vianna (2006) conducted a qualitative study to show the results of workshops held with health workers and public health users (raped women) aimed at raising these women's self-esteem and creating awareness among health workers who attend hem. Neuro-Linguistic Programming techniques were used to bring back life experiences which contributed to re-reading and to minimize causal factors of low self-esteem. Results showed that experiences lived at home and with loved and admired people and carrying experiences resulting from the rape were responsible for low self-esteem.

Conclusion and Recommendations

According to several studies the number of rape cases is increasing in India. The disturbing trends of increased attempts and rate of rape across various females of various age groups and states are also visible. Rape victims suffer with spectrum of physical and psychiatric disorders naming lower self-esteem, depression, victimization and sexual and physical health to name a few, resulting in higher health care use. In the domain of psychology, review of the literature indicates that rape is associated with multiple psychological disorders including anxiety, depression, PTSD, eating disorders, sleep disorders and low self-esteem.

The tailing after-effects of rape viz. social stigma, alienation and trust deficit are the layer of negative consequences of the trauma. Rape victims need extensive post-assault attention and understanding and may turn to multiple social systems for assistance. Approximately 26 per cent to 40 per cent victims report the assault to the police and pursue prosecution through the criminal justice system, 27 per cent to 40 per cent seek medical care and medical forensic examination and 16 per cent to 60 per cent obtain mental health services. Survivors experience diverse negative impacts of sexual assault; there is no list of typical "symptoms" they should exhibit. Such impacts affect not only the physical and mental health of survivors but also their interpersonal relationships with family, friends, partners, colleagues and so on. Further research is necessary to better understand the pathogenesis of psychiatric disorders in survivors of sexual assault. Research is also needed to determine evidence-based management of survivors of sexual abuse coping with long-term mental health outcomes.

The literature studied and various patterns and trends related to the rape victims examined along with the after-effects they experience, implies that the victims need a sophisticated and multi-pronged strategy encompassing the medical, physical, mental and legal intervention. The traumatic and inhuman crime warrants the need for the victims to be able to receive the medical intervention (physical and clinical), psychological assistance and legal follow-up in empathic, supportive manner, thus facilitating the urgently needed recovery process.

References

Abdullah, S., Salleh, A., and Abdul, S. (2011). Cognitive Distortion, Depression and Self-esteem among adolescent rape victims. *World Applied Science Journal, 67*(7), 1067-71.

Abraham, N., and Jewkes, R. (2005). Effects of South African men's are having witnessed abuse of their months during childhood on their levels of violence in adulthood. *American Journal of Public Health, 95*, 181-196.

Atkinson, B., Cathoun, K., Resick, P., and Elis, E. (1982). Victims of Rape: Repeated Assessment of Depressive Symptoms. *Journal of Counselling and Clinical Psychology, 50,* 96-102.

Bohner, G. and Lamprides, E. (2004). Expecting to meet a rape victim affects women's self-esteem. The moderating role of rape myth acceptance. *Group Processing and Intergroup Relations, 7*, 77-87.

Briere, J., and Jordan, C.E. (2014). Violence against women: outcome complexity and implications for assessment and treatment. *Journal of Interpersonal Violence*, 19 (11), 1252-1276.

Bulman, R.J. and Frieze I.H. (1983). Theoretical Perspective for understanding reactions to victimized understanding Reactions to victimization. *Journal of Social Issues, 39* (2), 195-22.

Choudhary, E., Merideth, S. and Bussente, R.M. (2011). Depression, anxiety and symptom profile among female and male victims of sexual violence. *American Journal of men's Health, 6* (1), 28-36.

Crime against women, *Crime in India 2012 Statistics,* National Crime Records Bureau (NCRB), Ministry of Home Affairs, Government of India, p. 81, archived from the original (PDF) on 16 January 2016.

Davey, S. (2020). Rapes in Society: An emerging public health problem of Indian Girls and Women, *Acta Scientific Women's Health, 2*(2).

Frank, F., Turner, S.M. and Duffy, B. (1979). Depressive Symptoms in rape victims. *Journal of Affective Disorder, 1,* 269-277.

https://www.reuters.com/article/us-india-rape-factbox/statistics-on-rape-in-india-and-some-well-known-cases-idUSKBN1YA0UV.

Jagori and Women, U.N. 2010 Report on the baseline survey. http/Jagori.org.

Kilpatric, D.G. (1985). The Sexual assault research Project: Assessing the aftermath of rape response, 8, 20-24.

Kilpatric, D.G. and Aciernnao, R. (2003). Mental Health Needs of Crime Victims Epidemiology and outcomes. *Journal of Traumatic Stress, 16,* 119-132.

Koss, M.P., Bailey, J.A., Yuva, N.P., Herrera, V.M., and Litcher, E.L. (2003). Depression and PTSD in survivors of male violence: Research and Training initiatives to facilitate recovery. *Psychology of Women Quarterly, 27,* 130-142.

Krate, B. (1998). Sexual aggression among adolescents. *Psychology of women Quarterly, 22*, 37-54.

Kumar, R. (2003). *The history of doing: an illustrated action of movements for women's rights and feminism in India, 1800-1990.* New Delhi: Kali for Women, 128.

Lora, P. and Sarah, P. (2014). *The Fear that Stalks: Gender Based Violence in Public Spaces*, Zubaan Books, 79.

Mathew, S., Jewkes, R., Abraham, N. (2011). I had a hard life: Exploring childhood adversity in the shaping of masculinities among men who killed an intimate partner in South Africa. *British Journal of Criminology, 51*(4).

McNair, D., Lor, M. and Droppleman, L. (1971). Manual Profile of mood states. San Diego, SA Education and Industrial Testing Service.

Murphy, S.A. (1988). Mediating effects of intrapersonal and social support on mental health and 3 years after a natural disaster. *Journal of Traumatic Stress, 1,* 155-172.

Patrica, A.R. (1993). The Psychological impact of rape. *Journal of Interpersonal Violence, 6* 223-255.

Perilloux, C., Duntley, J.D. and Buse, D.M. (2012). The costs of Rape. *Archives of Sexual Behaviour, 41*(5), 1099-1106.

Rawat, R. and Masthanaiah, T. (2015). Explosion of Rape Cases in India: A study of last One decade, *International Journal of Current Research, 7 (7),* 17976-17985.

Resick, P.A. (1988). *Reactions of female and male victims of rape and robbery.* A Finl report (Grant no-85-IJ-(X-0042) Washington D.C. National Institute of Justice.

Rothbaum, B.O., Merdock, T., Riggs, D.S. and Walsh, W. (1992). A prospective examination of Post-traumatic Stress Disorders in rape victims. *Journal of Traumatic Stress, 5,* 455-475.

Sinha, R.K. and Madan, V.K. (2013). The Dynamics of Rape in Modern Indian Society. *International Journal of Juridical Sciences, 4,* 81-87.

Sirnate, V. (2014). Good laws had bad implementation. *The Hindu*, Chennai, India. Retrieved 1 February 2014.

Staff Writer (9 may 2017). NCRB Data shows 955 rape victims in India known to offenders, Madhya Pradesh tops the list First Chennai, India. Retrieved 27 October 2017.

Vasundhara, S. (1 February 2014). Good laws, bad implementation. *The Hindu*. Chennai, India. Retrieved 1 February 2014.

Vianna, L., Bomfem, G.F., Chicone, G. Self-esteem of Raped Women. *Rev Latino-and Enermager 14*(2), 695-701.

17

Notions of Happiness in Indian Women of Middle Adulthood

Dhvani Patel and *Manisha Gauniyal*

Introduction

Emotions have not received the due attention in psychology mainstream for long, except largely by clinical and personality psychologists in their attempt to understand the negative and pathological side of emotions. The Indian construct of intelligence, although sharing similarities with the western construct, has additional characteristics as marked by the commoners' notion of intelligence. One of the competencies thought to be important to consider an individual as possessing intellectual capabilities, is emotional competence. Emotions to a large extent determine the ill-being and wellbeing of both, the society and the individual (Misra, 2014, p. 205). In their exploratory study, Srivastava and Misra (2001) found the lay persons' conceptualizations of intelligence being predominated by the socio-affective regulation of one's conduct, which in turn determined the wellbeing of the individual as well as the society.

As the wave of Positive Psychology movement took over the academia since the last two decades, focus has shifted from the negative and irrational nature of emotions to the positive and constructive side of emotions. Even before the advent of positive psychology movement, there had been experts in the psychology discipline who had emphasized on the positive side of human nature, such as the approaches of humanism and existentialism. It was the illness model of the then thriving clinical psychology that gave the impetus to the birth of community psychology as a field of significance which emphasized on the health model. Happiness, well-being and optimal functioning are the subject areas of positive psychology. Positive psychology appears to be distinct from past perspectives, in its aims and objectives, and its commitment to scientific methodology (Seligman & Ciskszenthmihalyi, 2014). In India, the positive psychology movement witnessed a surge of national level conferences on themes pertaining to positive psychology, creating a strong need to apply the principles of positive psychology to varied areas of psychology.

Women and the Developmental Trajectory of Happiness

As an advocate to the life span perspective on development, Carl Jung recognized the importance of middle age, which is famously quoted as "the afternoon of life" (Jung, 1933, p. 109 cited in Lachman, 2015). Until recently, scholarly work on middle years (roughly ages 40-59 years) has been sparse and largely overlooked. One of the reasons behind failing to gain scholarly interest is also identifying what is so significant and different in middle years when compared to the rest of the life stages that warrants a researcher's curiosity. Stereotypical conceptions of midlife resulting in myths about "midlife crises" need to be rigorously addressed since these pre-conceptions have a negative impact on the otherwise smooth transition of a young adult into middle age. Frijters and Beatton (2012) point out that happiness and life satisfaction reaches the lowest point at midlife, which was termed as the "u-bend". In contrast, other experts point out toward a linear increase in happiness as one moves from young adulthood to middle adulthood (Easterlin, 2006). Variations such as these, can be attributed to covariates akin to one's marital and occupational status. It seems fair to propose that scholars in the development research need to highlight the importance of wellbeing among the middle aged, who play a central role for both the young and the old (Lachman, 2015). Lachman, Teshale, and Agrigoroaei (2015) further highlight upon the crucial role that midlife plays to function as a bridge between the past and the present, between the young and the old, and between the family and societal roles.

Research has also pointed out on the type of positive affect that goes through changes as one ages. Young adults are seen to have an increased preference for high arousal positive state and middle age adults, young olds and old-olds are seen to incline more toward the low arousal positive affect (Scheibe, English, Tsai & Carstensen, 2013). Arousal affective states are also aligned with the tendency of people to have reactions toward the futuristic life: excitement (high arousal positive state) and/or for people to live the experience of the present state: peace and calm (low arousal positive state) ((Mogilner, Kamvar, & Aaker, 2011, p. 162 in Scheibe *et al.*, 2013). Kamvar, Mogilner, & Aaker (2009) concluded from a group of four studies that the meaning of happiness undergoes a shift as one ages.

As a young adult, happiness is associated with excitement and as one grows older, happiness becomes associated with feeling peaceful, resulting largely from the increase in social connectedness as one progress in age.

Marital status and happiness have often been twinned together. An across 17-nation study pointed out that marriage equally affects men and women to experience happiness, which is a function of increased financial satisfaction and an improvement of health (Stack & Eshleman, 1998). Arranged marriages in India have been an age old tradition which is still followed. The success of an arranged marriage, which is not necessarily a forced alliance, depends on the higher levels of marital satisfaction. Bowman and Dollahite (2013) point out that family and religious involvement are the key elements that result in marital satisfaction in arranged marriages among Indian couples.

India and Cultural Experiences of Happiness

Culture is a learned phenomenon, which portrays a set of shared attitudes, feelings and behaviour, enabling us to differentiate one cultural group from the other. One of the frequent classifications of culture as explored by anthropologists and social psychologists is individualism versus collectivism. While individuals in the individualistic culture experience emotions as "coming from within", those in the collectivistic culture experience emotions based on "relatedness with others" (Baron & Branscombe, 2012, p. 79). Biswas-Deiner, Tay, & Deiner (2012) noted that happiness can be majorly caused by "outside-in" or "inside-out" phenomenon. The "outside-in" perspective largely covers the nation's wealth and current economic state that result in the feeling of happiness for the Indians. The "inside-out" perspective includes all the factors that help individuals to interpret and make sense of the daily occurrences, which in turn will influence the experience of happiness. Since Indians are more of a group culture, it makes more sense to focus on the "inside-out" perspective to the study of happiness.

As the proportion of women working in the Indian labour force continue to show a steady decline, one questions as to how happy are the homemakers? Nathawat and Mathur (1993) concluded from their study that working women scored higher on general health, life satisfaction and self-esteem measures as compared to their non-working counterparts. However interestingly, non-working women had low scores on negative affect when compared to the working women. Working women striving to go beyond their homes, bare an addition of strained relations, guilty parenting and working overtime based on the disproportionate distribution of household chores on the home front. Homemakers on the other hand, may display a higher satisfaction from having fulfilled their role relationships, experiencing reduced stress resulting from zero burdens from role conflicts.

The Present Study

This is an explorative study aimed at gaining an insight into the 'happy moments' to understand how female homemakers in the middle adulthood construe happiness in their lives. There is an underlying assumption of being able to link the relational, social-cultural, and developmental factors that act as a force, jointly shaping the lived experiences of these female participants.

Method

The present study adopted the qualitative research method, using semi-structured in-depth interviews as a tool to gather information from the participants of the study.

Sample—The participants of the study included middle aged women (between the age range of 45-65 years) residing in India, belonging to the urban middle class. These women: (1) Homemakers not engaged in any form of economic or work-related activities, (2) Were married and had children (women who were single owing to varied reasons were excluded and women whose children had left home for further studies and/or jobs were also excluded), and (3) The knowledge of either English or Hindi. The tool was prepared in English and translated in Hindi, so participants fluent in any of these languages were considered as ideal sample. Since the study was on understanding the experiences of the middle-aged women, life situations like divorce, death of spouse, empty nest syndrome, had to be controlled in the selection of the participants for this study so as to not cloud the experiences of happiness in these women. Also, life experiences of working women are quite varied than those of home-makers; hence, conscious efforts were made to select participants who neither were currently involved in any form of economic activity nor had past history of having been engaged in any form of economic activity.

Tools—A semi-structured interview schedule was prepared by the researchers by carrying out an extensive literature review on happiness studies in order to ensure a complete coverage of varied aspects of happiness, ranging from understanding the basic explanations of happiness to expressions of happiness and relating some lived experiences of a recent 'happy moment'. A personal data sheet was also prepared for the purpose of seeking demographic details of the participants (for instance, age, education qualification, and details of family members, religion, and the like). The interview schedule was first constructed in English and translated into Hindi by a language expert and then verified by a Professor in Hindi. It was further given for expert validation to three experts from the field of social sciences for their inputs (one from psychology, one from sociology and one from education). A final draft of the interview schedule was prepared after incorporating the suggestions from the experts. Thereafter, the researchers' pilot tested the interview schedule to understand whether meaningful information is being generated from the set of questions asked. Some questions were reworded and few additional probing questions were added.

Procedure—The present study was a qualitative study exploring the parameters of happiness in middle-aged Indian women. For ease of rapport formation and disclosure, the participants were approached for prior permission. Snowball purposive sampling method was used for the selection of the study participants. Snowball sampling is an extensively used non-probability method to locate hidden population. This sampling method relies on the referrals made by the participants of the study, to identify other individuals who share similar characteristics with the participants and thereby fulfill the inclusion criteria of the research.

Each participant was approached either at their residence or at a place which they frequent (for instance, a park, or vegetable market). They were provided with information regarding the research and informed about the study requirements. Once they agreed to participate, a date and time was fixed and a consent form was signed by them, wherein they were informed that their confidentiality would be maintained and the interview would be recorded for data collection purposes only. The interviews were carried out in the home settings of the participants in order to make it convenient for the participants and also to enable them to freely engage in a meaningful conversation.

At the end of each interview, the researchers also maintained a journal for field notes, to capture their own subjective experiences and observations made during the interview. During the interviewing, there were a lot of nonverbal acts, venting of emotions and prolonged pauses that necessitate the need to highlight those, which may have further implications.

Interviews were carried out on ten participants, after which a decision was reached to discontinue interviewing more participants, since the researchers had reached saturation. Saturation is often used in qualitative research as a criterion to discontinue gathering more data, at a stage when the researcher fails to extract any further new information from the sample participants (Glaser & Strauss, 1967).

Analysis—Given the small sample size and the exploratory nature of the study, the data analysis was qualitative in nature. The responses from the interview were transcribed verbatim. Wherever Hindi was used, the translations were made, but certain utterances were kept in the original language to capture the nuances so culturally relevant. Using content analysis, the data was reduced and categories were formed. Emerging themes are discussed in the following section.

Results

This section is divided into two sub sections: I. Profile of the participants, II. Emerging themes from the qualitative content

Profile of the Participants

Ten female homemakers represented as the sample for this study. All the study participants were followers of Hindu religion, and have been residing in India. The average age of the participants was 50.5 years, with the youngest participant of 45 years and the oldest being of 61 years. In terms of educational qualification, only one had post-graduation degree, three with graduation degree, and rest were school dropouts at either grade 8, 10 or 12. With regard to family structure, two participants were living in a joint family system, residing with ten other family members. The rest of the eight participants belonged to the nuclear family system, with number of family members ranging from four to six. Number of years of wedlock ranged from 22 years to 42 years among the ten participants. A noteworthy feature is when asked for number of years of marriage, the female participants even recalled their own age when they got married. Five participants had two children, two participants having a single child, and two participants gave birth to five children. Age of the children varied considerably, with some being in early twenties and rest being in thirties.

Happiness is Family Bound

The responses of all the participants of the study reflected an uniformity in their view of the family as the main source of happiness. Happiness was thought to be strongly connected with the achievements of the children for some and also, the marriage of the grandchildren for one. As quoted by one of the participants, *"Mere sare bacche hai...kal ko poti ki shadi ho jaye uss mai khushi hai. Sab ka sath me rehna khushi hai"* (Unity and family solidarity were of utmost importance). Within the family, husband's health and ability to make a living was considered something to be grateful about (*husband apne kaam may busy rahi bus yeh he mere leya khushiya hai*). These middle aged women derived a significant amount of comfort from the ability to perform the routine activities of everyday life. The value of happiness was also equated with 'family time', a phenomenon which is gradually fading in this rapid paced technological living. One participant went on further to add that keeping the family members happy, is what brings happiness to her. There was a sort of dilemma and paradox, where on one hand, she readily defined happiness as "*apne hisab se jeena*", viz., living on one's own terms and then immediately, added "*aur family k members ko bhi kush rakhna*", that is, keeping the family members happy. While dwelling over what she had just said, she further added "*agar may unko pehley kush rakhu to mai apney ko pehley let go karungi, compromise karungi haa or mai ye he kartihu. Apneyko compromise kar k*", meaning that family happiness becomes the first priority and more often than not, she compromises her own happiness. This interestingly demonstrates the predicament that many women in the Indian tradition go through. Having been socialised from an early age, to keep others' needs first, be it the elders of the house, and more specifically the men of the household, and that followed by the needs of the brother(s) and the husband, for an Indian women the flow of happiness has many obstructions and curves, that often slow down the speed of this flow to bring to consciousness the experience of becoming aware of one's happy state and critically judging their own responses to fulfilment of their needs and desires. This brings to mind the notion of "*Lakshmana Rekha*" as popularly recited in *Ramayana*[1] where *Lakshmana* (Lord Rama's brother) draws a line (*Rekha*) to protect his brother's wife *Sita*. *Sita* must resist her temptations to cross the line, which when she does, brings a lot of misfortune and everyone suffers through

1. *Ramayana* is a Sanskrit Epic of Ancient India, in which that Maharshi Valmiki (Sage) narrates the life of Lord Rama, the Prince of Kosala.

the end. As compared to females of the 21st century, women born in the previous century, have been accustomed to having their existence within boundaries; boundaries that here extend from physical boundaries (four walls of the home) to psychological boundaries (containing oneself and one's emotions).

Expressing Happiness the Sharing Way!

Sharing of happiness as well as expressing happiness has also found to be largely defined by family ties. Most of the participants of the study (70%) share their happy moments with their spouses. As one participant responded with amusement, *"jab khush hoti hu tabh bhi or jab bahut gusasey may hoti hu tabh bhi* (laughing) *kyuki ab hamre pass ak dusare k sevay option nahi hein, vaha bhi or yaha bhi vo he hai jin se bol saktey hai he is the only option"*. This is indicative of the close bond that couples at middle age experience. Studies on marital happiness have also supported this phenomenon where couples, as they progress further in their marital relationships, over the years, learn to be with each other and become fond of each other. A probable explanation as indicative of what the participant quoted above, is that reduction in family size owing to death of grandparents, and also a minimising of demands posed by children once they get married and move ahead with their own lives, there is an observed positive shift toward one's spouse. Positive family relationships thus play an integral part in both causing happiness and sustaining it. Pagani, Parise, Donato, Gable and Schoebi (2020) researched on reactions toward partner's disclosure to positive wellbeing and conceptualised it as 'capitalization response'. Further, findings from their study revealed that partner's involvement and support in good times not only reinforced a positive couple identity but also contributed to the partner's relational wellbeing. Easterlin (2003) further points out that on an average, married people are consistently throughout the duration of their marriage happier than people who are not. Just as marriage affects happiness positively, dissolution of marriage affects happiness negatively.

20 per cent of the study participants enjoy sharing happy moments with their neighbours. One of the participants in sharing happiness states *"vase tho koi nahi or ha aas pas log hai jese padosi unkay sath bolti hut to mann halka ho jata hai* (*although no one is there, but the neighbours and I talk to them and it makes me relieved*)*"*. The close proximity with the neighbours enables the female participant to often share with them in situations where she cannot contain herself. Patel and Prince (2001)

note in their study on Goan Aging people that the caring tradition of the extended family is changing rapidly and that neighbours, as a part of community resources often act as a strong source of social support. 20 per cent of the study participants also fondly share their happiness with 'daughter-in-law'. Usha Menon (2012) points out on how women at this age, if fortunate, attain mature adulthood, as the senior-most women of the house, which provides them with opportunities for wellbeing. By experiences of wellbeing here is meant, centrality, dominance and coherence. Relation between mother-in-law and daughter-in-law has received very less attention from researchers, although the implications of it are many in a joint family structure. Marked by power struggles, it is considered rarest of the rare, when the relations between the mother-in-law and daughter-in-law are cordial. Sharing of happiness definitely paints a unique picture of this relationship.

Religiosity and Happiness go Hand in Hand

At different stages of the interview, the study participants revealed the pleasure they seek from engaging in religious activities like singing devotional songs, going for 'satsang' (in the company of spiritual people) and following the daily morning ritual of prayers to God. One of the participants is quoted as saying *"bas sanoshrakhneka... sab apne aap hojata hai jo naseeb me hota hai wohi miltnahai zabardasti kisi se le naisakte"*. This reveals the extent to which one is adjusting to what life has to offer. There is a strong faith in God and a firm belief in destiny. The Hindu concept of 'karma' comes into play here. As a devotee, one firmly believes what one gives is what one gets. Past research has echoed with the findings of this study to indicate toward a positive relation between happiness and religiosity (Maheshwari & Singh, 2009; Migheli, 2009; Singh, 2014).

Researchers' Note

An interesting phenomenon observed by the researchers was the venting of emotions, more often of remorse of having left something joyful or being unable to attain something in life. Two participants experienced catharsis, and the interviewer-interviewee relation turned into a counselor-client session. What seemed to the researchers was that the study participants had lesser people to talk to, and when asked, responded in a manner as if they had suppressed all those emotions. This finding points out to the fact that it becomes important for the community to provide alternatives to counselling to this age group. More research should be guided in this direction of understanding the mental health needs of the women in middle adulthood.

Conclusion

Several theoretical attempts have been made to understand the state of happiness. Haybron (2008) quotes happiness as "a paradigm of uncertainty", pointing out to the intangible and evanescent nature of happiness. Happiness is one of the most basic emotions but culture dictates how emotions are expressed in a given context. It was manifested from the participants' responses that happiness is primarily shared and expressed with the family, a reaction of "otherwise who else it can be?" Following our age old philosophy of "*Vasudhaiva Kutumbakam*", which means the whole world is one family, family values are considered important to be passed on from one generation to the other. The joint family system has been a unique feature of our Indian culture that finds proof in the responses emitted by the participants of the study. The findings of the study do not diverge from the past research on Happiness in the Indian context, although definitely add to the notion of how happiness is experienced in the middle age by women who are primarily home-makers. The responses of the participants indicate toward an experience of wellbeing rather than happiness, largely shaped by non-materialistic pursuits such as being able to spend time with family. Age as a factor also surfaced to determine the experiences that Indian female homemakers have, where happiness is akin to peace and rooted to social connectedness. Beyond social links, are found the religious ties that enhance the experience of a peaceful living.

References

Bowman, J.L., and Dollahite, D.C. (2013). "Why would such a person dream about heaven?" Family, faith, and happiness in arranged marriages in India." *Journal of Comparative Family Studies*, *44*(2), 207-225.

Biswas-Diener, R., Tay, L., and Diener, E. (2012). Happiness in India. In *Happiness across Cultures,* pp. 13-25, Springer, Dordrecht.

Easterlin, R.A. (2003). Explaining happiness. *Proceedings of the National Academy of Sciences*, *100*(19), 11176-11183.

Easterlin, R.A. (2006). Life cycle happiness and its sources: Intersections of psychology, economics, and demography. *Journal of Economic Psychology*, *27*(4), 463-482.

Frijters, P., and Beatton, T. (2012). The mystery of the U-shaped relationship between happiness and age. *Journal of Economic Behaviour and Organization*, 82, 525–542. doi: 10.1016/j.jebo.2012.03.008.

Glaser Barney, G., and Strauss Anselm, L. (1967). *The discovery of grounded theory: strategies for qualitative research*. New York, Adline de Gruyter.

Haybron, D.M., and Haybron, D. (2008). *The Pursuit of Unhappiness: The Elusive Psychology of Well-being*. Oxford University Press.

Kamvar, S., Mogilner, C., and Aaker, J.L. (2009). *The Meaning (s) of Happiness*. Graduate School of Business, Stanford University.

Lachman, M.E., Teshale, S., Agrigoroaei, S. (2015). Midlife as a pivotal period in the life course: Balancing growth and decline at the crossroads of youth and old age. *International Journal of Behavioural Development*, 39: 20–31. doi: 10.1177/0165025414533223.

Lachman, M.E. (2015). Mind the gap in the middle: A call to study midlife. *Research in Human Development*, *12*(3-4), 327-334.

Maheshwari, S., and Singh, P. (2009). Psychological well-being and pilgrimage: Religiosity, happiness and life satisfaction of Ardh–Kumbh Mela pilgrims (Kalpvasis) at Prayag, India. *Asian Journal of Social Psychology*, *12*(4), 285-292.

Menon, U. (2012). Hinduism, happiness and wellbeing: A case study of adulthood in an Oriya Hindu Temple Town. In: *Happiness Across Cultures*, pp. 417-434, Springer, Dordrecht.

Migheli, M. (2009). *Religiosity and Happiness: An ever winning couple? An answer from India* (No. 126). Institute of Public Policy and Public Choice-POLIS.

Misra, G. (2014). Psychology of emotions: Some cultural perspectives. *Foundations and Applications of Indian Psychology*, *2*, 205-221.

Nathawat, S.S., and Mathur, A. (1993). Marital Adjustment and Subjective Wellbeing in Indian educated housewives and working women. *The Journal of Psychology*, *127*(3), 353-358. Doi: 10.1080/00223980.1993.9915570

Pagani, A.F., Parise, M., Donato, S., Gable, S.L., and Schoebi, D. (2020). If you shared my happiness, you are part of me: Capitalization and the experience of couple identity. *Personality and Social Psychology Bulletin*, *46*(2), 258-269.

Patel, V., and Prince, M. (2001). Ageing and mental health in a developing country: who cares? Qualitative studies from Goa, India." *Psychological Medicine*, *31*(1), 29-38.

Scheibe, S., English, T., Tsai, J.L., and Carstensen, L.L. (2013). Striving to feel good: Ideal affect, actual affect, and their correspondence across adulthood. *Psychology and Aging*, *28*(1), 160.

Seligman, M.E., and Csikszentmihalyi, M. (2014). Positive psychology: An introduction. In: *Flow and the Foundations of Positive Psychology*, pp. 279-298, Springer, Dordrecht.

Singh, S. (2014). Well-being and emotion regulation in emerging adults: The role of religiosity. *Indian Journal of Positive Psychology*, *5*(1), 46.

Stack, S., and Eshleman, J.R. (1998). Marital status and happiness: A 17-nation study. *Journal of Marriage and the Family*, 527-536.

Srivastava, A.K., and Misra, G. (2001). Lay people's understanding and use of intelligence: An Indian perspective. *Psychology and Developing Societies*, *13*(1), 25-49.

18

Caring the Chronically Ill

Toll on Mental Health of Women Caregivers

Garima Singh and *Anubhuti Dubey*

Introduction

Caregiving may mean direct care of all types also including work done by paid workers such as nurses, social workers, and counsellors. But our focus is not on professional caregivers, but on family caregivers. Family caregivers are emotionally involved in the process of caregiving, thus although they may undertake caregiving as a responsibility still they may perceive a threat to their physical and psychological being. Thus, caregiving being associated with emotional, financial and social turmoil is a predisposition to stress in itself. In India, caregivers are taken for granted because it is culturally expected that the family would look after the ill person, regardless of what changes it means.

Caregiving, thus, can be better understood bringing into light the cultural norms, values and roles of society. In India, caregiving is a blend of cultural expectations, duty, love, and a positive attitude towards aging in general (Bhagat & Unisa, 2006; Gupta, 2000). So, reciprocity and certain subjective feelings in caregiving make way for positive feelings being involved with it and minimization of the caregiver burden. Institute on Medicine (2008) estimated that 90 per cent of long-term care in India is delivered by family members. However, in India, caregivers are taken for granted because it is culturally expected that the family will look after the chronically ill patients, regardless of what changes it means and what is their need for assistance and support. This is widely different from the cultural assumptions made in present literature, where caregivers seem entitled to "having a life" and respected for what they are doing. However, even Indian caregivers find their role difficult and even they perceive problems related to it.

Caregivers tend to find themselves facing and dealing with anger, resentment, guilt, depression, financial crunches, isolation and conflict with family and work, however, it was found that Indians whether living in America (NRCNAA, 2004) or elsewhere are less likely to raise their voice about their constraints to the same extent as the other culture population because caregiving is perceived as a part of family life and not as a "burden". It is governed by the Hindu philosophy of compassion and harmony.

The personal characteristics and nature of caregiver also plays a role in determining the impact caregiving has on the caregiver. Wright *et al.* (1993) found that caregiver's sex, ethnicity, education level, self-related health and relationship to the care receiver have been associated with the psychological well-being of the caregivers.

The majority of informal or family caregiving provided is by the female nobility of the society, may be as a mother, sister, daughter, daughter-in-law, friend or any other role. Even the literature on caregiving reveals a major 66 per cent of the caregivers being female. Not only as Indian caregivers, but female all over the world form the major population providing care to their disabled or chronically ill family members. The traditional and social demands established in the Indian culture are the reason that evokes the female caregiver's population. Also, the contemporary changes in the society demands women to equate in all aspects with men. So, women tend to embrace various responsibilities even crossing the domestic boundaries.

Objectives of the Study

The objective of the present study is to find the percentage and distribution of working women caregivers in the present population. Also, the study would aim to identify the pattern of stress in women caregivers.

Method

Sample: The main sample consisted of female caregivers who take care of people who are afflicted with any chronic disease (i.e., on bed for more than a month and are dependent on others for their daily chores and self-hygiene). The sample consisted of a total of 115 female caregivers caring for chronically ill patients drawn from some private hospitals in the city of Gorakhpur and Faizabad districts where the patients of heart diseases, cancer, diabetes and other chronic illnesses are treated and admitted. Amongst them 57 were caring for male patients and 58 were caring for female patients. Seventy eight caregivers were in the age range of 18-27 years.

Purposive method of sampling was used. In this study, the term caregiver refers to people 18 years of age or older who satisfy a number of eligibility criteria for selection. To be selected in the final sample, the subjects needed to qualify according to the criteria below:

(1) Subjects need to be caregivers of chronically ill patients.
(2) Subjects need to be taking care or responsibility of the patient for at least a month.

Measures used in the study: For the data collection, an interview schedule was prepared. The interview schedule was framed in Hindi, the Indian national language. Hindi is the main language spoken in the regions from where the sample has been drawn. Although many participants were comfortable conversing in their local dialect (Bhojpuri), interviews were conducted in Bhojpuri also.

The interview was open-ended semi-structured for which an interview schedule was created. The interview started with rapport building and obtaining demographic details. Demographic information like age, educational level, marital status, socio-economic status, relationship between the caregiver and the patient, and disease of the patient have been obtained. Thereby, the interviewer focused on the following question during the interview:

1. आपके परिवार के सदस्य की बीमारी को कितना समय हुआ तथा यह रोग कितना गंभीर है?
2. नित्य प्रतिदिन के कार्यों के लिए मरीज़ आपके ऊपर कितना आश्रित या निर्भर है?
3. आपके परिवार के सदस्य की बीमारी के बाद आपके जीवन में क्या परिवर्तन हुए हैं?
4. आप मरीज की देखभाल करने को कैसे एवं कितनी महत्वपूर्ण बीमारी मानते हैं?
5. मरीज की देखभाल के शुरुआती समय से लेकर अब तक की अपनी भावनाओं को बताएं।
6. मरीज की देखभाल से जुड़े अपने नकारात्मक अनुभवों (यदि हों तो) का वर्णन करें।

7. मरीज के देखभाल से जुड़े अपने नकारात्मक अनुभवों (यदि हों तो) का वर्णन करें।

Some participants required added explanation and probing during the interview. A self-reflexive approach for data collection helped the researcher to remain associated with the research participants. Most interviews lasted for 45 minutes to one hour.

Results and Discussion

Caregivers, and so do their patients do not form a homogenous group. In the present study, the interview was initiated by taking the essential demographic information, which is presented in tables below. When the data collection process was complete, each protocol was checked and rechecked for missing or false data. Thereby, the data was analysed by creating themes using thematic analysis process.

The data was obtained in the form of narratives using semi-structured open interview methods and observations. The semi-structured open-ended interview protocol was prepared with the help of pilot study. The narratives about the caregiving experiences from the caregivers have been obtained. To gain an in-depth understanding of the narratives, thematic analysis of the interview transcripts using manual coding techniques was done. Firstly, key direct quotes were identified, and common ideas were interpreted. Next, related patterns were combined into themes.

Thematic analysis as an autonomous qualitative approach is mostly labelled as a method for identifying, investigating and recording patterns (themes) within data (Braun & Clarke, 2006).

Thematic Data Analysis process applied for the present investigation is based on the Thematic Analysis (Braun & Clarke, 2006) which is presented below.

Thematic Data Analysis Process by Braun & Clarke (2006)

Phases	*Process done*
Familiarizing with data	Transcribing data, reading and re-reading the data noting down initial ideas.
Generating initial codes	Coding interesting features of the data systematically across the entire data set, collating data relevant to each code.
Searching for themes	Collecting codes into potential themes, gathering all data relevant to each potential.

Phases	Process done
Defining and naming themes	Ongoing analysis for refining the specifics of each theme and the overall story that the analysis tells, generating clear definitions and names for each theme
Producing the report	The final opportunity for analysis. Selection of vivid, compelling extract examples, find analysis of selected extracts, relating back of the analysis to the research question and literature, producing a report of the analysis

Source: Braun & Clarke, 2006.

On the basis of thematic analysis, seven major themes related to the caregiving experiences of the caregivers as well as their own perceptions and understanding of the illness had been emerged. These themes were the reflections of the feelings of caregivers as attached to the caregiving task.

The obtained data reveals the differences in age, family structure and the relation of caregiver with patient. Table 18.1 presents the age and socio-economic status of the caregivers.

Table 18.1: Age and Socio-economic status of the caregivers

Age (in years)	*N*
18-22 years	54
23-27 years	24
27-32 years	08
33-37 years	10
38-42 years	12
43-47 years	03
48-52 years	04
Socio-economic Status	*N*
Lower class	80
Middle class	29
Upper class	06

The table undoubtedly highlights that the majority of the caregivers were young adults (18-35 years) who were mostly serving their family members from the earlier generation. Table depicts that in the sample, most of the caregivers belong to lower class, some were from middle class, and a few caregivers were from upper class. The relationship between the caregiver and the patient also modifies the outcomes and perception of caregiving, so investigating it in the study was essential.

Table 18.2: Relation of caregivers with patients

Patient	*Caregiver*	*N*
Mother-in-law	Daughter-in-law	25
Husband	Wife	22
Mother	Daughter	20
Grandmother	Granddaughter	14
Father	Daughter	18
Uncle	Daughter	06
Daughter	Mother	04
Sister	Sister	03
Bhabhi	Sister-in-law	02
Father-in-law	Daughter-in-law	01

As it is clear from the Table 18.2, most of the caregivers are daughters-in-law, caring for their mothers-in-law, and then wives caring for their husbands, and also daughters caring for their mothers.

Demographic Details of Patients

The present study includes the caregivers of chronically ill patients and hence only those patient were included who were ill for at least a month. The chronically ill patient population is diverse as many diseases qualify for the criteria of being chronic. The demographics of the patient presented here would reveal so.

Table 18.3: Gender and Family type of the patients

Gender	*N*
Male	57
Female	58
Family Type	*N*
Joint	46
Single	69

Caregiving in India is a part of cultural responsibility towards family and thus the family structure also plays a significant role, the sample had single families more in number than joint families.

The findings suggested that the major part of sample of caregivers in the feminine nobility is daughters, daughters-in-law and wives. The average age of caregivers was 18 to 25 years and average duration of care giving in a single day is four to five hours and for most of the caregivers care giving was a 24×7 job for them, which had reduced their social mobility. However, most of the caregivers had uttered that their roles are a part of their lives or 'dharma'. Significant differences with regards to age, gender and relationship have been found in the Indian family caregivers.

Atienza and associates (2002) investigated 96 adult daughter caregivers who simultaneously occupied mother, wife and employee roles. Results showed evidence to support that dispositional optimism buffered i.e., moderated the effects of wife stress on depressive symptoms and life satisfaction. Dispositional optimism has served as beneficial resource that reduces the negative effect of wife stress on psychological well-being and contributes to adult daughter caregiver's well-being irrespective of stress experienced in specific social role including caregiving.

According to the study by Juster and Marin (2011), the intensity of chronic caregiving is allied to a number of health issues. The caregiving experience places a cumulative toll on the body and psychological strains the caregiving person. Moreover, the financial cost associated with family caregiving, is a significant factor in caregiving burden, both for male and female caregivers (Mishra, Mishra, *et al.,* 2016).

Gupta, Rowe and Pillai (2009) examined a sample of 263 primary caregivers of elderly in Allahabad city of Uttar Pradesh and found that although male caregivers' perceived burden depends only on the size of the role overload, for female caregivers, perceived burden depends on the inter-relationships between the size of the role overload and adherence to Asian cultural norms. The addition of novel responsibility, new combat to the social and personal relationships and other additional roles come up wrapped in the box of caregiving (Juster & Marin, 2011).

Indian families adopt the role of caregiving naturally as normative behaviour, when someone in the family falls ill of chronic diseases as threatening as cancer. But now the changing family pattern and structure have made this caregiving role challenging. In a study, Shivkumar (2017), adopting descriptive research design found that majority of family caregivers are female, aged between 35 to 45 years, education varying illiterate to post-graduation, adopted dual role voluntarily but finding it very difficult to cope with dual responsibility and mental health issues.

Spitze, Logan, Joseph, and Lee (1994) conducted study on a sample of 763 midlife (aged 40 to 65) men and women respondents. The objective of their study was to examine different roles (spouse, parent of minor co-resident child, parent of adult co-resident child, helper to parents, and helper to adult children) and their combinations for midlife adults and to consider how different roles and their interactions with each other affected psychological well-being (burden, distress, life satisfaction). The findings proposed that hours of help provided to parents were not associated with a difference in well-being among women; while among men, help to parents was associated with more distress. Combining employment with help to parents somewhat buffered the association of help to parents with distress for men-suggesting that the caregiver role and the work role do not tend to conflict for men, leading to poorer well-being. No significant interaction effect for this combination of roles for women also suggested that combining employment with helping a parent was not a major problem for women's well-being. It was also found in the study by Marks (1997) that if work and family conflict differences between caregivers and non-caregivers were eliminated, the caregiving role would also often lead to positive well-being benefits.

Caregivers move through minutes, hours, and years of stress to provide proper care to their ill counterparts. So, caregiving is an enduring experience that demands the attention and concern of the caregiver. When sharing this experience, the female caregivers report both positive and negative feelings. All the same, a number of facets of caregiving stress are recognized, caregivers do indulge in the task of caregiving due to varied cultural values and norms. Such cultural affections make the caregivers capable of identifying even positive aspects to the process of care giving (Cohen, Colantonio & Vernich, 2002; Kramer, 1997). Caregivers feel compassion with patients that helps them to carry out the caregiving task with positive vibes of reciprocity and duty, as stated in the narration: *"aatma ko santushti rehti hai jitna thik hote jate hai"*(Feel satisfaction when recovery is fast). Cassell (2012) considered compassion to be an emotion that is vital process of connecting with others by identifying with them and providing them with motivation and sense of relief in case of any kind of suffering. According to Batson, *et al.* (2009), compassion in a collectivist culture rears a sense of prosocial behaviour in its members. In Indian context, being a collectivist culture, the caregivers took over the task of caring for a family member as a compassion which leads to positive perception of the caregiving task and thus reduced stress in them.

The hamper of their positive experiences in spite of the caregiving stress included improved prognosis of patient, belongingness with the patient, satisfaction and happiness in caring, time spent with patient, fighting spirit of patient and enhanced knowledge of medicine. The affirmative spirits of the caregiving experience have been reflected in the following verbatim of the female caregivers: *"bahut manatey hai, theek nahi huye to* (Adores me a lot, if he doesn't get well...)(*cries*)*"; "sabse acchi feeling to hya hi hai ki dekhbhaal kar rahe*" (The best feeling is that we are taking care); *"hamesha ghar se durrahe, ab kam se kam bahut si batein karne ko milta hai"*(I was always away from home, now atleast I get to talk to him).

Although many positive aspects are linked to it, caregiving in general discourse is commonly perceived as a burden. It is considered that the caregiving task in itself acts as a source of burden, be it physical, mental, social or financial burden. Caregiving for women especially imposes restrictions on social participation, family involvement, personal goals, and health. Nevertheless, considerable caregiving literature specifies that caregiving is related with psychological distress (e.g., Pinquart & Sorensen, 2003). The caregivers, in their narrations, give account of sadness and distress in their caregiving experience, related to the care-recipient: *"bahut taklif mein tha pura parivar bimari ke bare mein janke"*(The family was distressed after getting to know about the illness) "*shuru mein toh koi rasta nazar nahi aata tha*" (In the beginning there was no way out).Being a daily job, caregiving leads to irritability and hopelessness in the caregivers. The caregiver report of their own irritating behaviour: *"kabhi kabhi man ub jata hai"* (At times the mind seems boring); *"baar baar bulane se accha toh mar jate"* (instead of calling repeatedly, it was better if he dies). The slow recovery process and prolonged illness leads to hopelessness in the patient, as reported in the following verbatim of the caregivers: "*kabhi umeed khatam si ho jatihai*"(At times there is no expectation); *"dawa lagta hai koi asar hi nahi karrahi"*(It seems medicine has no effect). While negative experiences have been reported by the caregivers, but the majority in the present caregiver population do report of no negative feelings being associated with the caregiving experience, they clearly state: "*kuch bura nahi hai man mein*" (There is nothing negative about it); *"sab theek hi tohhai"*(Everything is going well).

Both positive and negative experiences being related to the caregiving task, the caregivers do majorly talked about faith in God. They mention that: *"sudhar jaise hua use man mein astha badh gayi hai"* (With recovery, faith in God increased), *"bhagwan sath de gatoh sahi hoga"*(If God helps, all would be well). The faith in God is so strong that sometimes they believe more in prayers than in the medical treatments for recovery: *"sabki dua hai ki aaj pehle se bahut thik hai"*(It is because of the prayers that recovery is happening).

In nutshell, it could be inferred from the narratives of the female caregivers that they do adopt the caregiving role due to the responsibility and obligation existing in the tradition, but with time the caregivers perceive stress, i.e., physical, psychological, social and financial stress, during the caregiving task. Howsoever, the narratives also revealed that the pattern of stress in the caregivers is such that they overpower such stress with their reasons of reciprocity and duty towards the family member. Lin, Rong and Lee (2013) similarly established in their study the positive facets of caregiving. Casado, *et al.* (2012) found in their study too that obligation is considered as a cultural caregiving motive which reduces subjective burden of caregiving.

The caregiving population worldwide reflects that women do form the major caregivers. As mentioned by Morrow-Howell, Rozario, & Hinterlong (2004) given the role of women as caregivers in the Asian Indian context, women are generally more likely to provide care to the elderly and therefore more likely to experience perceived caregiver burden than males.

References

Anand, K.S., Dhikav, V., Sachdeva, A., and Mishra, P. (2016). Perceived caregiver stress in Alzheimer's disease and mild cognitive impairment: A case control study. *Annals of Indian Academy of Neurology*, *19*(1), 58.

Atienza, A.A., Stephens, M.A.P., and Townsend, A.L. (2002). Dispositional optimism, role-specific stress, and the well-being of adult daughter caregivers. *Research on Aging*, *24*(2), 193-217.

Barer, B.M., and Johnson, C.L. (1990). A critique of the caregiving literature. *The Gerontologist*, *30*(1), 26-29.

Bayliss, E.A., Bonds, D.E., Boyd, C.M., Davis, M.M., Finke, B., Fox, M.H., and Lind, C. (2014). Understanding the context of health for persons with multiple chronic conditions: Moving from what is the matter to what matters. *The Annals of Family Medicine*, *12*(3), 260-269.

Berg-Weger, M., Rubio, D.M. and Tebb, S.S. (2001).Strengths-based practice with family caregivers of the chronically ill: qualitative insights. *Families in Society, 81*(3), 263-272.

Bhagat, R.B., and Unisa, S. (2006). Ageing and dependency in India: A new measurement. *Asian Population Studies*, *2*(2), 201-214.

Brody, E.M. (1990). *Women in the middle: Their parent care years.* New York: Springer.

Burrow, A.L., O'dell, A.C., and Hill, P.L. (2010). Profiles of a developmental asset: Youth purpose as a context for hope and well-being. *Journal of Youth and Adolescence*, *39*(11), 1265-1273.

Burton, L.C., Zdaniuk, B., Schulz, R., Jackson, S., and Hirsch, C. (2003). Transitions in spousal caregiving. *The Gerontologist*, *43*(2), 230-241.

Coon, D.W. (2012). Resilience and family caregiving. *Annual Review of*

Gerontology and Geriatrics: Emerging Perspective on Resilience in Adulthood and Later Life (Hayslip & Smith, eds.). New York: Springer.

Cox, C., and Monk, A. (1993). Hispanic culture and family care of Alzheimer's patients. *Health and Social Work, 18*(2), 92-100.

Del, Pino., Casado, R., Pérez., Cruz, M., and Frías., Osuna, A. (2014). Coping, subjective burden and anxiety among family caregivers of older dependents. *Journal of Clinical Nursing, 23*(23-24), 3335-3344.

Evercare (2006). *Caregivers in Decline: A Close-up Look at the Health Risks of Caring for a Loved One.* Retrieved from http://www.EvercareHealthPlans.com/Caregiver.

Glaser, J.K.K., Dura, J.R., Speicher, C.E., and Glaser, R. (1991). Spousal Caregivers of Dementia Victims: Longitudinal Changes in Immunity and Health. *Psychosomatic Medicine,* (53), 345-362.

Gupta, R. (2000). A path model of elder caregiver burden in Indian/Pakistani families in the United States. *The International Journal of Aging and Human Development, 51*(4), 295-313.

Higginson, I.J., and Sen-Gupta, G.J.A. (2000). Place of care in advanced cancer: a qualitative systematic literature review of patient preferences. *Journal of Palliative Medicine, 3*(3), 287-300.

Irvin, B.L., and Acton, G.J. (1997). Stress, hope, and well-being of women caring for family members with Alzheimer's disease. *Holistic Nursing Practice, 11*(2), 69-79.

Juster, R.P., and Marin, M.F. (2011, March). The Stress of Caregivers. *Mammoth Magazine* (10).

Lee, S., Colditz, G.A., Berkman, L.F., and Kawachi, I. (2003). Caregiving and risk of coronary heart disease in U.S. women: A prospective study. *American Journal of Preventive Medicine*, (24), 113-119.

Levine, C., Reinhard, S., Feinberg, L.F., Albert, S., and Hart, A. (2003). Family caregivers on the job: Moving beyond ADLs and IADLs. *Generations, 27*(4), 17-23.

Lin, F., Rong, J., Lee, T. (2013). Resilience among caregivers of children with chronic conditions: a concept analysis. *Journal of Multidisciplinary Healthcare,* (6), 323-333.

MacLean, M.J., Kelley, M.L., Arthur, M., and Stones, M. (2001). Palliative care in rural Canada. *Rural Social Work, 6*(3), 63-73.

Marin, M.F., Lord, C., Andrews, J., Juster, R.P., Sindi, S., Arsenault-Lapierre, G., and Lupien, S.J. (2011). Chronic stress, cognitive functioning and mental health. *Neurobiology of Learning and Memory, 96*(4), 583-595.

Marks, N.F. (1997). Does it Hurt to Care? Caregiving, Work and Family Conflict, and Midlife Well-being. *Child and Family Studies*, Madison.

Mehrotra, S., and Sukumar, P. (2007). Sources of strength perceived by females caring for relatives diagnosed with cancer: An exploratory study from India. *Supportive Care in Cancer, 15*(12), 1357-1366.

Murthy, R.S. (2016). Caregiving and caregivers: Challenges and opportunities in India. *Indian Journal of Social Psychiatry*, *32*(1), 10.

Pinquart, M., and Sorensen, S. (2003). Differences between caregivers and non-caregivers in psychological health and physical health: A meta-analysis. *Psychology and Aging*, *18*(2), 250.

Poulin, M.J., Brown, S.L., Ubel, P.A., Smith, D.M., Jankovic, A., and Langa, K.M. (2010). Does a helping hand mean a heavy heart? Helping behaviour and well-being among spouse caregivers. *Psychology and Aging*, *25*(1), 108.

Rozario, P.A., Morrow-Howell, N., and Hinterlong, J.E. (2004). Role enhancement or role strain: Assessing the impact of multiple productive roles on older caregiver well-being. *Research on Aging*, *26*(4), 413-428.

Sahoo, S., Brahma, P.K., and Mohapatra, P.K. (2010). Burden of caregiver's among the mentally ill and diabetic patients: A comparative study. *The Orissa Journal of Psychiatry,* 39-47.

Savage, S., and Bailey, S. (2004). The impact of caring on caregivers' mental health: A review of the literature. *Australian Health Review, 27* (1), 103-109.

Shaji, K.S., Smitha, K., Lal, K.P., and Prince, M.J. (2003). Caregivers of People with Alzheimer's disease: A qualitative study from the Indian 10/66 Dementia Research Network. *International Journal of Geriatric Psychiatry*, *18*(1), 1-6.

Singh, G., and Dubey, A. (2016). Mental Health and Well-being of Caregivers: A Review of the Literature. *The International Journal of Indian Psychology, 3 (4),* 57, 98.

Spitze, G., Logan, J.R., Joseph, G., and Lee, E. (1994). Middle generation roles and the well-being of men and women. *Journal of Gerontology*, *49*(3), S107-S116.

Srivastava, G., Tripathi, R.K., Tiwari, S.C., Singh, B., and Tripathi, S.M. (2016). Caregiver burden and quality of life of key caregivers of patients with dementia. *Indian Journal of Psychological Medicine*, *38* (2), 133.

Tseng, C.N., Huang, G.S., Yu, P.J., and Lou, M.F. (2015). A qualitative study of family caregiver experiences of managing incontinence in stroke survivors. *PLoS One*, *10*(6), e0129540.

19

Ageism, Psychological Capital and Life Satisfaction

A Study on Elderly Women

Suchismita Pramanik and *Nandita Das*

Introduction

The concept of Ageism was first propounded by Butler. According to Butler ageism is the negative attitudes of others as well as the old people toward themselves and the process of aging (Butler, 1980). However, Palmore (2001) suggested ageism can be of both positive and negative. Prejudice against age is a common type of prejudice and it was found from a study young men experience more ageism and depression than old female (Lyons *et al.*, 2017). Rupp *et al.,* (2005) found ageism is more noticeable among young males but it is evident that both male and female experience ageism (Levy & Banaji, 2004). If we take cultures into consideration people from individualistic as well as collectivist culture hold negative stereotypical attitude towards elderly (Cuddy *et al.*, 2005).

When people move toward the process of aging they started taking themselves away from the young age group which makes them to feel negative towards their own age, this phenomenon is termed age "self-ageism" (Bonder, 2009). Many times the stigma attached to aging is, it makes people unattractive, dependent, incompetent and emotional (Atchley, 1997). Old people are taken as dependent, slow, sick, emotionally not stable, stubborn in many societies (Schaefer, 1983).

Ageism can be very detrimental for the old age groups. Findings suggested that negative attitude can affect the motivation level, self-efficacy of the old adults (Levy, 1996) and may increase the tendency to have cardiovascular diseases (Levy *et al.*, 2000). Ageism was found positively correlated with poor mental health, depressive symptoms and health problems among elderly (Lyons *et al.*, 2017). Result from the previous study also show that perception about age discrimination is significantly related with symptoms of depression amongst the elderly (Ayalon, 2016).

Correlates of Life Satisfaction among the Elderly

It is believed that satisfaction with life gradually decreases with increasing age. Old age has always been associated with different types of problem ranging from physiological to psychological issues. However many times the senility phase of life is also associated with gaining more life experience and emotional regulations and competencies (Kunzmann *et al.*, 2000). There are many factors responsible to lead successful aging and achieve subjective wellbeing as well as life satisfaction. Researches in the related area of aging have always fascinated on the wellbeing of individual as they grow old. In consideration to this Social gerontology was found as a branch to explore the effect of aging process and its relation to life satisfaction of an individual (Lawton, 1975; Neugarten *et al.*, 1961). It has found that psychological wellbeing and life satisfaction doesn't get affected by the social and biological changes during old age (Mercier, Peladeau & Tempier, 1998).

A research have done to examine the role of gender in life satisfaction among elderly and result found that female to have high in life satisfaction compared to males (Vinsi, 2014; Macia *et al.*, 2015). The results of a similar study found that financial condition, good interpersonal relation are the main predictors of life satisfaction in old age (Macia *et al.*, 2015). Result from a study on life satisfaction across life span has found satisfaction with life is more during 40 to early 70 years of age and after 70 years it started decreasing (Baird *et al.*, 2010). In contradiction to this Prenda and Lachman (2001) reported a positive association between age and life satisfaction.

Lewinsohn, Redner, and Seeley (1991) examined the association between life satisfaction and psychosocial variables and found many psychosocial variables are highly associated with life satisfaction. The person with greater life satisfaction are found to be more involved in activities, socially skilled, happy with the company of others and more optimistic over negative aspects of their life (Bulman & Wortman, 1977). Priyanka and Mishra (2013) found there is no significant difference between old people staying in urban and semi-urban areas in relation with life satisfaction.

It was also found from the result of a study that greater functional status during old age is related to higher life satisfaction among the elderly population (Markides & Martin, 1979). Studies have reported that subjective perception about one's health is highly linked to life satisfaction (Berg *et al.,* 2006; Hamashima, 1994). Findings suggested physical health has hardly any relationship with lower life satisfaction (Puvill *et al.,* 2016) but Choudhary (2015) found there is a significant negative relationship between physical health and life satisfaction among old. On the other hand, it was found that poor mental health is significantly related to low life satisfaction (Puvill *et al.,* 2016) which is consistent with the finding of Choudhary (2015). Adams *et al.,* (2016) found that "depressive symptoms and perceived stress" are negatively related with life satisfaction, whereas social support was found to be a significant predictor of high life satisfaction.

Joseph *et al.* (2014) had done a study to examine life satisfaction among the aged who are staying in institutions. The result from their study found that more than half of the participants expressed a moderate psychological well-being as per test score. Steel *et al.* (2008) found future expectations and person's temperament are the moderators of life satisfaction. In addition to this findings also show that good marital relationship is found to be positively associated with life satisfaction.

Psychological Capital and the Elderly

Psychological capitals (psycap) are the internal tendencies of an individual which emphasizes more on positivity over negativity. It helps to cope better with adverse situations in our life by using positive qualities of an individual. Positive psychological capital includes hope, optimism, self-efficacy and resilience.

Self-efficacy

Self-efficacy is the belief of an individual, on his or her ability to complete a task (Bandura, 1997). A research study was done to find out the predictors of self-efficacy among old people. The result revealed that physical activity and social involvement was the significant predictors of self-efficacy (Perkins *et al.*, 2008). Findings showed that the elderly who are high in perceived self-efficacy and who involve in physical activity have more satisfaction with life and low in depressive symptoms (Luszcynska *et al.*, 2005). Result shows that self-efficacy is a strong predictor of successful aging among the elderly population (Kim, 2013). Studies have found that elderly have more self-efficacy than young adults (Artistico, Cervone & Pezzuti, 2003).

Resilience

Old age resilience has been defined as flexibility and ability to cope in adverse situation (Staudinger, Marsiske & Baltes, 1993). Many elderly are high in overall wellbeing despite their illness and problematic situation. In some cases elderly adults are found high resilient than young people (Nygren *et al.*, 2005; Netuveli *et al.*, 2008) and high resilience is positively related with successful aging, less mortality risk, less depressive symptoms and quality of life among elderly (Netuveli, 2008).

Findings from the study of Mamta and Sharma (2013) revealed that resilience, self-efficacy and wellbeing are positively correlated and these relationships are significant. Moreover they also found that resilience and self-efficacy are significant predictors of wellbeing (Pezent, 2011). A study by Zhang *et al.* (2017) examined resilience of empty-nest old people. Result found three types of group characteristics in resilience of the empty-nest elderly and they named it "high resilience group, low pressure resilience group and low resilience group". The proportions of these groups are 26.6 per cent, 40.4 per cent and 32.9 per cent respectively. Moreover the results also revealed that age, marital status, relationship with children, education level and physical exercise has significant effect on "high resilience group", on the other hand education level, gender, physical exercise and relationship with children has significant effect on the "low pressure resilience group" compared to the "low resilience group".

Zhao *et al.* (2018) aimed to study the mediated effect of resilience between loneliness and depressive symptoms, and the moderating effect of social support on the mediation model. Result found the relationship between loneliness and depressive symptoms was partly conciliated by resilience. They also noticed that with high social support, the impact of loneliness on depressive symptoms through resilience was weaker.

Li, Theng and Foo (2015) studied the relationship between social support, resilience and geriatric depression among Chinese elderly. The finding suggested that both resilience and social support is negatively related with geriatric depression.

Result from a study by Melendez *et al.* (2018) shown that older adults with Alzheimer disease have lower level of resilience and psychological wellbeing than elderly with mild cognitive impairment and healthy adults.

Studies also showed resilience is positively related with high social engagement, optimism, high psychological and physical health and functional independence (Hardy *et al.*, 2004; Lamond *et al.*, 2009; Schure *et al.*, 2013; Wells, 2009) and higher level of resilience is found to be negatively related with chronic pain and depressive symptoms (Schure *et al.*, 2013). Similar findings suggested that resilience positively correlated with family functioning and quality of life, life satisfaction among elderly (Hayat, Khan & Sadia, 2016), survival or low mortality rate among elderly (Shen & Zeng, 2010). Moreover resilience is found to be a significant predictor of happiness, life satisfaction and physical health (Fullen, Richardson & Granello, 2018).

Melendez *et al.* (2015) analyzed the effectiveness of instrumental reminiscent to enhance adaptive capacity and resilience among older adults. Instrumental reminiscent programme involves recalling the effectiveness of successful coping strategies in the past or present. Result found reminiscent programme is highly effective to improve adaptive capacity and resilience to meet adverse situation among elderly.

Optimism

Optimism is the tendency to expect positive thing to occur in future. Optimist persons are more likely to follow healthy behaviour and it helps individual to adapt in the stressful situation and (Conversano *et al.* 2010). Optimism is found to be highly correlated with "hedonic wellbeing" (Gallagher & Lopez, 2009). Research finding suggested that when the old people hold positive attitude towards aging despite the negativity associated with getting old, the aging process will be continuing as positive (Keller, Leventhal, & Larson, 1989). It has been noticed that optimism helps to improve physical functioning and depressive symptoms among elderly people (Wurm & Benyamini, 2014). Bain *et al.* (2003) found optimism is significantly associated with quality of life of the aged.

Rationale of the Study

Numbers of studies have been conducted on elderly people and old age problems. Problems related to loneliness, depression, social isolation etc. and in relation to their mental health and attitudes of younger adults towards old age group. One of the emerging issues of old age is ageism which affects the entire life course of the old as well as younger people. Though researchers have look forward towards the old age problems but ageism is still overlooked by the researchers. Very few researches have been found on ageism in western as well as Indian context. In country like India women are often left behind and taken as dependent and burden to the family. So this matter creates curiosity to know the journey of women toward successful aging. From the above literature review no such study has been found in the relationship between human positive psychological capital and self-ageism and its effect on their life satisfaction. Therefore the present study attempts to find out the inter-correlation among ageism (benevolent & hostile), psycap and the life satisfaction among elderly women. For the present study only optimism, self-efficacy and resilience are taken to measure psycap.

Objectives of the Study

The objectives of the present study are to examine the relationships between ageism (benevolent, hostile ageism), psychological capital (optimism, resilience, and self-efficacy) and life satisfaction among elderly women.

Method

Design: The present study adopted a correlational research design, aimed at finding out the inter-correlation between benevolent ageism, hostile ageism, psychological capital and the life satisfaction among elderly.

Participants: Total numbers of 30 elderly women were selected through convenient sampling method from three districts of Odisha (Khordha, Puri and Balasore). The participants for the present study were among the age group of 60 years and above.

Tools

Ambivalent Ageism scale: Ambivalent ageism scale was developed by Cary, Chasteen and Remedios (2016). This scale consists 13 items in which 4 items measure hostile ageism and 9 items measure benevolent ageism. The subjects are supposed to read each item carefully and indicate his/her degree of agreement or disagreement on a seven-point rating scale. The S's response to each items are scored 1, 2, 3, 4, 5, 6 and 7 for strongly disagree, disagree, slightly disagree, neither agree nor disagree, slightly agree, Agree, Strongly agree respectively.

The Satisfaction with Life Scale (SwLS): The satisfaction with life scale was developed by Diener *et al.* (1985). It has five items that assess an individual's global judgement of life satisfaction as a whole. The respondent indicates his/her response in a seven-point rating scale where 1 is strongly disagree, 2 is disagree, 3 is slightly disagree, 4 is neither agree nor disagree, 5 is slightly agree, 6 is disagree, 7 is strongly agree.

Psychological Capital: The psychological capital includes optimism, self-efficacy and resilience. Brief Resilience Scale was developed by Smith *et al.*, (2008), Life-Orientation Test was developed by Scheier *et al.*, (1994) and the General Self-efficacy scale (GES) was developed by Ralf Schwarzer & Matthias Jerusalem (2013). The respondent responds his/her agreement in a five-point rating scale. The responses for each item was scored 1, 2, 3, 4 and 5 for strongly disagree, disagree, neither agree nor disagree, agree and strongly agree respectively.

Procedure: Total number of 30 respondents were taken from different places in Odisha. Rapport was initiated with them and informed consent was taken verbally from them before starting the data collection process. All the data were collected individually. The instructions were given properly to everyone and clear all the doubts regarding the questionnaire and the research. Then the researcher asked each item to the subject personally and indicated their responses in the questionnaire. After completing the questionnaire the researcher thanked them for their cooperation.

Results and Discussion

The inter-correlation analysis among components of ageism, i.e. benevolent ageism and hostile ageism; psychological capital and life satisfaction was performed and the obtained correlation matrix has been presented in Table 19.1.

Table 19.1: Inter-correlation matrix in the dimensions—ageism, life satisfaction and psychological capital

	Benevolent ageism	*Hostile ageism*	*Psychological Capital*	*Life satisfaction*
Benevolent ageism	1			
Hostile ageism	-.167*	1		
Psychological Capital	.269**	-.178*	1	
Life Satisfaction	.266**	-.185*	.357**	1

Note: **P <. 01; *P < .05.

The result shows that there is a positive relationship between psychological capital and life satisfaction (r = .35, P < .01). This means psychological capital and life satisfaction among elderly population increasing and decreasing together. The psychological capital and life satisfaction are the part of subjective well-being; Psychological capital includes positive aspect of human life for example, hope, optimism, resiliency and self-efficacy. All these dimensions are helpful for better psychological functioning of the individuals. Though life satisfaction includes physical, psychological and social satisfaction of an individual but psychological factor always plays an important role to determine both physical and social factor. Previous studies had done in the specific dimensions of psychological capital and findings suggests that resilience, hope are related to positive emotional functioning and resilience helps to enhance the psychological well-being (Pezent, 2011). However the present study used the combinations of optimism, self-efficacy and resilience. Though the result is not significant but it also shows a positive correlation between psychological capital and life satisfaction.

Result also shows that hostile ageism is negatively correlated with life satisfaction ($r = -.18$, $P < .05$) and Psychological Capital ($r = -.17$, $P < .05$). In fact, There is no supportive study has been found on the relationship between Psychological capital and life satisfaction. Life satisfaction is linked with positive aspect of human life whereas hostile ageism is related to negative attitude. Moreover, life satisfaction is a part of positive psychological well-being therefore, there is negative correlation between ageism and life satisfaction. This means when life satisfaction increases the ageism decreases and vice-versa.

From the inter-correlation matrix it can be also noticed that benevolent ageism is positively associated with life satisfaction ($r = .26$, $P < .01$) and Psychological Capital ($r = .26$, $P < .01$). It means benevolent ageism; Psychological Capital and life satisfaction are increasing and decreasing together. However, none of these relationships were statistically significant.

Conclusion

The current study was done in order to find out the inter-correlation between ageism (benevolent and hostile), psychological capital and life satisfaction among elderly women. The study was conducted on the total number of 30 older women. All the participants were administered the ambivalent ageism scale, life satisfaction scale and the psychological capital scale.

Findings revealed that there is positive correlation between benevolent ageism, psychological capital and life satisfaction and negative correlations are found between hostile ageism, Psychological capital and life satisfaction among the elderly women.

Due to urbanization break-up in the joint family system the generation gap is widening day by day. So ageism or negative attitude towards older people is becoming more prominent. In order to have a more balanced and caring family as well as social structure these negative attitudes needs to be modified, because the negative attitudes make the elderly feel more dependent and isolated. The findings of the present study will help in delineating the negative perception and attitude towards old age by providing adequate counselling to the elderly. Intervention package can be designed to improve psychological capital, which will help to lead the elderly toward successful aging. The current study was done with very less number of participants which doesn't represent the true characteristics of the population. Therefore, it is suggested to include more participants for a desirable outcome. Moreover study does not take into account other intervening variables like duration of staying with old people, other age group, place of domicile, personality etc. which could have an effect on the variables. In addition to this study is purely a quantitative research so there may the social desirability effect and fixed response set is always there.

References

Adams, T.R., Rabin, L.A., Da Silva, V.G., Katz, M.J., Fogel, J., and Lipton, R.B. (2015). Social Support Buffers the Impact of Depressive Symptoms on Life Satisfaction in Old Age. *Clinical Gerontologist, 39*(*2*), *139–157.* doi:10.1080/07317115.2015.1073823

Artistico, D., Cervone, D., and Pezzuti, L. (2003). Perceived self-efficacy and everyday problem solving among young and older adults. *Psychology and Aging, 18*(1), *68–79.* doi:10.1037/0882-7974.18.1.68

Atchley, Robert, C. (1997). *Social Forces and Aging: An Introduction to Social Gerontology*, New York; Wadsworth Publishing Co.

Ayalon, L. (2016). Perceived Age Discrimination: A Precipitator or a Consequence of Depressive Symptoms? *The Journals of Gerontology Series B: Psychological Sciences and Social Sciences,* gbw101. doi:10.1093/geronb/gbw101

Bain, G.H., Lemmon, H., Teunisse, S., Starr, J.M., Fox, H.C., Deary, I.J., and Whalley, L.J. (2003). Quality of Life in healthy old age: relationships with childhood IQ, minor psychological symptoms and optimism. *Social Psychiatry and Psychiatric Epidemiology, 38*(11), 632–636. doi:10.1007/s00127-003-0685-5

Baird, B.M., Lucas, R.E., and Donnellan (2010). Life Satisfaction Across the Lifespan: Findings from Two Nationally Representative Panel Studies. *Social Indicator Research, 99,* pp. 183–203. DOI: 10.1007/s11205-010-9584-9.

Bandura, A., 1997. Self-efficacy: The Exercise of Control. New York: W.H. Freeman.

Berg, A.I., Hassing, L.B., McClearn, G.E., and Johansson, B. (2006). What matters for life satisfaction in the oldest-old?. *Aging and Mental Health, 10*(3), 257-264.

Bulman, R.J., and Wortman, C.B. (1977). Attributions of blame and coping in the real world: severe accident victims react to their lot. *Journal of Personality and Social Psychology, 35*(5), 351.

Butler, R.N. (1980). Ageism: A Foreword. *Journal of Social Issues, 36*(*2*), *8–11.* doi:10.1111/j.1540-4560.1980.tb02018.x

Choudhary, A. (2015). A study of life satisfaction and health in old age. *International Journal of Science and Research* (*IJSR*), *4*(9), 2319-7064.

Conversano, C., Rotondo, A., Lensi, E., Della Vista, O., Arpone, F., and Reda, M.A. (2010).Optimism and its impact on mental and physical well-being. *Clinical Practice and Epidemiology in Mental Health: CP and EMH, 6*, 25.

Cuddy, A.C., Norton, M.I., and Fiske, S.T. (2005). This old stereotype: the pervasiveness and persistence of the elderly stereotype. *Journal of Social Issues, 61*, 267–285.

Fullen, C.M., Richardson, E.V., and Granello, H.D. (2018). Comparing successful aging, resilience, and holistic wellness as predictors of the good life. *Educational Gerontology*, 44 (7), 459-468.

Gallagher, M.W., and Lopez, S.J. (2009). Positive expectancies and mental health: Identifying the unique contributions of hope and optimism. *The Journal of Positive Psychology, 4*(6), 548-556.

Hamashima, C. (1994). The quality of life in aged people. *Nippon Eiseigaku Zasshi* (*Japanese Journal of Hygiene*), *49*(2), 533-542.

Hardy, S.E., Concato, J., and Gill, T.M. (2004). Resilience of community dwelling older persons. *Journal of the American Geriatrics Society, 52*(2): 257–262.10.1111/j.1532-5415.2004.52065.x

Hayat, Z.S., Khan, S., and Sadia, R. (2016). Resilience, Wisdom, and Life Satisfaction in Elderly Living with Families and in Old-Age Homes. *Pakistan Journal of Psychological Research*, 31 (2), 475-494.

Josph, *et al.* (2014). Life satisfaction among inhabitants of selected old age home at Chandigarh: A cross-sectional survey. *Delhi Psychiatric Journal, 17*, 2.

Keller, M.L., Leventhal, E.A., and Larson, B. (1989). Aging: The lived experience. *International Journal of Aging and Human Development*, 29, 67–82.

Kim, H.K. (2013). Factors affecting successful aging among male elders in Korea. *Journal of Convergence Information Technology, 8*(14), 341.

Kunzmann, U., Little, T.D., and Smith, J. (2000). Is age-related stability of subjective well-being a paradox? Cross–sectional and longitudinal evidence from the Berlin Aging Study. *Psychology and Aging, 15*, 511–526.

Lamond, A.J., Depp, C.A., Allison, M., Langer, R., Reichstadt, J., Moore, D.J., and Jeste, D.V. (2009). Measurement and predictors of resilience among community-dwelling older women. *Journal of Psychiatric Research, 43* (2), 148-154. doi: 10.1016/j.jpsychires. 2008.03.007.

Lawton, M.P. (1975). The Philadelphia Geriatric Centre Morale Scale: A revision. *Journal of Gerontology, 30*, 85-89.

Levy, B.R. and Myers, L.M. (2004). Preventive health behaviours influenced by self-perceptions of aging. *Preventive Medicine, 39*, 625–629.

Levy, B.R. (1996). Improving memory in old age by implicit self-stereotyping. *Journal of Personality and Social Psychology, 71*, 1092–1107.

Levy, B.R., Hausdorff, J., Hencke, R. and Wei, J.Y. (2000). Reducing cardiovascular stress with positive self-stereotypes of aging. *Journals of Gerontology: Psychological Sciences, 55*, 205–213.

Lewinsohn, P.M., Redner, J., and Seeley, J.R. (1991). The relationship between life satisfaction and psychosocial variables: New perspectives. *Subjective well-being: An Interdisciplinary Perspective, 21*, 141-169.

Li, J., Theng, L.Y., and Foo, S. (2015). Does psychological resilience mediate the impact of social support on geriatric depression? An exploratory study among Chinese older adults in Singapore. *Asian Journal of Psychiatry, 14*, 22-27.

Luszcynska, A., Gutierrez-Dona, B., Schwarzer, R. (2005). General self-efficacy in various domains of human functioning: Evidence from five countries. *International Journal of Psychology, 40*, 80-89.

Lyons, A., Alba, B., Heywood, W., Fileborn, B., Minichiello, V., Barrett, C., Dow, B. (2017). Experiences of ageism and the mental health of older adults. *Aging and Mental Health, 1–9.* doi:10.1080/13607863.2017.1364347

Macia, E., Duboz, P., Montepare, J.M., and Gueye, L. (2015). Exploring life satisfaction among older adults in Dakar. *Journal of Cross-cultural Gerontology, 30*(4), 377-391.

Mamta and Sharma, N.R. (2013).Resilience and Self-efficacy as Correlates of Well-being among the Elderly Persons. *Journal of the Indian Academy of Applied Psychology, 39*(2), 281-288.

Markides, K.S., and Martin, H.W. (1979). A causal model of life satisfaction among the elderly. *Journals of Gerontology, 34*(1), 86-93.

Melendez a, C.J., Fortuna, B.F., Sales, A., and Mayordomo, T. (2015).The effects of instrumental reminiscence on resilience and coping in elderly. *Archives of Gerontology and Geriatrics, 60*, 294-298.

Melendeza, C.J., Satorresa, E., Redondoa, R., Escuderob, J., and Pitarquec, A. (2018). Wellbeing, resilience, and coping: Are there differences between healthy older adults, adults with mild cognitive impairment, and adults with Alzheimer-type dementia? *Archives of Gerontology and Geriatrics, 77*, 38-47.

Mercier, C., Peladeau, N., and Tempier, R. (1998). Age, gender and quality of life. *Community Mental Health Journal, 34*(5), 487-500.

Netuveli, G., Wiggins, R.D., Montgomery, S.M., Hildon, Z., and Blane, D. (2008). Mental health and resilience at older ages: bouncing back after adversity in the British Household Panel Survey, *Journal of Epidemiology and Community Health,* 62 (11), 987-991.

Neugarten, B., Havighurst, L., and Tobin, S. (1961). The measurement of life satisfaction. *Journal of Gerontology, 16*, 134-143.

Nygren, B., Alex, L., Jonsen, E., Gustafson, Y., Norberg, A., and Lundman, B. (2005). Resilience, sense of coherence, purpose in life and self-transcendence in relation to perceived physical and mental health among the oldest old. *Aging and Mental Health, 9* (4), 354-362.

Palmore, E. (2001). The Ageism Survey: First findings. *The Gerontologist, 41,* 572.

Perkins, J.M., Multhaup, K.S., Perkins, H.W., and Barton, C. (2008). Self-efficacy and participation in physical and social activity among older adults in Spain and the United States. *The Gerontologist*, *48*(1), 51-58.

Pezent, G.D. (2011). Exploring the Role of Positive Psychology Constructs as Protective Factors Against the Impact of Negative Environmental Variables on the Subjective Well-being of Older Adults. Doctoral dissertation. Texas A & M University, Texas.

Prenda, K.M., and Lachman, M.E. (2001). Planning for the future: A life management strategy for increasing control and life satisfaction in adulthood. *Psychology and Aging, 16,* 206–216.

Priyanka and Mishra (2013): Differences in life satisfaction of elderly people in urban and semi-urban families of Lucknow (U.P.). *Journal of Humanities and Social Science, 16*, 28-32.

Puvill, T., Lindenberg, J., de Craen, A.J.M., Slaets, J.P.J., and Westendorp, R.G.J. (2016). Impact of physical and mental health on life satisfaction in old age: A population-based observational study. *BMC Geriatrics, 16(1)*. doi:10.1186/s12877-016-0365-4

Rupp, D., Vodanovich, S. and Crede, M. (2005). The multidimensional nature of ageism: Construct validity and group differences. *Journal of Social Psychology, 145,* 335–362.

Schaefer, R.T. (1983), *Sociology*, New York, McGraw-Hill Book Co.

Schure, B.M., Odden, M., and Goins, T. (2013). The association of resilience with mental and physical health among older American Indians: the native elder care study. *Am Indian Alsk Native Ment Health Res, 20*(2), 27–41.

Shen, K., and Zeng, Y. (2010).The association between resilience and survival among Chinese elderly. *Demographic Research, 23*, 105-116.

Staudinger, U.M., Marsiske, M., and Baltes, P.B. (1993). Resilience and levels of reserve capacity in later adulthood: perspectives from life-span theory. *Developmental Psychopathology, 5* (4), 541-566.

Steel, P., Scmidt, J., and Shultz, J. (2008). Refining the relationship between personality and subjective well-being. *Psychological Bulletin, 134*, 138–161.

Vinsi, S.M. (2014). A Comparative Study to Assess the Life Satisfaction Level among Male and Female Geriatrics Living in Selected Old Age Homes of Indore City. *International Journal of Health Sciences and Health, 4*(5), 241-243.

Wells, M. (2009). Resilience is rural community-dwelling older adults. *The Journal of Rural Health, 25*(4), 415-419.Doi: 10.1111/j.1748-0361.

Wurm, S., and Benyamini, Y. (2014). Optimism buffers the detrimental effect of negative self-perceptions of ageing on physical and mental health. *Psychology and Health, 29*(7), *832–848.* doi:10.1080/08870446.2014.891737

Zhanga, J., Zhanga, J.P., Chengb, Q.M. Huangc, F.F., Lic, S.W., Wangc, N.A., and Suc, P. (2017). The resilience status of empty-nest elderly in a community: A latent class analysis. *Archives of Gerontology and Geriatrics, 68,* 161-167.

Zhaoa, X., Zhanga, D., Wua, M., Yanga, Y., Xiea, H., Lib, Y., Jiaa, J., and Sua, Y. (2018). Loneliness and depression symptoms among the elderly in nursing homes: A moderated mediation model of resilience and social support. *Psychiatry Research, 268,* 143-151.

20

Breaking the Silence: A Counter to the Menstrual Menace in India

Aishwarya Jaiswal, Tushar Singh and *Yogesh Kumar Arya*

In August 2017, a 12-year-old schoolgirl in Tirunelveli (Tamil Nadu) killed herself by jumping off her home's rooftop. Her death note read that she didn't realize the mistake for which she was tortured by her Class VII school teacher, and was left with no other option rather than dying. Girl's family alleged it to be a stance of "period shaming". The girl's mother alleged that her daughter was sternly rebuked and upbraided by the female (26 years) school teacher for her experience of menstruation in the class (of 52, with 12 girls and 40 boys) and, was further humiliated by making her exhibit the menstrual stains she had on her uniform in front of the entire class without being considerate about even boys being present there. The school management too failed to provide the girl with a sanitary napkin (SN) and she was given a duster cloth to use instead. Such gestures pushed the girl in depression and forced her into the dire consequence of committing suicide. To our shock, this was just in succession to another shocking instance of period-shaming that occurred in April 2017 in Muzaffarnagar's (Uttar Pradesh) Kasturba Gandhi Girls Residential School where a residential school's warden, infuriated by the specs of blood in the hostel washroom, allegedly forced some 70 school girls aged between 8-14 years to strip and sit naked in the classroom for menstrual blood 'check', that resulted in the parting of around 35 students from the school. Interestingly, such instances saw no reduction with the change of calendar. November 2018 was again a witness to the incidence of death of 14-year-old Thanjavur (Tamil Nadu) Vijayalaksmi, who on account of an archaic tradition of domiciliary segregation of menstruating femme fell to the annihilations of cyclone Gaja. Likewise, young girls attending Sail Government Inter College in Rautgara village (Uttarakhand) were forced to skip school during their menstrual cycle as a temple dedicated to local deity Chamu Devta fell on their way to school, which in regard of locals would be desecrated if women on their periods passed by it. Till the 1960s women of all ages were allowed entry into the famous Sabarimala Temple dedicated to Lord Ayyappan in Kerala. However, after that menstruating age women were barred entry into the temple premises. It has been possible only after the ruling by the supreme judicial authority of the nation that women have been, of recent, gained re-entry into the temple.

It has again been possible after women fought for their rights and were granted legal permission by the supreme judicial authority of the nation. Not only is this, but the existence of Gaokor – a thatched hut outside the village where girls and women were banished during menses also a dreadful actuality to believe. Gaokor usually lacks basic facilities such as a proper bed, kitchen, electricity, etc., and the appearance of wild animals isn't uncommon there. Girls and women have reportedly suffered harassment and have even died from snakebites while staying in the gaokors. The National Human Rights Commission in 2015 dubbed this practice as a "serious violation of the human rights of women" and instructed the governance of the Maharashtra state to intervene and eradicate the practice of gaokar. However, the instances don't limit to the few outlined here and the number of such happenings is on an upsurge.

Menstruation has always been a taboo in India. These instances once again highlighted the age-old (Vedic period, c. 1500–600 BCE) menstruation-related stigma, prejudice, and discrimination that prevails across each stratum of the Indian society, irrespective of caste, religion and/or geographical bounds. Since this phenomenon occurs monthly, it becomes highly disruptive for the lives of the girls and women who are subjected to such practices. Before proceeding with the actual issue, let's have a glance at what is menstruation.

Menstruation

Every month a sexually mature (12- 45 years) female's ovary releases an egg cell that, through the fallopian tube, travels to the uterus. The uterus prepares for a possible pregnancy by developing a uterine lining made of tissue and blood vessels (endometrium). If the egg isn't fertilized and pregnancy does not occur, the uterine lining is shed and it exits the body through the vagina as a mixture of blood and tissue over a course of 3 to 7 days. This is called menstruation or a period.

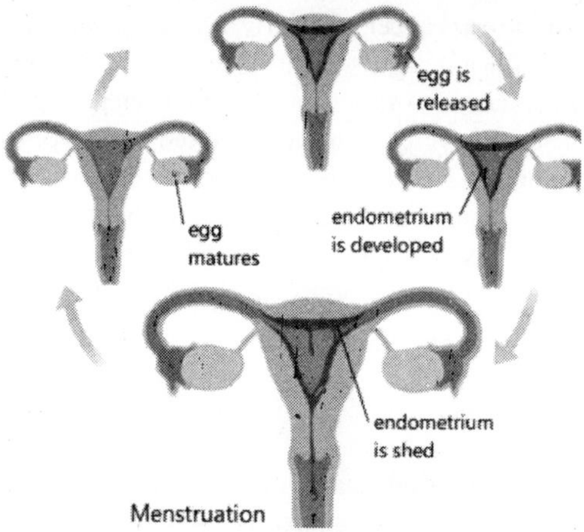

Fig. 21.1: The Menstrual Cycle. Adapted from Menstrupedia

The cycle starts over again with an egg that begins to mature in one of the ovaries. This cycle is called the menstrual cycle and is generally 25 to 35 days long. Menstruation is a hormonal process, any irregularity in which, probably results in females encountering associated physical and psychological health issues.

The Global Scenario

Menstruation forms a critical part of millions of female's physical, psychological, social and cultural lives, worldwide. It is remarkable is that these instances aren't just limited to the Indian subcontinent but rather affect most South Asian regions. In Nepal, there is a practice 'Chaupadi' which forces menstruating women and girls to sleep outside their house often in a cowshed. Afghan women are prevented from washing their hair or having a shower during periods on the pretense that it will render them infertile. Japanese women were disallowed from being sushi chefs as it believed that menstruation affects their sense of taste. The reports from Western nations further confirm period shaming and period-based discriminatory practices being a pretty global phenomenon.

Research commissioned by THINX (2008), a company providing innovative period solutions, found that 58% of women in the United States have undergone embarrassment owing to periods and 42% of them have also been subjected to period shaming. Women in Bolivia are prevented from discarding SN waste in bins on the pretense that it might lead them to consequences as dire as cancer. Similarly, a survey commissioned by Plan International UK (2017), a girls' rights charity in 2017 found that 48% of girls in the age bracket of 14 to 21 years have been period-shamed. Over the years, this natural cycle has been converted into a cycle of shame for women undergoing it. It is for this reason that most women fail to report the period-related complications and problems, be it in terms of lack of basic amenities or physical symptoms, they undergo. Though the stigma surrounding menstruation is a pretty global phenomenon, it has an even exclusive prevalence in India.

The Paradox in India

Every year, the Assadh month (June-July) of the traditional Hindu calendar witnesses a four-day long grand gathering and festival "Ambubachi Mela" in an around the Kamakhya Devi temple of Guwahati, Assam to celebrate the annual menstrual cycle of Kamakhya Devi, who is worshipped in the form of female genitalia that is believed to be the reproductive portion of mother earth herself. The mela witnesses a torrent of Sadhus, Sanyasis, and devotees getting indulged in ascetic modes of devotion such as jugglery, tantra, etc. For the first three days, entry into and practice of religious activities near the sanctum sanctorum of the temple is prohibited as the goddess is believed to be undergoing her menstrual phase. Festivities with the same core belief and different names are witnessed across states. For instance, in Karnataka, it is termed as Keddasa while in Odisha it called Raja Parva (menstruation festival). The paradox faced by the nation is that, while goddesses are worshipped and celebrated for menstruating, ordinary girls and women are made to feel ashamed owing to the same. In spite of pretext being the same, the treatments are so atypically non-conforming.

Biologists from eminent universities and education centres acclaim that stigmatization of menstruation shall be seen as a denial of women's basic human right to manage their menstruation safely. Sabrang India (December 2018) mentioned that the biologists opine that any form of menstruation-based discrimination against women is a glaring breach of the core principles of the Indian Constitution and the Universal Declaration on Human Rights. The same has been agreed upon by other international organizations working for menstrual health management (MHM). What adds to the dilemma is that the family itself teaches the period stigmas and other societal institutions perpetuate it. The severity of the issue necessitated a consideration of the historical and religious roots that led to the arousal of stigma surrounding menstruation in the Indian context.

Riches to Rags: Tracing the Regression

The conception of menstruation has attracted an explicit divide in the present times. While one sect firmly and uncritically adheres to varied menstruation restrictions without bothering to examine the essence of such practices, the other sect blindly and mechanically rejects those menstruation practices on the notion of modernization and feminism. There also exists a middle line of those who, based upon their personal beliefs and convenience, adhere to varying degrees of such menstrual practices and restrictions. The packaging of the menstrual regulations as forbidden practices and superstitions has made the current generation perceive them in highly negative connotations. Certain ancestral ideologies defaming the menstrual process, passed down and warped through generations, continue to detrimentally impact the present-day women. As the time is ripe to target the propagators of period-related stigma, this study undertook to trace the historical roots that led to the degraded status of the menstrual process that was once associated with rituals and divinity.

The *Rig-Veda*, one of the four most sacred Hindu texts, acclaims that Lord Indra, the Hindu deity regarded as the King of Heaven slew Vritra, a three headed dragon depicted as the demon of droughts with a thunderbolt, unleashing streams of water, prosperity, and progeny. However, Indra encountered guilt on killing Vritra as he was the son of a god. Indra rushed to nearby women for comfort and protection. The women said that they would own culpability on Indra's behalf if he promised them the blessing of healthy offspring. The scripture says that it is Indra's guilt that appears as menstruation every month. The story acclaims that it is the guilt of Indra that monthly appears as menstruation. *Yajurveda Taittiriya Samhita* (2.5.1) also narrates a similar story where Indra incurred the sin (Paapa) of Brahmahatya (the slaying of a Brahmana) on account of killing Vishvaroopa, the second teacher of the Devas. Indra was able to free himself from this act of Adharma, only when the earth, the trees, and the women agreed to take one-third of the Brahmahatya papa. As a result of this, women began to menstruate once every 28-30 days. In return, Indra gave women the boon that they will be able to give birth to children after their menses.

Vasishtha Dharmashastras divulges that the menstrual excretion month by month takes away a women's sins. The Hindu scriptures like *Angirasa Smriti* (Verse 35, 37), *Vashishta Dharma Sutra* (5.5, 5.6), *Baudhayana Dharmasutra* (2.2.4.4), *Parashara Smriti* (7. 16-17), *Sushruta Samhita* (Sharirasthana 2.24, 2.25), *Stridharmapaddhati* of

Tryambakayajvan describe menstruation as a temporary phase (lasting 3 days and nights) of Ashaucha i.e. ritual impurity wherein women shall avoid running, exercising, carrying out household activities and eating meat. They are also advised not to engage in holy/sacred activities. Refrainment from daily rituals such as bathing and combing, and application of cosmetic products such as collyrium and perfume, and the practice of self-adorning activities alike massage have also been suggested in the Ayurvedic (e.g., *Sushruta Samhita* [Sharirasthana 2.24]) and scared (e.g., *Yajurveda Taittiriya Samhita* [Verse 2.5.1], *Vashishta Dharma Sutras* [5.6]) texts. Though the Hindu texts don't explicitly state to segregate menstruating women, most of them (e.g., *Charaka Samhita* [Sharirasthana 8.4], *Brihadaranyaka Upanishad* [6.4.13], Yajurveda Taittiriya Samhita [Verse 2.5.1], *Vashishta Dharma Sutras* [5.6]) have prescribed certain tenets desiring varied degrees of exclusion that women shall practice during their periodic cycles. Avoidance of intimate relations and sexual intercourse during menses has also been prescribed in the *Yajurveda Taittiriya* (Verse 2.5.1), *Kashyapa* (Sharirasthana 5.5) and *Sushruta* (Sharirasthana 2.31) *Samhitas*.

However, contrary to the modern view that de-roots menstruation to negative notions, the archaic Hindu tradition promoted a productive and reasonable conception of menses and regarded it as a monthly time of privilege, rest, austerity, and self-purification. Celebrations like - Ritu Kala Samskara, Manjal Neerattu Vizha (Tamil Nadu), Xoru Biya (Assam), Yoni Puja, Raja festival (Orissa), The Keddasa festival (Karnataka), etc. also accentuate this fact. Even the ritualistic regulations and restrictions imposed upon women were nowhere meant to delimit them or subject them to any disparity but were rather meant to honor their feminine process. In the past, mundane Karmic obligations used to be physically consuming and thus restrictions in a way were a spiritual retreat for women. However, over generations, the rituals of the past have become a distorted taboo of the present that women are made to mechanically follow across religions. This work further details the varied conceptions of menstruation that are found in ancient scriptures and the probable logic behind such conceptions along with the regulations and restrictions associated with them.

The (Mis)conceptions surrounding Menstruation

In spite of being the worst sufferers, most women themselves refrain from standing against the flawed practices that they are subjected to.

This is mainly because the faulty conceptions surrounding menstruation have become more of a well-ingrained belief system. Even at times the mother who is the first person the girl contacts on having her periods for the first time, shame away from talking in this regard. A study reported in India Spend (2018) also found that 70% of mothers themselves believed periods to be "dirty" and rarely discussed period hygiene with their daughters. A report by Water Supply and Sanitation Collaborative Council (WSSCC, 2012) even held that the conversation related to period management seemed almost non-existent between mothers and daughters in India. This report clarifies that to date menstruation is a less-discussed theme even within same-sex individuals.

Van Eijk et al. (2016) in a study utilizing systematic review and meta-analysis found that in India 77% of girls are restricted from religious participation during their monthly cycles and, only 55% of them considered menstruation as normal. Kumar and Srivastava's (2011) poll study found that women themselves believed that during monthly cycles their body emits a smell or ray that has the power to turn food bad. The trend of associating menstrual blood with impurity and pollution has led women to be banned from kitchens, temples, and other public spaces while on their periods. Singh (2006) in his study "Place of Menstruation in the Reproductive Lives of Women of Rural North India."

Found that in the rural society people still relate menstruation with evil spirits and even regard the cloth used for menstrual blood absorption as "the most vulnerable object and a potent agent which might be used for casting evil eyes/magic on someone". This is also one of the reasons that women make all attempts to hide/conceal the rag/pad, to the extent of burying them. Garg and Anand (2015) in their study found that in some parts of India menstruating women are not allowed into communal baths for the first few days of their cycle. Also, the idea that whatever a menstruating woman touches will be ruined is commonplace. For instance, if she touches a cow, it will become infertile; if she uses, she will pollute the water.

The Taboos and Restrictions associated with Menstruation

While the religions like Buddhism and Sikhism saw menstruation as a normal body functioning process (Yip, 2016) and didn't impose any restriction on women, the leading religions of Islam, Christianity (Ahmed, 2016; Fonrobert, 2002), Judaism, and Hinduism regard menstruating women as 'unclean'. These religious views and teachings suggest that menstruating women shall be segregated during this duration of time. Although much has been done to promote awareness about menstrual hygiene, in terms of making operational improvements to building menstruation-related infrastructure, most women fail to access them on account of their inability to break the silence on the 'period blood' stigma which is drowning them. Menstruation is just not a biological process in India but has become a means of perpetuating gender discrimination. The period-linked superstitions and cultural taboos that stake menstruating women's health and safety are yet to be penalized under Indian law. Thus, discussion and awareness related to menstrual hygiene are important. For this to happen, it is first important to identify the major taboos relating to menstruation that are prevalent in the Indian society. Some of the most rampant and unreasoned menstrual taboos and restrictions that exist in India are enlisted below.

Taboos surrounding menstruation in India	***Restrictions placed upon women in India***
• Menstrual blood is magical.	• Menstruating women shall not enter religious places.
• What women shed during menses is their sins.	• Bleeding women shall not wash their hair for at least the first two days of their periods.
• Menstruating women possess special powers.	• Menstruating women shall not sleep on the same bed as their husbands.
• The holy *Tulsi* (basil) plant shouldn't be approached during periods.	• Menstruating women shall not water plants.
• It was on account of taking a part of Lord Indra's sin that women menstruate.	• Menstruating women shall not go to communal baths as the water will then be polluted.
• Menstruating women are impure, dirty and/or cursed.	• Menstruating women shouldn't be allowed to touch pickles, which might else rot.
• A menstruating woman should not be touched.	• Menstruating women shall use separate utensils and not enter the household kitchen.

• Any sort of contact with menstruating women shall be forbidden.	• Virgins should not use tampons.
• Menstruating women shall be forbidden from households for the first three nights.	• Pickles, curd, tamarind, and other sour foods shall be avoided as they could disrupt the menstrual flow.
• A woman must be "purified" before being allowed to return to her family after menses.	

Exploring the Logical Angle

These conceptions and suggestions put forth by the historical and religious texts have now attained extreme versions and, are supplemented by awkward logic. For instance, avoidance of household and other activities involving physical exertion have led to women made to stay in separate menstrual huts away from household. The avoidance of cooking food has taken the notion that the touch of menstruating women will pollute certain edible items (for example, pickles) and will make them rot. Refraining from sacred activities has taken a form as seen in the Sabarimala instance where the women of reproductive ages are completely barred from entering temple campuses. Also, the false notions such as—the holy basil plant would rot if it is touched by a woman in her menses have come to exist. During the past, women already had issues managing their menstrual blood and so restrictions on self-adorning activities would probably have been to provide their time for rest and self-care and prevent them from facing any further inconveniences. The advice of avoidance of sexual contact with a woman has reduced down to women been made to sleep on separate beds during menses, or in a separate room if allowed to stay within the house, or on the floor with a mattress that shall be used as a cushion during day time. Also, the suggestions to avoid food that wasn't easily digestible have been taken over by the dietary restrictions that demand the avoidance of sour foods (such as pickles, curd, tamarind, etc.) which may otherwise disrupt the periodic flow.

This section presents the logic for laying down the menstrual restrictions, as stated in the ancient texts. One very obvious reason would have been to provide women with a period of rest. This has been drawn from the instances of menstrual celebration and the treatment meted out to the popular goddesses during that period. Like, during the Ambubachi festival in Assam, the Kamakhya Devi temple is shut for three days to provide rest to the menstruating Goddess. Similar practices are observed in Karnataka's Keddasa fest where mother earth is awarded rest for three days on the pretense of undergoing her earthly menstrual cycle. Likewise happens in Odisha's Raja Parva (menstruation festival). As the monthly discharge brings pain, stress, and discomfort for most women, the aim of refraining them from most bodily as well household activities would have been to prevent them from overexerting themselves in the physically demanding household tasks of the past. Also, there was non-availability of options such as SNs that make the management of blood and public mobility of women easy, so staying away from crowded and public spaces would have been recommended.

As per some, menstruating women are themselves a living goddess and hence their entry into temples would lead to a disbalance or disequilibrium in the temple's energy. Scholar Janet Chawla too supports this proposition. In her paper "Mythic Origins of Menstrual Taboo in Rig Veda", she quotes historian Narendra Nath Bhattacharya who opines that in the past many Indian cultures considered menstruation as an auspicious phenomenon and treated menstruating women like goddesses. He further states that the popular belief was that during this period the fertile earth and woman must rest, be venerated and celebrated. Also, the menstrual blood was served as offering to the goddesses.

Most parts of our country abide by the teaching of the *Bhagwat Gita*, a great wisdom scripture that is also regarded to be the Bible of Hinduism. The chapter XIV of the Gita mentions the existence of three Gunas relating to the mind, emotions, and daily life of all existing beings. They include - sattva (goodness, constructive, harmonious), rajas (passion, active, confused), and tamas (darkness, destructive, chaotic) and are central to the Hindu philosophy. Hinduism regards menstruation as a complicated psycho-physiological phenomenon wherein women are exposed to heightened physical, vital and mental rajasic conditions. Hindu texts regard such a state as that of ritualistic impurity and thus refrain women from following some of the mundane activities. This indicates that on probable logic behind different forms of segregation women were made to observe during their monthly cycles would have been due to their heightened rajasic condition that could also over time lead to imbalances in the physiological and subtle processes of those around them. The constraints imposed upon mobility into public spaces and places of worship, might also probably be due to the same reason. As it's believed that menstruating women are high on *Rajas guna* dissipate enormous energy and are open to the reception and absorption of energies, their visit to crowded places or those with huge gatherings such as temples might make them liable towards the absorption of negative energies as well. Further, religious chants were meant to balance out body's energies and visiting places, where chants were made, could lead to excessive energy build-up in women.

The chapter XVII of the *Bhagwat Gita* emphasizes the concept of '*Tapas*', which involves the practice of varied austere physical and spiritual refrainment in an attempt to attain sacred and/or secular life goals, material welfare, and spiritual emancipation. The restrictions on the washing of hair or the application of fragrances or other beauty enhancing products and the wearing of ornaments over eyes or body could have been to enable women, who are known for special inclination towards beauty, to have better control over their senses and physical bodies. Ancient Ayurvedic texts lay a lot of emphasis on the three doshas—*Vata*, *Pitta*, *Kapha*—as essential to maintaining a balanced lifestyle. *Vata* is associated with a voluntary and involuntary movement, circulation, and transportation energies within the body. *Pitta* regulates metabolism, digestion, emotion, and mental experiences. *Kapha* has a role in bringing stability, stamina, and grounding to the body along with providing nourishment and protection to the body parts. When it comes to the dietary restrictions, Ayurveda states that the digestive fire (*Jathara-Agni*) of women are very weak during the menstrual phase and their all three primary doshas are more susceptible to become vitiated, thus they shall avoid any such edible item that flares up the digestive fire and causes an imbalance to the doshas.

Similarly, restrictions relating to sleeping patterns might be to detach them from material comforts, lust, and attachment to sexual pleasures. *Manusmriti* (4.40-41) states that sexual intercourse with menstruating women shall be prohibited as the child born out of such intercourse would be liable to early death, and also such intercourse could adversely affect the male's energy, strength, and vitality. However, this advice has been distorted in the present times, where even touching or sleeping on the same bed with a menstruating woman is debarred. Rajarshi Nandy, a spiritualist, in his article "Sabarimala Discreet, Not Discriminatory" mentions that even the yogic literature advice the menstruating women to not perform Yoga or any religious activities by the logic that these activities might have a damaging impact over their life-force known as "Prana Vayus". There are five types of it and each is associated with the regulation of distinct body parts and activities. Women, to prevent any dysregulation in their *Apana Vayu* (the force associated with download and outward flow of bodily energy) that governs the prime eliminative body functions such as urination excretion, and menstruation, and thereby suffer unpleasant physiological conditions, shall prohibit from yogic and other prescribed functionalities and activities. However, the logical control of the past, because of being blindly adorned and not being thought of and explained rationally, have lost meaning. They now exist in a version that adds to the torment of girls and women.

The Current State

MMXIX, the 19th year of the 3rd millennium's first century, has witnessed a heightened realization that menses aren't just a woman's but a human issue and thus we need to break the culture of shame and silences that prevails around menstruation. There have been global campaigns such as "Breaking the Silence", digital campaigns such as Happy To Bleed, paid menstrual leave for women employees by two Indian companies, period-positive protest by some 5 million women via forming 385-mile human wall, foundation of women empowerment NGOs such as Myna Mahila Foundation, of which Duchess of Sussex Meghan Markle is an ally, creation of websites such as Menstrupedia, release of movies such as Padman which is based on the true story of low-cost SN making machine invented by Arunachalam Muruganantham, the taking up of the #PadManChallenge by Bollywood celebs, launch of #YesIBleed social media campaign by Minister for Women and Child Development Maneka Gandhi, and setting up of strong examples by people like Miss Kiran Gandhi who ran her first London Marathon by deciding to bleed freely and highlighted the tussles that millions of women undergo.

Although India has come a long way and the nation that saw banning advertisements on SNs in 1990 has shown appreciation for a full-fledged feature film raising menstrual menace of women in 2018, the stigma surrounding menstruation is still strongly prevalent in India and is largely an unsurfaced issue.

Though the government initiatives such as The Right of Children to Free and Compulsory Education Act (2009), the Rashtriya Kishore Swasthya Karyakram, the Sabla programme, the National Rural Livelihood Mission, the Swachh Bharat Mission, and the Swachh Bharat: Swachh Vidyalaya (SB: SV), and the Gender Issues in Sanitation guidelines (2017) have taken up the task of promoting menstrual hygiene management in India, taboos surrounding menstruation prevent women from even seeking medical guidance if encountered with any menstruation-linked health issue. The impact that period shame has on women's health could be well understood by going through the Ministry of Health surveys (2002; 2005; 2008; 2012) that found low awareness and poor menstrual hygiene management among most Indian women make them fall prey to the preventable menstrual hygiene problems. For instance, two-third of the 60,000 annual cases of cervical cancer deaths in the nation occur due to poor menstrual hygiene. Around 120 million menstruating youths in the nation undergo either menstrual dysfunctions such as short or prolonged periods, anemia, reproductive tract infections, or psychological issues such as shame, embarrassment, and anxiety. A country analysis of menstrual health sponsored by the Bill and Melinda Gates Foundation found that around 71% of girls in India had no knowledge about menstruation till their menarche and felt shocked, fear, anxiety, guilt, and frustration during menstruation. As per UNICEF report (2014), 79 % of girls and women in Tamil Nadu, 66% in Uttar Pradesh, 56% in Rajasthan, and 51% in West Bengal were unaware of menstrual hygiene practices. The ordeal doesn't end here. While for the majority of women periods mark a hurried visit to the washroom with SN clutched clandestinely or hidden in paper bags, most women even lack this basic facility. According to the World Health Organization (WHO), India in 2018 had 355 million menstruating women. Only 12 percent of menstruating women in India use sanitary napkins (The Neilson Company and NGO Plan India survey, 2011) while the rest 88% rely on newspapers, plastic, dried leaves, rag cloths, ash, hay and wood shavings, etc. (FSG, 2016). A Rutgers study reported by IndiaSpend (June 2017) also found that 89% of Indian women used cloth for menstrual blood absorption and only 7% used sanitary napkins. This fact is further accentuated by the fact that India comprises less than 1.5% of the global feminine hygiene product market (Donald W. Reynolds National Center for Business Journalism, 2018).The National Family Health Survey (NFHS-4) released in 2015-16 revealed that just seven of India's 36 states and union territories had women (above 90%, aged 15-24 years) utilizing hygienic protection during menstruation. Surprisingly, between 2014-15, Rajasthan, Punjab, and Kerala reported more than 25% decrement in the utilization of SNs by women. A 2017 survey found a lack of access to sanitary essentials at menarche among 43% of Indian girls, and 36 % of them experienced discomfort in purchasing them in the presence of other customers (Deccan Chronicle, 2018). The National Health Mission's 10th common review mission (2016) found that SNs delivered in Odisha, Rajasthan and Kerala had quality issues. Also, they ran out of stock in the states of Jammu and Kashmir, Arunachal Pradesh, Bihar, and Maharashtra, and there were no distributions at all in Chhattisgarh (Comptroller and

Auditor General, 2015). This is also supplemented by the fact that India has one of the lowest penetrations of SNs in the world.

An article by The Better India in May 2017 reported that women in certain parts of the country even lack proper sanitation facilities, which have a close connection with menstrual hygiene. The article mentioned that even to date women such as those from villages in Lalitpur district of UP and Daringbadi district of Odisha lack private bathing spaces and are forced to bath in open, which places them in extremely unhygienic conditions. The lack of awareness and facilities have made undergoing hysterectomy (after having two or three children) a norm for the women working as cane-cutters in the Beed district of Maharashtra. Omidvar and Begum (2011) in their study on unmarried South Indian women found that the normal daily chores of 75% of adolescent girls were affected owing to their experience of dysfunctional menstruation. An India-based survey study by AC Neilsen (2011) involving 1,033 women in their reproductive ages and 151 gynecologists found that women using unhygienic materials for blood absorption during the period have 70% more reported incidences of Reproductive Tract Infection (RTI). WHO reports indicate that the reported cervical cancer deaths in India are twice the global average for the same. Close to 30% of the total cervical cancer death occurrences are reported to occur in India, and doctors attribute these to the poor period hygiene practices prevalent across the nation. Even the psychological problems aren't uncommon. The Neilsen (2011) survey also found that around 75% of the women who participated in his study revealed not being psychologically prepared for periods. Dasra, an NGO, in 2014 reported that the lack of proper menstrual hygiene management facilities led to school dropouts amongst around 23 million girls.

The Consequences

The silence surrounding menstruation has led to a lack of awareness on the issue and has also fueled the blind following of the ages-old deformed beliefs, restrictions, and superstitions. As period stigma, by itself, and in conjunction with the lack of awareness, accessibility and facilities are contributing towards the deteriorated health (both physical and psychological), functioning and menstrual hygiene management of the reproductive age females in the country, there is a pressing need shatter these. The box below gives a brief outline of the problems that most adolescent girls and adult women of reproductive ages encounter owing to their monthly cycles.

Problems		
Common Menstruation-related	**Poor Hygiene-related**	**Psychological**
• Cramps • Pain • Anemia • Short/scanty periods (Hypomenorrhea) • Infrequent bleeding (Oglimenorrhea) • Heavy and prolonged periods (Anemia Menorrhagia) • Bloating, headaches, moodiness, etc. (Premenstrual Syndrome) • Hormonal disorders, e.g., Polycystic ovary syndrome (PCOS), etc.	• Vagina Infections (Bacterial or Fungal) • Urinary Tract Infections • Skin problems such as Dermatitis • Susceptibility to cervical cancer • Bacterial vaginosis (BV) that predisposes the female to sexually transmitted infections • Complications in pregnancy • Loss of fetus • Proneness to infertility • Toxic Shock Syndrome	• Fear • Anxiety • Shame • Guilt • Embarrassment • Frustration • Mood Swings • Depression • Agony • Horror

Advocacies to Counter Menstrual Menace

Stigma and shame surrounding menstruation have turned a monthly biological process of concern into a hidden public health issue. The portrayal of periods as a cycle of shame has made numerous girls and women stay mute on the cycle-related physical, sexual and psychological health complications they undergo. Though many awareness-raising programmers' have been proposed and conducted, the wall of silence surrounds the issue still makes most reproductive age females struggle with understanding their bodies and the transformations therein. An Oxford University report published in 2016 even held that not much researches have been conducted to examine the actual ground-level performance of the programs introduced to facilitate menstrual management in India. This work highlights some of the activism desired on the part of the government and the non-government bodies, the society, and the psychologists to address the problems arising out of the menstrual menace. The table below pinpoints some suggestions, desired advocacies, and efforts by different bodies that could aid in the better management of menstrual stigma.

Government Organizations	Non-Government Organizations (NGOs)	Society	Psychologists
Attempts shall be made to alleviate 'period poverty'- a lack of sanitary products, and other essentials like toilets with clean water due to the financial constraints in the region.	Public awareness and support for the health management efforts introduced by the govt. bodies shall be promoted.	Societal outlook, attitude, and shared belief towards menstruation being impure and unclean shall change. The seriousness of the problem shall be realized else all govt. and NGO efforts surrounding it would be rendered unworthy.	It is for the psychologists to raise people's cognizance that the psychological health concerns and mental well-being surrounding menstruation hold relevance parallel to the physical health and well-being concerns.
Periodic evaluation of the programs introduced to improve menstrual hygiene shall be conducted.	In coordination with Govt. bodies, educative workshops for girls and women, especially those residing in a rural locale, shall be conducted.	Normalcy shall be created around the talk concerning periods. The misinformation surrounding menses could not be countered unless the issue is discussed as openly as any other normal body process.	The foremost and highly prevalent psychological challenges and mental health issues encountered by females shall be identified and appropriate modules for proper intervention shall be drafted.
It is for the government bodies to, in association with concerned authorities and organizations, introduce menstrual health awareness-raising programs.	Grassroot level analysis concerning the females' needs during their menstrual cycles shall be carried out.	Women, particularly mothers, shall not shy away on discussing menses issues with their family members, especially their daughters. The relevance of this phenomenon in a girl's life shall be emphasized.	The psychological issues encountered by young girls is quite different in nature and intensity to those encountered by women. Effective results desire that the psychologists while drafting counseling programs and strategies shall have into consideration the developmental needs and dilemmas of females of varying age-brackets.

Government Organizations	Non-Government Organizations (NGOs)	Society	Psychologists
The products and facilities provided to improve menstrual health management shall undergo a periodic check.	NGOs shall serve as a link between the menstruating women and the concerned authorities in helping women avail the facilities introduced for their betterment.	More start-ups aimed at providing low-cost and high-quality pads shall come up. Involving women in local ventures would be even effective in bringing grassroots changes.	Young girls, especially in schools, shall be counseled for psychological or cognitive vulnerability factors such as anxiety, sadness, tension, affect lability, etc. All their misinformation and maladaptive beliefs concerning periods shall be identified and clarified.
Impartment of sex education shall be made compulsory in all schools. It shall further be checked that the curriculum is taught effectively.	Raising the menstrual blood absorbent's penetration to all classes and categories of reproductive age girls and women shall be strived at.	Women shall strive for financial independence so that they have higher jurisdiction in matters concerning them and self-care products aren't perceived as a financial burden.	The socio-cultural context, acting as an external stressor, shall be targeted for extensive modifications. Group counseling and community training programs shall be organized in collaboration with govt. and non-govt. bodies.
The installation of Automatic sanitary napkin dispenser machines shall be made mandatory in all educational organizations and workspaces.	NGOs shall educate women about the difference between hygienic and non-hygienic menstrual practices.		Irrespective of the mode and nature of propagation, the positives associated with this natural phenomenon shall be highlighted.
The key decision-makers of the region, e.g., panchayat members of a village, shall be assigned the responsibility of ensuring effective implementation of government plans and policies concerning menstruation and female health.	NGOs shall make women cognizant about the short-term and long-term costs and consequences of practicing inappropriate menstrual hygiene management.		

Government Organizations	Non-Government Organizations (NGOs)	Society	Psychologists
	Attempts shall be made to sensitize not only women but also the men of the village. Right from the elderly to the young boys shall be involved in all talk or efforts surrounding menstrual awareness.		

Thus, in sum, all efforts are targeted at teaching a relatively period-phobic society the ways to normalize the period talk. The silence around the issue shall be broken and it shall be promoted as a topic of open discussion just like any other normal body processes. In most rural parts of the Indian subcontinent, there exists a lack of period education to the extent of a hazard. Awareness-raising and educative workshops for women, especially for those residing in rural locales, shall be organized. Attempts shall be made to include boys and men as allies and supporters in the 'period talk'. The studies, globally, have found that male counterparts have period shamed their menstruating female friends and colleagues. As the issue doesn't anymore remains a girl's thing or girl's issue, it becomes essential to involve, educate and sensitize men towards it. The schools shall provide menstrual education to young girls of reproductive age. Young girls shall be made aware of the menarche to prevent them from panic or fear during their first menses. The actual science behind this biological process of shedding blood shall be explained to the growing girls. They should be made conscious that each month it is their uterine wall linings that they shed and not any sin. The deteriorating consequences that result from unhygienic menstrual processes like urinary/reproductive tract infections, bacterial vaginosis, etc. shall be highlighted to make girls and women realize the gravity of the problem. Special attention shall be paid on teaching women about safe and unsafe menstrual products (sanitary napkins, tampons, etc.) disposal techniques. Having an insight into the short-term and long-term impacts that could result from unhygienic practices during menstruation will help in the better implementation of the MHM programs along with preventing the mechanical following of not-so-desirable unhygienic practices.

Raising menstrual blood absorbent's penetration to all classes and categories of reproductive age girls and women by increasing their availability, accessibility, and affordability. For instance, the installment of sanitary pad-dispensing machines in the washrooms of schools, colleges, and workplaces could be a significant step forward. Also, the manufacturing of low-cost good quality absorbents will enable women from weaker economic sections to all avail them, rather than regarding them as a financial burden. Attempts shall be made by concerned government authorities and associated stakeholders shall attempt at eliminating the 'period poverty'—a lack of sanitary products, and other essentials like toilets with clean water due to financial constraints in the region. The government bodies shall monitor the effective implementation of the programs introduced to facilitate menstrual health care. Constant quality checks of products and services provided by the programs shall be conducted. In case the programs aren't fulfilling their purpose, the concerned authorities shall take apt actions. In the provision of sanitation facilities, special regard shall be given to the design of toilets and washing areas as there is ample data that not only absence but also the poor design of toilets has limited so may girls. Also, frequent surveys or poll studies shall be conducted to assess the impact of the already introduced programs and get an insight into the further reforms and facilities desired. The NGOs and social activists involved therein shall co-ordinate with the government bodies in their efforts towards better MHM and awareness. We need more people like Urmila Chanam, a health activist-cum-journalist, who launched the Break the Silence campaign and educated around 6000 in 9 states about menstruation in an attempt to shatter the menstrual myths and taboos. The activists shall conduct more community-based training in villages to acquaint people with accurate information on the issue. Also, awareness and educative sessions shall be organized in the schools so that girls can generate a better understanding of the phenomena and distinguish between what constitutes a normal or abnormal period, and if there are encountering any such problems that desire medical consultation. This will build up a support system for girls. All attempts to fill the huge void that exists in terms of correct information relating to periods shall be made.

Attempts at involving the locals, especially women, shall be made. This can be done through springing up of more startups and local ventures looking to build viable feminine care businesses. This applies more to the rural locale where the awareness level and the penetration of menstrual blood absorbents are comparatively lower. This would serve varied purposes, the more important being to empower the women. This won't just help them become more independent but would also prove a facilitator in bringing about grass-root level changes in menstruation-related perceptions and practices. Easy and widespread penetration of period products and services would also follow. It is critical to involve the prime decision-makers such as the older women and members of the panchayat, both male and female, to create an enabling atmosphere for promoting MHM.

Ultimately, there shall be a realization that the psychological health and well-being of menstruating women need equal attention as their physical health. Open discussion on topics relating to menstrual complications shall be encouraged. As period shaming impacts the female's self-concept, self-esteem, and emotional health as well, attempts at providing psychological support to the girls and women shall be considered an equally critical component.

The Positives

So far, there has been a trend towards discussing more on the disadvantages and discomforts that accompany periods. Even before experiencing them, most girls are made to believe about its negative repercussions. Arguments are being laid forth by activists to stop negative portrayal of periods, and start with highlighting the meaningfulness it holds in a girl's or women's life. As the attitude formation at the time of menarche will have a long-term bearing on a girl's body-image, psyche, and reproductive health, she shall be educated about both the merits and complications associated with the process. the importance of cycles in providing a bringing a physical and emotional detox and bringing new life to existence shall be cherished.

Conclusion

Menstrual taboos are a harsh but actual reality. Even so, various moves are being made to counter them, it is still for women to realize that the ultimate power of transformation lies with them. As women at the receiving end, it's chiefly them who have to become self-assured as opposed to being self-ashamed. They shall take a step forward towards the direction of change, make themselves comfortable with discussions surrounding periods and, feel free to discuss it just as they do any other bodily process. Those who have adequate scientific knowledge and awareness about the menstrual phenomena must encourage others with limited knowledge, so that the blind circulation of taboos could be brought to a halt and, from now, proper instructions could be passed on to the younger generation for a healthier life for our women populace.

References

Ahmed, B. (2015, June 20). Bloody Hell: Does Religion Punish Women for Menstruating? Retrieved December 25, 2019, from Vice website: https://www.vice.com/en_us/article/7bdbw9/bloody-hell-menstruating-while-religious-235

Almost half of girls aged 14-21 are embarrassed by their periods | Plan International UK. (2017). Retrieved December 25, 2019, from Plan International UK website: https://plan-uk.org/media-centre/almost-half-of-girls-aged-14-21-are-embarrassed-by-their-periods

Discrimination over menstruation a breach of human rights: Indian Biologists | SabrangIndia. (2018). Retrieved December 25, 2019, from SabrangIndia website: https://sabrangindia.in/article/discrimination-over-menstruation-breach-human-rights-indian-biologists

Fonrobert, C. E. (2002). Menstrual purity: Rabbinic and Christian reconstructions of biblical gender. Stanford University Press.

Garg, S., & Anand, T. (2015). Menstruation related myths in India: strategies for combating it. *Journal of family medicine and primary care*, 4(2), 184–186. doi:10.4103/2249-4863.154627

George, R. (2013). Celebrating Womanhood: How Better Menstrual Hygiene Management Is the Path to Better Health, Dignity and Business: Break the Silence. WSSCC: Geneva, Switzerland.

https://archive.indiaspend.com/author/ojaswi-rao. (2017, June 19). Shame, Taboo Resulting In Unhygienic Menstrual Practices Across Much of India. Retrieved December 25, 2019, from IndiaSpend-Journalism India |Data Journalism India|Investigative Journalism-IndiaSpend website: https://archive.indiaspend.com/cover-story/shame-taboo-resulting-in-unhygienic-menstrual-practices-across-much-of-india-13221

https://www.facebook.com/goonj.org. (2017, May 30). Let's Break the Silence: 4 Simple Ways to Spread Awareness About Menstrual Hygiene. Retrieved December 25, 2019, from The Better India website: https://www.thebetterindia.com/102475/menstrual-hygiene-invisible-women/

https://www.facebook.com/nithin.sridhar.54. (2016, July 12). Hindu View of Menstruation- IV: Menstruation from Yogic perspective | IndiaFacts. Retrieved December 25, 2019, from IndiaFacts website: http://indiafacts.org/hindu-view-menstruation-iv-menstruation-yogic-perspective/

https://www.facebook.com/rajarshi.nandy.1. (2016, January 20). Sabarimala Discreet, Not Discriminatory » Sirf News. Retrieved December 25, 2019, from Sirf News website: https://www.sirfnews.com/sabarimala-discreet-not-discriminatory/

Kumar, A., & Srivastava, K. (2011). Cultural and social practices regarding menstruation among adolescent girls. *Social Work in Public Health*, 26(6), 594-604.

Nearly half of US women have experienced 'period shaming' | MHDay. (2018). Retrieved December 25, 2019, from Menstrualhygieneday.org website: https://menstrualhygieneday.org/nearly-half-us-women-experienced-period-shaming/

Omidvar, S., & Begum, K. (2011). Menstrual pattern among unmarried women from south India. *Journal of natural science, biology, and medicine*, 2(2), 174–179. doi:10.4103/0976-9668.92329

On Spot. (2014). "Improving Menstrual Health and Hygiene in India." Report. Dasra, Kiawah Trust, and USAID 114.

Performance Audit of Tribal Sub-Plan (2011-12 to 2013-14), Ministry of Human Resource Development, Ministry of Health & Family Welfare and Ministry of AYUSH Report of the Comptroller and Auditor General of India Union Government (Civil) Report No. 33 of 2015 (Performance Audit) Education and Health Sector (Selected Schemes/Central Autonomous Bodies). (n.d.). Retrieved from https://cag.gov.in/sites/default/files/audit_report_files/Union_Performance_Tribal_Sub_Plan_33_2015.pdf

Soumyabrata Gupta. (2018, August). An Indian woman spends about Rs 300 per month in buying sanitary pads. Retrieved December 25, 2019, from Deccan Chronicle website: https://www.deccanchronicle.com/lifestyle/health-and-wellbeing/030818/an-indian-woman-spends-about-rs-300-per-month-in-buying-sanitary-pads.html

Singh, A. J. (2006). Place of menstruation in the reproductive lives of women of rural North India. *Indian Journal of Community Medicine*, 31(1), 10.

Saptarshi Dutta. (2018, May 28). 23 Million Women Dropout of School Every Year When They Start Menstruating In India | *Women's Day*. Retrieved December 25, 2019, from NDTV-Dettol Banega Swasth Swachh India website: https://swachhindia.ndtv.com/23-million-women-drop-out-of-school-every-year-when-they-start-menstruating-in-india-17838/

Sravan Pallapothu (2018, July 4). Shoddy Sanitary Napkins Impact Menstrual Hygiene Drive |. Retrieved December 25, 2019, from IndiaSpend website: https://www.indiaspend.com/shoddy-sanitary-napkins-impact-menstrual-hygiene-drive-27299/

van Eijk, A. M., Sivakami, M., Thakkar, M. B., Bauman, A., Laserson, K. F., Coates, S., & Phillips-Howard, P. A. (2016). Menstrual hygiene management among adolescent girls in India: a systematic review and meta-analysis. *BMJ* open, 6(3), e010290. doi:10.1136/bmjopen-2015-010290

What is menstruation? (2019). Retrieved December 25, 2019, from Menstrupedia.com website: https://www.menstrupedia.com/articles/girls/whats-menstruation

Why menstruation is a nightmare for many women in India - Firstpost. (2014, May 31). Retrieved December 25, 2019, from Firstpost website: https://www.firstpost.com/living/why-menstruation-is-a-nightmare-for-many-women-in-india-1550781.html

Yip, A. K. (2016). The Ashgate research companion to contemporary religion and sexuality. Routledge.

Yoshita Rao. (2018, April 15). Feminine hygiene market to reach $36 billion; here's what's in store for India... Retrieved December 25, 2019, from DNA India website: https://www.dnaindia.com/just-before-monday/report-just-business-period-2604902

21

Machocracy in Lyrics: A Gizmo towards Vilification of Women

Aishwarya Jaiswal, Tushar Singh and *Yogesh Kumar Arya*

Technological advancements in the second half of the twentieth century have transfigured the current generation's musical access. All kinds of music are available all the time to all people just at the touch of a switch. Cheap and widely-available audio equipment has made possible the fast and large-scale distribution of music. Global estimates indicate that people are spending more time listening to music than ever before. Right from waking up in the morning to exercising in the gym, or from traveling to the workplace to working there, people are continuously listening to musical songs. Music has now become ingrained in our everyday life. Even applications allowing the production of music and recording of songs into one's voice. Music demonstrably has a strong influence on an individual's physiological movement, mood, emotional, cognitive and behavioral responses. It alleviates boredom, anxiety, and pain, and promotes relaxation, well-being, self-esteem, productivity and overall quality of life. Music has also been found to be intimately related to society. Music facilities social communication and group identity formation.

However, the continual availability of music has developed a tendency towards taking it for granted. As the beneficial aspects of music are increasingly demonstrated in health, psychology and other fields, there is a heightened need to consider the quality of music that is rendered to the society. Across nations, the music industry now counts amongst the top income generators. Thus, music, more than being a personal choice thing has become an important national economic health issue. As most people are exposed to musical lyrics on an everyday basis, the leading messages within music hold the ability to permeate into the listener's consciousness. If the messages in music follow discriminatory themes such as sexism or racism, they are most likely to have a disadvantageous impact on society.

The preceding years have witnessed a revolutionizing success for the rap industries. Rap wasn't anymore regarded a taboo and got widespread public acceptance. However, most lyrical compositions under this musical theme are saturated with misogyny, and thereby spread messages that objectify and demean women. This work states a few instances of misogynistic lyrics as observed in the Indian scenario and then progresses towards the probable impact that rising misogyny in lyrics has for the society in general and women in particular.

The Changed Scenario

Most of us are no exception to dancing to popular catchy beats or the so-called "items songs" without being much interested in what is being conveyed. The 'item' term is usually a reference to the performers of the dance, usually females. These days most of the item songs are performed by actors holding celebrity status. Item numbers are very much a part of Indian cinema and continue to be so even after decades. Close attention to the lyrics of these compositions reveals that they are nice tuned use of repulsive words, where demeaning messages are wrapped in a shiny cover. Actually, at most times the entire theme of the song along with its title talks about women as sex objects and shame them of their sexuality. What's more interesting is the fact that most of these item songs don't have anything to add to the movie's plot. The rising trend towards rap has come wrapped with dual meaning and misogynistic lyrics that hypersexualize and demean women. The idea of non-consensual intimacy and violence with women is also glorified. Bestsellers usually consist of those songs and albums that have degrading and abusive lyrics. This has been the reason that some researchers (e.g., McLeod et al. 1997; Thompson et al. 1990) have highlighted the need to censor such lyrics. However, in spite of earning the reputation of being sexist and misogynistic, surprisingly, this dimension of music hasn't received much scholarly regard. It is problematic that the major consumers of such lyrics are the youth, and most of them don't regard these lyrics as simply lyrics meant for entertainment and rather draw significant conclusions from them. Before proceeding with other aspects of the issue, a clear understanding of what misogyny means is important.

What is Misogyny?

Misogyny is an ideology that objectifies women as things owned, used or abused by men. It inherently disdains women and promotes hatred against them. Though it might take different guises depending on socioeconomic and other factors, it is characteristically pervasive. In the lyrical context, it involves the support and justification of the oppressive ideas about women, with their glamorization and humorization being common. This ideology supposes women to be trouble or burden for men and the sole purpose of their existence is for sexual purposes. It manifests in varying forms ranging from blatant defamation, stereotypical characterizations, to mild innuendos, but what's archetypal about them is the derogatory image of women they project. Adams and Douglas (2006) held that for any lyrical composition to be regarded as misogynic, it shall have the following six themes, all of which reduce women to a subgroup unworthy of love and respect.

- Characterization of women as exploiting and using men, just for having materialistic pleasures such as money, gifts, expensive cars, etc.
- Characterization of women as a cause of trouble for men.
- Depiction of women as usable and dischargeable.
- Description of women as being inferior to or "beneath" men.
- Derogatory comments on women, particularly of sexual nature.
- Statements indicating the use of force and violence against women, particularly in intimate relations.

Examples of Misogynistic Lyrics

Popular music is full of stereotypical hints at women, who are presented as low-grade, marginalized, trivialized and subordinate to their male counterparts. Derogatory images of females were always far more common than lyrical compositions demeaning women. Even the researches dating back to the late 1980s (e.g., Vincent, Davis & Boruszkowski, 1987) found that majority of rock music lyrics and visuals presented women in traditional sex role (e.g., domestic roles, subservient, and nurturing) and 'condescending manners (e.g., victim, unintelligent, sex object). Even a decade later, surveys found no difference in the way women were portrayed in lyrical compositions (Alexander, 1999; Andsager and Roe 1999). It is, to date, an uncommon practice to portray women as in any way superior to men. However, in modern times, the lyrics have gone to become more explicit and straightforward in conveying radically mixed messages about women's persona and their role in society.

Bollywood cinema has many times glorified the use of force over a woman as a form of romance, thereby further contributing to the parochial mentality of the Indian society. Women have been since long portrayed at sex objects aiming to please and entertain men. The scenes of women, dressed in glittery clothes, dancing amongst the drunkards, smugglers, drug dealers, mafia dons, etc. isn't uncommon. While we have inspiring movies like "Kahaani", "Neerja" and "Dangal" depicting strong women, we also have embarrassing songs with lyrics like *Saree Ke Fall Sa* (R... Rajkumar), *Hai Tujhpe Right Mera* (Phata Poster Nikla Hero), and many more. There has been a continual trashy and misogynistic portrayal of "heroines" in Bollywood. Presented below are few of the Bollywood and Punjabi songs and album titles who had lyrics loaded with, intended or unintended, misogynistic messages.

Sexy Sexy Mujhe Log Bole (Khuddar), *Tu Cheez Badi Hain Mast Mast* (Mohra, and recreated in Machine), *Ankhiya Na Maar* (Ek Khiladi Ek Haseena), *Choli Ke Peeche Kya Hein* (Khalnayak), *Choot* and *Brown Rang* by Honey Singh, *Kudi Menu Kehndi* by Hardy Sandhu, *Chikni Chameli* (Agneepath), *Fevicol Se* (Dabangg 2), *Halkat Jawani* (Heroine), and *Chammak Challo* (Ra.One), *Sheila ki Jawaani* (Tees Maar Khan), *Aa Re Pritam Pyare* (Rowdy Rathore), *Munni Badnaam Hui* (Dabangg), *Ooh Lala* (The Dirty Picture), *Khaali Peeli* (Phata Poster Nikhla Hero), *Pinky Hai Paise Walo Ki* (Zanjeer), *Chamia No. 1* (Zilla Ghaziabad) and lots more.

However, not everyone is convinced with the Bollywood's ardent admiracy of such derogatory songs and the portrayal of women therein. The kicking off of campaigns such as #GaanaRewrite and #NotMusicToMyEars in 2017 well substantiate this fact. The endorsement of sexist and violent ideas and behaviors in rap music has led to a collective effort to define this type of music as audio pornography (Lynxwiler & Gay, 2000).

Tracing the Roots: Indian Classics Examined

One from an older generation would like to argue about the western influence on our music and ignorance of our treasures of classical fine arts. However, an examination of the classical Indian music reveals that misogyny is nothing new to Indian music compositions. It's just that their form has changed to be more straight-forward.

Initially, Indian classical music had a more mechanical structure – Dhrupad – which contained purely deity-based verses, and the music was just a means of worship. Afterward, the north side of the country got under the influence of Muslim rulers—Sultans, Nawabs, Mughals, Nizam, etc. Indian music artists embraced the change as they were for the first time allowed to express themselves through the Khyalgaayki (Khyal meaning 'thought'). The melodic compositions called 'Bandish' began to be based on the theme Khyal. While very little bandish in Hindustani classical music is based on themes relatable to everyone, like nature, etc., most were Hindu religion-based. Amongst that also, most parts were occupied by those based on Radha and Krishna. The rest focused on the love of some unknown woman who is desperate to seek the attention of her intended. Even the lyrics in famous bandishes such as Raga Hameer, Puriya Dhanashree, Todi and Malkans posit that women possess extremely low self-esteem, facing atrocities, and can't do anything about a situation where their husband is the source of their trouble. And it is not very surprising in India that a woman is not supposed to do anything other than pleasing the man in her life and always depend on a man in the first place. So, in almost all the bandish lyrics, a woman is depicted as someone desperate to please her man. The man, however, is highly notorious and is extremely ignorant of this woman. She has nothing interesting to do. Looking at the ratio of male and female classical singers (males being dominant), it is highly ironic to see a male singer singing all this on behalf of that helpless woman, and a female singer singing those lyrics, not caring about the hidden insult in them. Even the lyrics that followed, for example, Thumri, in spite of having an honorary place in the Hindustani classical music status doesn't have very desirable lyrics. Some such examples include the lyrics in Raag Sindhura and Raag Tilak Kamod that are sung to date.

Why Misogyny – The Sources

Researchers like Weitzer and Kubrin (2009) hold the music industry, the local environment, and the larger gender relations as the major social prompters of the negative portrayal of women in contemporary rap songs. It is, thus, basically to promote the larger gender order that legitimates subordination of women, that reproduction of misogynistic content surfaces. It's then just another promotional aspect of the larger hegemonic masculinity ideology that substantiates male's hegemony and dominance over women, as something is ordinary and accepted. Next, that comes in a row is in the corporate pressures and interest in enhancing selling records. The explicitness in rap composition has proportionate linkages with their recorded sale. Record industry moguls encourage provocative and edgy lyrics as it maximizes their sales. Thus, at most times the rappers disregard the socio-political messages they are conveying to respond to the pressures from the elites in the music industry and boost their sales. Artists are encouraged to become hardcore, and artists going against the grain are without any delay marginalized. This simultaneously also indicates the preference of targeted audiences for these lyrics. Some rappers in their interview revealed that their focus is on violence and misogyny die to the fact that the audience appreciates such themes. Thus, rappers are coming up with more and more misogyny-saturated lyrics not to assert their masculinity (as believed by some), but to demonstrate their authenticity as rappers.

What's the Big Deal?

In December 2012, India's capital witnessed a brutal gang-rape of a medical student on a moving bus. It was after this incident that rap and pop singer Honey Singh (popularly called YoYo Honey Singh) was severely criticized for the use of visibly abusive and abrasive content in his songs. Social Networking sites were flooded with criticism of rappers whose songs promoted rape culture, assaults, domestic violence, and murder. Popular stereotypes Punjabis degrades women. Even the censor board was questioned on why the disturbing lyrics disguised behind the catchy beats and hummable music is ignored. Questions were raised on why the stringent attitude that is withheld for the portrayals of nudity, social messages, and inessential details on the silver screen, isn't applied to the subliminal and overt misogyny in these widespread rap songs. An online petition was also circulated to stop women's objectification in mainstream pop culture.

Different generations have made varying attempts to counter misogyny and rape. Millennials have also promoted the notion of affirmative consent, in their effort to prevent and end the culture of assault and rape. The changing of the mindset has, at every step, demanded the refusal of acceptance to any notion or practice that promotes assault and rape culture. However, pop music has been comparatively less thoughtfully attended compared to other practices. This is majorly because it isn't mostly considered in the substantive light, and is popularly took to be meant only for fun, entertainment, and dance.

The Psychological Angle

Cable (2017) by pointing out the similarities between intrusive songs and involuntary memories highlighted the complete possibility of unwillingly

supportive partner, etc. that are equally relevant to modern women. The unrealistic portrayal and generalization of women are detrimental, as it has reinforced a culture of demonizing and disrespecting women. This can be seen in the everyday examples we read in newspapers where men use Bollywood ways of stalking women to express their love, and then blame either the women or the popular movies and songs as an excuse for their behaviour.

Alleviating the Impact

One point of the argument is that rappers shall take responsibility for not dehumanizing women. However, at the same time, we are cognizant that rap artists and music creators have the liberty to rap about and post-visuals of anything they want. Unfortunately, sex and even more vulgarity are what sells the most. Still, it is advised that rap artists shall realize the importance they hold in society and the progression of civilization. Little vigilance on their part could largely contribute towards the improvement of people's common mental set and behavior towards women. As hip-hop influences the lives of many associated with it, it should be taken care that the supporters of this genre draw benefits out of it and aren't instead targeted or victimized.

However, in the face of severe disregard from the hip-hopper's end, censor should come into action. It is the responsibility of the censor authorities and their related bodies to take a note of the messages that rap songs are conveying at large, and that they don't prove to be disadvantageous to any section of the society. But even censorship is half the solution.

The major portion of responsibility is with the consumers of rap music. It is for them to be sensible to the messages being conveyed in the top-hits of the time, and be conscious of not subconsciously integrating the vocabulary, expression, thoughts, judgments, and actions into their being. Consistent auditory exposure to words that express double standards on women can have concrete effects on society's mentality about them. To promote a culture of respect for women, songs with negative undertones about females shall be disregarded. Already a host of educational institutions such as the women's colleges affiliated with Delhi University (DU), one of India's top educational institutions, have banned singers whose songs contain abusive and sexist messages, from performing on their campus. They argue that it is a paradox to preach women empowerment and equality in class and practice women's objection during college fests. Thus, both the lyrical virtuosos and the consumers of misogyny-drenched music shall partake in creating a more socially equitable place that prevents women's disenfranchisement.

References

Adams, T. M., & Fuller, D. B. (2006). The Words Have Changed but the Ideology Remains the Same: Misogynistic Lyrics in Rap Music. *Journal of Black Studies*, *36*(6), 938–957. https://doi.org/10.1177/0021934704274072

Alexander, S. (1999). The gender role paradox in youth culture: An analysis of women in music videos. *Michigan Sociological Review*, 13, 46-64.

Andsager, J. L. and Roe, K. (1999). Country music video in country's year of the woman. *Journal of Communication*, 49(1), 69-82.

Barongan, C., & Nagayama Hall, G. C. (1995). The influence of misogynous rap music on sexual aggression against women. *Psychology of Women Quarterly*, 19, 195-207.

Breines, J., Crocker, J., & Garcia, J. (2008). Self-objectification and well-being in women's daily lives. *Personality and Social Psychology Bulletin*, 34, 583-598. doi:10.1177/0146167207313727

Cable, C. (2017). I sing of misogyny and sexual assault: Rape culture in contemporary American pop music. Unpublished dissertation submitted to the University of Iowa. Available at https://ir.uiowa.edu/cgi/viewcontent.cgi?article=1070&context=honors_theses

Calogero, R. M., & Pina, A. (2011). Body guilt: Preliminary evidence for a further subjective experience of self-objectification. *Psychology of Women Quarterly*, 35, 428-440. doi:10.1177/0361684311408564

Carr, E. R., & Szymanski, D. M. (2011). Sexual objectification and substance abuse among young adult women. *The Counseling Psychologist*, 39, 39-66. doi:10.1177/0011000010378449

Fried, Carrie B. 1999. "Who's Afraid of Rap." *Journal of Applied Social Psychology* 29: 705-721.

Gay, R. K., & Castano, E. (2010). My body or my mind: The impact of state and trait objectification on women's cognitive resources. *European Journal of Social Psychology*, 40, 695-703. doi:10.1002/ ejsp.731

Lynxwiler, John and D. Gay. 2000. "Moral Boundaries and Deviant Music." Deviant Behavior, 21:63-85.

Martino, Steven, Rebecca Collins, Marc Elliott, Amy Strachman, David Kanouse, and Sandra Berry. (2006). Exposure to degrading versus nondegrading music lyrics and sexual behavior among youth. *Pediatrics* 118:430-41.

Mcleod, D. M., Eveland, W. P., & Nathanson, A. I. (1997). Support for Censorship of Violent and Misogynic Rap Lyrics: An Analysis of the Third-Person Effect. *Communication Research*, *24*(2), 153–174. https://doi.org/10.1177/009365097024002003

Muehlenkamp, J. J., Swanson, J. D., & Brausch, A. M. (2005). Self-objectification, risk taking, and self-harm in college women. *Psychology of Women Quarterly*, 29, 24-32. doi:10.1111/j.1471-6402.2005.00164.x

Peat, C. M., & Muehlenkamp, J. J. (2011). Self-objectification, disordered eating, and depression: A test of mediational pathways. *Psychology of Women Quarterly*, 35, 441-450. doi:10.1177/0361684311400389

Rudman, Laurie and M. Lee. 2002. "Implicit and Explicit Consequences of Exposure to Violent and Misogynous Rap Music." *Group Processes & Intergroup Relations*, 5:133-150.

Thompson, M. E., Chaffee, S. H., & Oshagan, H. H. (1990). Regulating pornography: A public dilemma, *Journal of Communication*, 40(3), 73–83.

Tiggemann, M., & Kuring, J. (2004). The role of body objectification in disordered eating and depressed mood. *British Journal of Clinical Psychology*, 43, 299-311. doi:10.1348/0144665031752925

Tiggemann, M., & Williams, E. (2012). The role of self-objectification in disordered eating, depressed mood, and sexual functioning among women: A comprehensive test of objectification theory. *Psychology of Women Quarterly*, 36, 66-75. doi:10.1177/0361684311420250

Timmerman, L. M., Allen, M., Jorgensen, J., Herrett-Skjellum, J., Kramer, M. R., & Ryan, D. J. (2008). A review and meta-analysis examining the relationship of music content with sex, race, priming, and attitudes. *Communication Quarterly*, 56(3), 303–324. doi:10.1080/01463370802240932

Vincent , R. C. , Davis , D. K. , & Boruszkowski , L. A. (1987). Sexism on MTV: The portrayal of women in rock videos. *Journalism Quarterly* , 64 , 750 – 754 .

Volpato, C. (2011). Deumanizzazione: Come si legittima la violenza [Dehumanization: How violence is legitimated]. Roma-Bari, Italy: Editori Laterza.

Weitzer, R., & Kubrin, C. E. (2009). Misogyny in Rap Music: A Content Analysis of Prevalence and Meanings. *Men and Masculinities*, *12*(1), 3–29. https://doi.org/10.1177/1097184X08327696

Wester, Stephen, Cynthia Crown, Gerald Quatman, and Martin Heesacker (1997). The influence of sexually violent rap music on attitudes of men with little prior exposure. *Psychology of Women Quarterly* 21:497-508.

22

Gender Disadvantage

Mental Health Risk Factors

Anubhuti Dubey

Even after the passage of two decades of this very hyped 21st century, the new millennium, the half of the population i.e. females of any age of most of the societies around the globe are struggling to receive what they deserve to be in terms of status, power, voice, physical and mental health. And from the last few months the world is facing a pandemic due to novel corona virus, COVID-19. This virus had been affecting a large segment of population around the globe directly. It has direct effects on those who are infected by virus or those who are treating it or those who are in administration and governance or those whose businesses are affected or those whose jobs and other works are affected. However, little has been discussed about the more subtle and far-reaching impact of this pandemic. The widespread effects on the mental health of individuals, particularly on those who are already the marginalized, like poor, homeless women and children, pregnant women, women already facing domestic violence, women working in informal sectors, unskilled women labourers, people living in shelter homes and refugee camps, and any group or community marginalized based on gender, caste, ethnicity, sexual orientation, other infectious disease like HIV. This COVID-19 might be an immediate threat to our physical health, but not contacting the virus isn't quite enough to be free from its deadly grasp. It wouldn't be unfair to say that the disease being silent killer—planting seeds of fear, anxiety, uncertainty, panic and a host of other emotions in the minds of human beings, that just seems to increase with each passing day. World Health Organization present regional Director for Europe, Hans Kluge confirmed that countries are reporting up to 60 per cent increase in emergency calls by women subjected to violence by intimate partner in April 2020 compared to last year. The United Nations agency for Sexual and Reproductive Health

(UNFPA) has estimated that there would be 31 million cases of domestic violence worldwide if lockdowns continue for another six month (*The Hindu*, May 7, 2020).

In view of the pandemic, Indian government had declared total lockdown of country on March 22 which was extended to May 31, 2020. In India, the first signs of the problem of domestic violence were appeared in data provided by the National Commission of Women (NCW) in mid-April, which suggested an almost 100 per cent increase in domestic violence during the lockdown. They highlight that it could be just a tip of the iceberg, as women from the underprivileged communities have no means to reach out. It's not just about the numbers but also the psychological and social impact that the lockdown would have on women. For women, the lockdown has also resulted in the increase in what is called as "unpaid work" at home. The cooking time has increased as all family members are at house. Young girls are more vulnerable during the time of COVID-19 as families are attempting to marry off many minors. Karnataka State Commission for Protection of Child Rights Chairperson Antony Sebastian has recently highlighted the recent spike in such marriages.

In the psychological researches, gender studies had very limited scope and impact on contrary to that of researches in other social sciences on gender. In her review article Vindhya (2007) identified three major themes of psychological researches in 1990-2000, these are work-family interface; mental health of women; and violence against women. Though work-family linkages and their effect on women's mental and physical health has been on the centrestage of psychological researches mostly on women coming from academic institutions such as university departments. The other two themes, related to women's mental health and violence against women, have been tracked by women's advocacy group researchers. Apart from these three areas, another important area highly examined in psychological world is the interface of reproductive health and psychological well-being such as premenstrual distress, menopause, pregnancy; developmental research such as midlife and aging, marriage, motherhood and widowhood; and gender stereotyping such as prejudice and gender-linked attributions. Hence, in psychology two streams of researches on women issues can be traced—one is 'academic' or mainstream psychological research, and second is advocacy/activism-based research (Vindhya, 2007).

Gender is a crucial determinant of mental health and mental illness. However, the researchers had focused more on the morbidity associated with mental illness than the gender-specific determinants and mechanisms to facilitate, promote and protect mental health and foster resilience to stress and adversity. Gender reveals the disparity in power and control men and women have over the socioeconomic features of their mental health and lives, social standing, status, handling and care in society as well as their vulnerability and exposure to specific mental health risks. To understand the pattern and prevalence of mental disorders among women and to recognize the socio-demographic associations of mental disorders and to underline the gender bias in mental health services hospital data, community surveys and secondary analysis of epidemiological studies have been utilized (Chakraborty, 1990; Davar, 1999, 2001; Jaswal, 2001; Vindhya *et al.*, 2001).

However, the epidemiological investigations failed to provide a coherent picture of mental disorders among women. They make dubious suppositions and draw methodologically debatable inferences on the condition of women's mental health (Davar, 1995).

Davar (1999) did a gender-sensitive analysis of epidemiological research in India, first of its kind and confirmed that the studies conducted so far had interpreted the greater representation of male patients recorded in hospital data as due to the greater stressful burden associated with the male role in Indian society. Keeping in mind the gender perspective, Davar (1999) reasoned that making these types of inferences are flawed as they fail to notice the higher prevalence of mental disorders in women registered from community surveys. The worldwide trend also suggests the same. The existing gender bias in access to health care services can't be overlooked. Based on this same set of data, Davar also constructed a profile of women's mental disorder which suggested no gender differences in severe mental disorders that have a biological basis, but women were found to be at least twice as frequently ill as men in the case of common mental disorders such as unipolar depression, anxiety and somatization disorders whose etiology is connected to psychosocial causes. Consequently, disorders that disproportionately affect women are seen to be linked to psychosocial causes such as their position in society and the work they do, rather than to biological/organic factors alone.

Up till now, ample research evidence hint of greater prevalence of depression, somatoform and dissociative disorders in hospital settings (Vindhya *et al.*, 2001) and somatic, anxiety and depression complaints among women in primary health care settings (Patel *et al.*, 1999; Sachi Devi, 2003). Association between reproductive illnesses such as gynecological morbidity and common mental disorders among urban poor women in particular (Jaswal, 2001) is also established by research findings. The recurrent prevalence of common mental disorders (e.g. depression and somatoform disorders) in women is attributed to social circumstances on women's lives. Consequently, inequity in schooling and higher education, financial possessions, access to health and legal services, the lopsided load of care-giving within family, and several forms of physical, psychological and sexual abuse across the life span is social factors that place women at greater risk of these disorders (Davar, 1999). Although the sexual assault and gender violence rate in India is very high but only a few studies have documented the severity and impact of psychological trauma like shock, fear, disbelief, denial, guilt and humiliation, anxiety, depression and suicidal attempts (Purewal & Ganesh, 2000; Ramanathan, 1996) resulting from such violence. The effects of gender-based violence are likely to be particularly high impact and contribute to health disparities for marginalized survivors of gender based violence. The impact of gender based violence is seen in the form of both fatal and nonfatal outcomes for women. Fatal outcomes include homicide, suicide, maternal mortality, and AIDS-related deaths. Studies from India consistently indicate a relatively high prevalence of intimate partner violence. Kumar and associates (2005) reported that 40 per cent of the 9938 Indian women they studied reported intimate partner violence in their marriage. Varma and colleagues (2007) found that physical violence was reported by 14 per cent of pregnant women in the past year, psychological abuse by 15 per cent, and sexual coercion by 9 per cent.

Gender specific risk factors for common mental disorders that inexplicably affect women include gender-based violence, socioeconomic disadvantage, low income and income inequality, low or subordinate social status and rank and unremitting responsibility for the care of others. The high prevalence of sexual violence against women and the resultant high rate of Post Traumatic Stress Disorder (PTSD) following such violence leave long term, cumulative impact on mental health and this psychosocial adversity has not been adequately investigated. Economic and social policies that cause sudden, disruptive and severe changes to income, employment and social capital that cannot be controlled or avoided, significantly increase gender inequality and the rate of common mental disorders. Even the present pandemic caused by COVID-19 is also led women in turbulent situation, a rise in human trafficking, and all sorts of violence against women as assumed by social activists and social workers. Hence, more such studies are needed to understand the demography of various types of violence faced by women of all ages, its impact and also the personality and social advantages of coarser.

Gender Bias and Treatment of Mental Disorders

Gender bias occurs in the diagnosis and treatment of psychological disorders. Medical professionals are apt to diagnose depression in women compared with men, even when they have alike scores on standardized measures of depression or show same symptoms. Female gender is a significant predictor of being prescribed mood altering psychotropic drugs.

Gender disparities exist in patterns of help seeking for psychological disorder. Women are more likely to look for help from and reveal mental health problems to their primary health care physician or the alternative healers of their native villages while men are more likely to seek specialist mental health care and are the principal users of inpatient care.

Gender stereotypes regarding emotional problems in women and alcohol problems in men emerge to reinforce social stigma and limit help seeking along stereotypical lines. They are stumbling blocks to the correct identification and treatment of psychological disorder.

Despite these differences, most women and men experiencing emotional distress and/or psychological disorder are neither identified nor treated by their doctor.

Violence related mental health problems are also poorly identified. Women are reluctant to disclose a history of violent victimization unless physicians ask about it directly. A critical gender gap in access to health care services in developing countries has already been well-documented (Dasgupta *et al.*, 1995). Although the pattern of gender differences in access to mental health care services is relatively under-researched. There is a paucity of data as psychological service providers in the form of counseling centers for both the victimized women and those responsible are meager or confined to the metro cities.

Depression, anxiety, psychological distress, sexual violence, domestic violence and escalating rates of substance use affect women to a greater extent than men across different countries and different settings. Demands created by their multiple roles, gender discrimination and associated factors of poverty, hunger, malnutrition, overwork, all sorts of abuse, coalesce a reason for deficient mental health of women. A positive correlation between the frequency and severity of such social factors and the frequency and severity of mental health problems in women is found. Moreover, ruthless life events that cause a sense of loss, inferiority, humiliation or entrapment can predict depression.

Not only access to mental health services is difficult for women but those available in primary health care are also discriminatory (Dubey,

2014; Tripathi & Dubey, 2013). Mostly, the communication between health workers and women patients is extremely authoritarian, making a woman's disclosure of psychological and emotional distress difficult, and often stigmatized. When women dare to disclose their problems, many health workers tend to have gender biases which lead them to either over-treat or under-treat women.

Conclusion

Further researches are needed to understand the protective factors within social milieu which save women against developing mental health problems. However, some research evidences suggest that having sufficient autonomy to exercise some control in response to severe events; access to some material resources that allow the possibility of making choices in the face of severe events and psychological support from family, friends, or health providers is powerfully protective. Nevertheless, extensive research should be done to put together the data on the prevalence and causes of mental health problems in women and encourage the formulation and implementation of health policies that address women's needs and concerns from childhood to old age. Moreover, the competence and sensitivity of primary health care providers should be enhanced through training and interventions to distinguish and treat mental health consequences of domestic violence, sexual abuse, and acute and chronic stress in women. Also, set up of more 'women in need' helplines with appropriate personnel for safety, counselling and wellbeing are required as those working are insufficient in number and unequipped to handle the rise in the number of cases and for providing the right kind of counselling support for women and girls. These helplines are also not widely known to all and are not advertised by police and government at regular intervals.

References

Chakraborty, A. (1990). *Social Stress and Mental Health: A Social-psychiatric Field Study of Calcutta*. New Delhi: Sage.

Davar, B.V. (1995). Mental Illness in Indian Women. *Economic and Political Weekly*, *30*(45), 2879–86.

Davar, B.V. (1999). *Mental Health of Indian Women: A Feminist Agenda*. New Delhi: Sage.

Davar, B.V. (ed.) (2001). *Mental Health from a Gender Perspective*. New Delhi: Sage Publications.

Dubey, A. (2014). The Psychology of Women Health. *Gorakhpur Social Scientist*, Vol. V (1&2), 57-62.

https://www.thehindu.com/news/international/coronavirus-lockdown-surge-in-domestic-violence-says-who/article31529111.ece

https://www.deccanherald.com/specials/insight/coronavirus-crisis-no-lockdown-for-domestic-violence-829941.html

Jaswal, S. (2001). Gynaecological Morbidity and Common Mental Disorders in Low income Urban Women in Mumbai. In: B.V. Davar (ed.) *Mental Health from a Gender Perspective,* pp. 138–54. New Delhi: Sage.

Kumar, S., Jeyaseelan, L., Suresh, S., and Ahuja, R.C. (2005). Domestic violence and its mental health correlates in Indian women. *British Journal of Psychiatry,* 187, 62-7.

Patel, V., Araya, R., de Lima, M., Ludermir, A. and Todd, C. (1999). Women, Poverty and Common Mental Disorders in Four Restructuring Societies. *Social Science and Medicine, 49*(3), 1461–71.

Purewal, J. and Ganesh, I. (2000). Gender Violence, Trauma, and its Impact on Women's Mental Health. *The Indian Journal of Social Work, 61*(7), 542–57.

Ramanathan, S. (1996). Violence against Women. *International Medical Journal 3*, 145–48.

Sachi Devi, K. (2003). Common Mental Disorders in Primary Health Care Settings: A Study of Socio-Demographic Correlates. Unpublished doctoral dissertation, Andhra University, Visakhapatnam, India.

Tripathi, K.M. and Dubey, A. (2013). Role of education in health and wellbeing of rural women. *Indian Journal of Social Science and Organization Behaviour, 2*(1), 22-27.

Varma, D., Chandra, P.S., Thomas, T., and Carey, M.P. (2007). Intimate partner violence and sexual coercion among pregnant women in India: relationship with depression and post-traumatic stress disorder. *Journal of Affect Disorder, 102*(1-3), 227-35.

Vindhya, U. (2007). Quality of Women's Lives in India: Some Findings from Two Decades of Psychological Research on Gender. *Feminism and Psychology, 17*(3), 337-356.

Vindhya, U., Kiranmayi, A. and Vijayalakshmi, V. (2001). Women in Psychological Distress: Evidence from a Hospital-based Study. *Economic and Political Weekly*, *36*(25), 4081–7.

Index